T0263866

Therapy for Severe Psoriasis

Therapy for Severe Psoriasis

JASHIN J. WU, MD

Los Angeles, CA, USA

STEVEN R. FELDMAN, MD, PhD

Departments of Dermatology,
Pathology, and Public Health Sciences
Wake Forest School of Medicine
Winston-Salem, NC, USA

MARK G. LEBWOHL, MD

Department of Dermatology
Icahn School of Medicine at Mount Sinai
New York, NY, USA

ELSEVIER

ELSEVIER

1600 John F. Kennedy Blvd.
Ste 1800
Philadelphia, PA 19103-2899

Therapy for Severe Psoriasis
ISBN: 978-0-323-44797-3

Notices

Knowledge and best practice in this field are constantly changing. As new research and experience broaden our understanding, changes in research methods, professional practices, or medical treatment may become necessary.

Practitioners and researchers must always rely on their own experience and knowledge in evaluating and using any information, methods, compounds, or experiments described herein. In using such information or methods they should be mindful of their own safety and the safety of others, including parties for whom they have a professional responsibility.

With respect to any drug or pharmaceutical products identified, readers are advised to check the most current information provided (i) on procedures featured or (ii) by the manufacturer of each product to be administered, to verify the recommended dose or formula, the method and duration of administration, and contraindications. It is the responsibility of practitioners, relying on their own experience and knowledge of their patients, to make diagnoses, to determine dosages and the best treatment for each individual patient, and to take all appropriate safety precautions.

To the fullest extent of the law, neither the Publisher nor the authors, contributors, or editors, assume any liability for any injury and/or damage to persons or property as a matter of products liability, negligence or otherwise, or from any use or operation of any methods, products, instructions, or ideas contained in the material herein.

Library of Congress Cataloging-in-Publication Data

A catalog record for this book is available from the Library of Congress

Content Strategist: Russell Gabbedy
Content Development Specialist: Colleen Viola
Design Direction: Renee Duenow

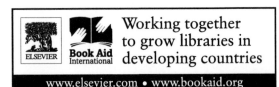

To my loving wife, Stephanie,
who understands and allows my pursuits as
an academic dermatologist.
To my parents,
who instilled in me the value of hard work and perseverance:
thank you for all that you have given me.

Jay

To the many people working to make the lives of psoriasis patients better—including our National Psoriasis Foundation, the many experts who've taught us so much about psoriasis, the researchers who've helped us understand the disease, the people who have developed the drugs that make patients' lives better, and the dedicated payers who help patients get access to treatment—and to the patients who have put their trust in us to care for them, we dedicate this book to them.

Steve

Mark

Contributors

EDITORS

JASHIN J. WU, MD
Los Angeles, CA, USA

STEVEN R. FELDMAN, MD, PhD
Departments of Dermatology, Pathology, and Public Health Sciences
Wake Forest School of Medicine
Winston-Salem, NC, USA

MARK G. LEBWOHL, MD
Professor and Chair
Kimberly and Eric J. Waldman Department of Dermatology
Icahn School of Medicine at Mount Sinai
New York, NY, USA

AUTHORS

JOHANN E. GUDJONSSON, MD, PhD
Frances and Kenneth Eisenberg Emerging Scholar
Taubman Medical Research Institute
Assistant Professor
Department of Dermatology
Director of Inpatient and Consultation Dermatology
University of Michigan
Ann Arbor, MI, USA

PETER W. HASHIM, MD, MHS
Clinical Dermatopharmacology Fellow
Department of Dermatology
Icahn School of Medicine at Mount Sinai
New York, NY, USA

DANE HILL, MD
Center for Dermatology Research
Department of Dermatology
Wake Forest School of Medicine
Winston-Salem, NC, USA

MICHAEL KELLY-SELL, MD
Department of Dermatology
University of Michigan
Ann Arbor, MI, USA

HENRY W. LIM, MD
Chairman and Clarence S. Livingood Chair
Department of Dermatology
Henry Ford Hospital
Detroit, MI, USA

ELAINE J. LIN, MD
Department of Dermatology
University of California—Davis
Sacramento, CA, USA

LAUREN M. MADIGAN, MD
Department of Dermatology
Henry Ford Hospital
Detroit, MI, USA

CATHERINE NI, MD
David Geffen School of Medicine
University of California—Los Angeles
Los Angeles, CA, USA

JOHN K. NIA, MD
Clinical Dermatopharmacology Fellow
Department of Dermatology
Icahn School of Medicine at Mount Sinai
New York, NY, USA

AMIT OM, BS
Center for Dermatology Research
Department of Dermatology
Wake Forest School of Medicine
Winston-Salem, NC, USA

SANDRA PENA, BS
Center for Dermatology Research
Department of Dermatology
Wake Forest School of Medicine
Winston-Salem, NC, USA

SHIVANI P. REDDY, BS
University of Illinois College of Medicine
Chicago, IL, USA

VIDHI V. SHAH, BA
University of Missouri–Kansas City School of Medicine
Kansas City, MO, USA

ANJALI S. VEKARIA, MD
Resident
Department of Dermatology
Icahn School of Medicine at Mount Sinai
New York, NY, USA

Foreword

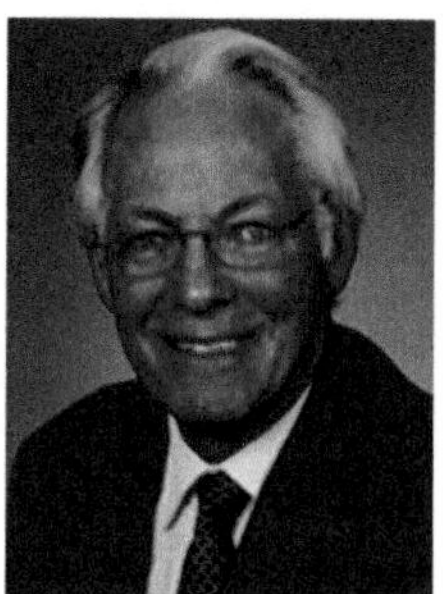

Alan Menter, MD

Psoriasis is a common, immune-medicated, genetic disorder affecting up to 2% of the world population with significant interracial variation, being far less common in Africa, Asia, and North America Indians than in Scandinavian countries, Northern Europe, and the Americas. Men and women, boys and girls, are equally affected, with the majority of patients developing their disease before the age of 40.

Psoriasis shares much of its ancient history with leprosy, with Biblical references to leprosy likely representing actual psoriasis. Hippocrates in fact described a series of skin disorders under the heading "Lopoi," Greek for epidermis, which possibly included both psoriasis and leprosy. The term "psoriasis" was derived from the Greek for epidermis, which possibly included both psoriasis and leprosy. The term "psoriasis," derived from the Greek "psora" meaning "itch," was first used by Galen (133-200 AD). Sixteen centuries later, Robert Willan (1757-1812) published the first true description of psoriasis in 1808.

Psoriasis is not "one disease." It has a vast array of clinical phenotypes with the classic "plaque" form being the commonest. It can vary from a few discrete areas of activity, such as the scalp, elbow, and knees, to generalized cutaneous involvement with various forms, shapes, and sizes of individual lesions. In addition, numerous other phenotypical manifestations can include guttate, erythrodermic, inverse, and palmar-plantar forms, either individually or in association with the classic plaque-type disease. Chapters in this book address multiple classes of therapy currently available for the treatment of psoriasis, together with investigational new drugs and the advent of biosimilar agents.

Our knowledge of the genetics and immunopathogenesis of psoriasis has exploded over the past two decades to the extent that psoriasis now has to be considered a systemic disease for a significant percentage of patients having other organ involvement, including the joints. Thus, more than 40 genes have been shown to be associated with psoriasis. However, a much smaller number of genes are associated with psoriatic arthritis, throwing into doubt the actual specific association between psoriasis and psoriatic arthritis. The severity of cutaneous inflammation is frequently "mirrored" systemically in the bloodstream with potential negative sequelae for the heart, especially the coronary vasculature, as well as the liver, including steatohepatitis. In addition, psoriasis has been shown to be statistically associated with a relatively long list of other comorbidities, including obesity; with the full spectrum of the metabolic syndrome, including obesity, hypertension, diabetes mellitus, and hypercholesterolemia; and with hypertriglyceridemia. Other conditions, including sleep apnea, chronic obstructive pulmonary disease, and renal disease, are also linked to psoriasis.

Psoriasis likewise has a major effect on patients' quality of life with social and personal interactions frequently disrupted due to the visible nature of the disabling condition, leading to depression, fatigue, and indeed a higher likelihood of suicidal ideation, especially in younger patients.

It is thus incumbent on all dermatologists with an interest in the fascinating disorder not only to assess each and every psoriatic patient's total skin surface, head to toe, at each consultation but also to evaluate for comorbidities, including psoriatic joint disease and psychosocial issues. Collaboration with colleagues in other specialties, including cardiology, endocrinology, hepatology, general internal medicine, and family practice, is frequently indicated for the betterment of the health of the psoriatic population as a whole. In patients with less severe psoriasis, who account for approximately 75% of the psoriatic population, topical agents are the treatment of choice in the overwhelming majority. For the remaining 25% with moderate to severe psoriasis, the wide array of systemic therapies, both oral and injectable, offers the opportunity to maximize the benefits of treatment to our psoriasis population, both short term and long term, while also reducing the impact of the multiple comorbidities associated with the more severe forms of psoriasis. Thus, the future for our psoriasis population is exciting indeed.

Alan Menter, MD
Chair, Department of Dermatology
Clinical Professor of Dermatology
University of Texas Southwestern Medical School
Dallas, TX, USA

Preface

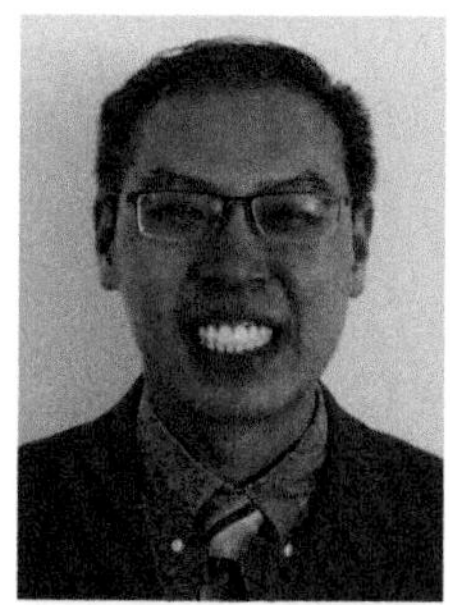
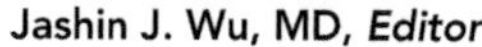

Jashin J. Wu, MD, *Editor*

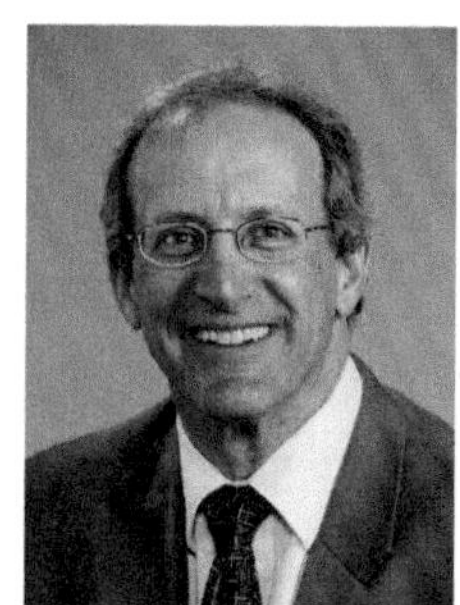

Steven R. Feldman, MD, PhD, *Editor*

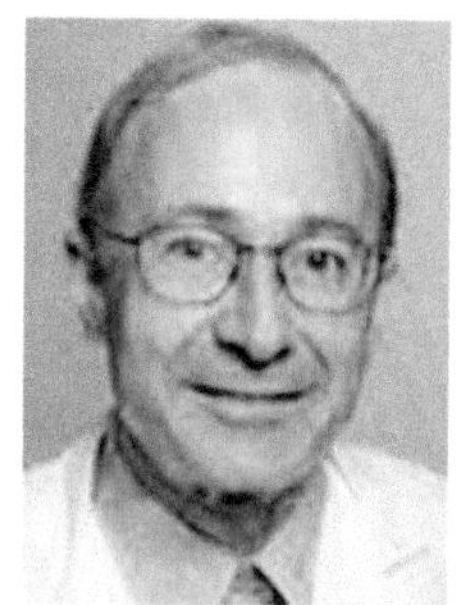

Mark G. Lebwohl, MD, *Editor*

The first edition of *Therapy for Severe Psoriasis* fills the need for an up-to-date resource for the rapidly changing treatment arena for severe psoriasis. Highlights of this book are chapters devoted to newly approved therapies such as apremilast, secukinumab, ixekizumab, and biosimilars. This is the golden era for treating patients with severe psoriasis. As more and more medications are approved, each wave seems to demonstrate higher efficacy with minimal adverse events. It is hoped that this textbook summarizes and guides the dermatologist in learning and choosing among the myriad of options.

The lead authors of each chapter are world leaders in their fields regarding their topics, and we thank them and their coauthors in developing comprehensive but readable chapters. The opening chapter gives an updated overview of psoriasis, including epidemiology, pathogenesis, and clinical findings in each of the subtypes of psoriasis. Each chapter devoted to therapy has a concluding paragraph that frames the therapy in their own "expert" algorithm of when to use the treatment. The final chapter gives an insight into therapies in the pipeline that may be approved in the near future.

We hope that this textbook serves as both a reference book and a practical guide in treating patients with severe psoriasis. We look forward to further advances in therapy for severe psoriasis in the coming years, and we plan to update this textbook with a second edition in a few years' time.

ACKNOWLEDGMENTS

The editors thank Russell Gabbedy, Colleen Viola, Louise Cook, and others at Elsevier for their steady support over the 6-month period of writing, revising, and editing this textbook. The editors acknowledge the patients who allowed their photos to be used for educational purposes like this and also for giving the authors inspiration in developing strategies to treat their severe psoriasis.

Jashin J. Wu, MD

Steven R. Feldman, MD, PhD

Mark G. Lebwohl, MD

Contents

Therapy for Severe Psoriasis

CHAPTER 1

Overview of Psoriasis

Michael Kelly-Sell, MD, Johann E. Gudjonsson, MD, PhD

KEYWORDS

• Psoriasis • Plaque psoriasis • Clinical subtypes • Pustular psoriasis • Nail psoriasis
• Comorbidities

KEY POINTS

- Today, psoriasis is a global disease causing significant impairment in quality of life, disfiguring morbidity, and increased mortality.
- Psoriasis affects men and women equally. Two-thirds of patients are thought to have mild disease, and one-third of patients are thought to have more severe involvement.
- Psoriasis is found in practically all racial groups and is thought to affect approximately 2% of the world's population.
- Psoriasis may appear at any age, but it most commonly presents between the ages of 15 and 30.
- Over the last 20 years, many of the immunologic drivers of psoriasis have been uncovered, and this research has been translated to the clinic with the development of increasingly powerful but selective biologic drugs targeting these immune pathways.

Psoriasis was first described by the ancient Greeks, Hippocrates and Galen, and grouped together with leprosy. The term psoriasis was derived from the Greek "psora" which means an, "itch, mange, scab." In the early nineteenth century, Robert Wilan and Hebra refined the description of psoriasis and distinguished it from leprosy. In 1879, Koebner described the appearance of psoriatic lesions at sites of injury, called the "Koebner phenomenon." Today, psoriasis a global disease affecting 125 million people across the world and causing significant impairment in quality of life, disfiguring morbidity, and even mortality. In the late twentieth century, basic science research demonstrated that psoriasis is an immune-mediated polygenic disorder that can be triggered by various environmental triggers. Over the last 20 years, many of the immunologic drivers of psoriasis have been uncovered, and this research has been translated to the clinic with the development of increasingly powerful but selective biologic drugs targeting these immune pathways. This increased understanding of the immunology of psoriasis has led to remarkable improvements in the treatment of psoriasis and makes it an exciting time to care for patients with psoriasis.

EPIDEMIOLOGY

Psoriasis affects male and female patients equally. Two-thirds of patients are thought to have mild disease, and one-third of patients are thought to have more severe involvement. Psoriasis is found in practically all racial groups and is thought to affect approximately 2% of the world's population. Although psoriasis is a global disease, there are some regional variations in prevalence, with rates varying from 0.4% in Asians to 2.6% in the United States and 2.9% in Denmark. In Africa, there is a higher prevalence in East Africans as opposed to West Africans, which may help explain racial differences within the United States. Interestingly, a study of 26,000 South American Native Americans did not document a single case of psoriasis.

AGE OF ONSET

Psoriasis may appear at any age, but it most commonly presents between the ages of 15 and 30. An earlier age of onset and family history have been associated with particular HLA class I antigens, most notably *HLA-Cw6*. Based on this finding, Henseler and Christophers[1] proposed that 2 different forms of psoriasis exist: type I psoriasis, with onset before the age of 40; and type II psoriasis, with age of onset after the age of 40. Both types of psoriasis respond similarly to treatment.

Cause and Pathogenesis

The root cause of psoriasis remains unknown. However, research is beginning to link the complex genetic, biochemical, and immunologic abnormalities that underlie the disease. These changes can be seen in both psoriatic lesions and normal-appearing skin of psoriatic patients.

There is strong evidence suggesting at least a partial genetic basis in psoriasis. Genome linkage studies in the 1990s identified a locus termed *psoriasis susceptibility 1 (PSORS1)* in the major histocompatibility complex (chromosome 6p21.3), home of the HLA genes.[2] Many HLA markers have been associated with psoriasis, but HLA-Cw6 has constantly demonstrated the highest relative risk for psoriasis in Caucasian populations.[3] HLA-Cw6 is also strongly associated with early onset, guttate psoriasis, and psoriatic arthritis. However, only about 10% of HLA-Cw6 carriers develop psoriasis and the *PSORS1* may account for only one-third of the genetic liability to psoriasis.[4] In recent years, additional genetic risk variants have been identified for psoriasis, with more than 60 genetic loci identified to date. These findings confirm the polygenic nature of psoriasis and also its heterogeneity because most patients carry different combinations of these risk variants, and this may influence clinical course of the disease as well as therapeutic responses.

DEVELOPMENT OF A LESION

Psoriasis is characterized clinically by red and scaly plaques sharply demarcated from normal skin. Histologically, it is characterized by marked proliferation of keratinocytes, altered epidermal differentiation, and proliferation of endothelial cells accompanied by an influx of a variety of inflammatory cells. The development of a psoriatic lesion is a complex and multicellular process that involves keratinocytes, T cells, dendritic cells, macrophages, mast cells, endothelial cells, and neutrophils. Cytokines and growth factors initiate and sustain inflammation in this process through pathways that involve cells of both the innate and the acquired immune systems. Initial pinhead-sized macular lesions show edema and mononuclear cell infiltrates within the upper dermis. The overlying epidermis becomes spongiotic, and there is a focal loss of the granular layer. As the plaque matures, the epidermis becomes thickened in the center with increasing parakeratosis, capillary elongation, and perivascular infiltration of various types of immune cells. Mature psoriatic lesions contain elongated and uniform rete ridges with thinning of the epidermis overlying the dermal papillae. The tips of the rete ridges may become clubbed with dilated, tortuous capillaries in the dermal papillae. There is typically confluent parakeratosis and hyperkeratosis.[5] More inflammatory cells are present with CD4+ T cells and dendritic cells in the upper dermis and CD8+ T cells in the epidermis. Neutrophils are commonly seen in psoriatic lesions and form characteristic collections in the spinous layer (spongiform pustules of Kogoj) and in the stratum corneum (Munro microabscesses). Eosinophils are not seen in psoriasis, unless the disease is drug induced.

T CELLS

The role of T cells in psoriasis was first documented in the 1980s, and the last 30 years of scientific and clinical research on psoriasis have further highlighted their role in the pathophysiology of the disease. The latest biologic medications for psoriasis target T-cell immune pathways, and their ability to clear plaques underlines the importance of the T-cell pathways these medications target.

In 1984, Dr Baker and colleagues[6] were the first to show a correlation between the eruption of psoriatic skin lesions and the epidermal influx and activation of T cells. Subsequently, deletion of epidermal T cells was shown to predate resolution of psoriatic plaques in patients on phototherapy.[7] In 1986, cyclosporine was shown to be highly efficacious in treating psoriasis due to its blockade of T-cell function.[8] Ten years later in 1996, activated autologous T cells initiated psoriatic lesions when injected into uninvolved psoriatic skin transplanted onto severe combined immunodeficient mice.[9] This showed that T cells were sufficient to induce a psoriatic process. More recently, using xenograft models where human skin is grafted onto immunodeficient mice, trafficking of T cells to the epidermis, particularly CD8+ T cells, was shown to be critical for development of psoriatic plaques, highlighting the importance of these cells in psoriasis.

Psoriatic lesions are typified by T helper 1 (Th1) polarized CD4+ cells and T cytotoxic 1 (Tc1) polarized CD8+ T cells producing interferon (IFN)-γ, which is the dominant cytokine profile of psoriatic lesions.[10] IFN-γ drives the production of interleukin-12 (IL-12) and IL-23 by dendritic cells. IL-23 supports and expands CD4+ T cells, and likely CD8+ T cells, that produce IL-17 and/or IL-22, whereas IL-12 promotes development of

Th1 and Tc1 cells. The secretion of IL-17 and IL-22 by these cell types likely maintains the chronic inflammation in psoriasis,[11,12] but the exact role of IFN-γ in this process is still unclear. T cells also contribute to the production of tumor necrosis factor-α (TNF-α), but TNF-α is a potent proinflammatory cytokine, the main role of which may be to amplify the effect of other cytokines, including IFN-γ and TNF-α. Biologic medications targeted at inhibiting these inflammatory mediators, including TNF-α, IL-12/IL-23, and IL-17, have shown great efficacy in treating psoriasis, underlining the important role this molecule plays in driving the disease.

MACROPHAGES AND DENDRITIC CELLS

Macrophages are important phagocytic cells that reside under the basement membrane, adjacent to proliferating keratinocytes, and are important in the early development of psoriatic lesions. They express Factor XIIIa and secrete the chemokine MCP-1 (CCL2).[13] They are an important source of TNF-α, inducible nitric oxide synthase, and IL-23.[13,14] It has been shown in mouse models that the selective elimination of macrophages leads to prompt improvement of psoriatic lesions.[15]

Dendritic cells have an important role in both priming the adaptive immune response and inducing self-tolerance. Subtypes of dendritic cells, such as Langerhans cells, dermal dendritic cells, and myeloid dendritic cells, help drive the Th1, Th17/Th22 polarization of psoriatic plaques. In particular, myeloid dendritic cells help make IL-12 and IL-23 cytokines that promote Th1 and Th17 differentiation and responses, respectively.[16] In a psoriatic plaque, myeloid dendritic cells can be increased up to 30-fold as compared with uninvolved skin and make up about 80% to 90% of the dendritic cells.[17]

NEUTROPHILS

Although neutrophils are a common histopathologic finding in the upper epidermis of psoriatic lesions, they do not seem to a have a significant role in lesional development in chronic plaque psoriasis, although they have a key role in pustular variants of psoriasis.

UNINVOLVED PSORIATIC SKIN

Normal-appearing skin of patients with psoriasis has been shown to have subclinical biochemical changes that lead to subtle histologic findings. Lipid biosynthesis is predominantly affected with measurable changes in the levels, constitution of phospholipids, free α-amino acids, and hydrolytic enzymes. These changes lead to histopathologic findings that can be identified on microscopic examination and have been termed "histochemical parakeratosis."

CLINICAL FINDINGS

History

In approaching a patient with psoriasis, it is important for the clinician to obtain a thorough personal, family, and social history because it often will influence the choice of therapeutic agent. Relevant information includes the age of onset of psoriasis and whether psoriasis is present in any close relatives, because both a younger age of onset and a positive family history have been associated with more widespread and recurrent disease.[18] In addition, the prior course of disease and frequency of relapses should be recorded, because there is significant variability in the clinical presentation of disease and the disease may change from one clinical phenotype to another (Box 1.1). In some patients, the disease frequently relapses, and this has been associated with more severe disease with rapidly enlarging lesions covering significant portions of the body surface.[19] Other patients have more chronic, slowly developing lesions with only occasional recurrences.

The presence or absence of joint symptoms should be recorded—such as painful, warm, or swollen joints. Any of these complaints are concerning for psoriatic arthritis and prompt a more thorough evaluation. It is important to remember that osteoarthritis is common and frequently coexists with psoriasis.

BOX 1.1
Clinical subtypes of psoriasis

- Chronic plaque psoriasis (psoriasis vulgaris)
  - Psoriasis geographica
  - Psoriasis gyrata
  - Annular
  - Rupioid
  - Ostraceous
  - Elephantine
- Guttate psoriasis (eruptive psoriasis)
- Small plaque psoriasis
- Flexural (Inverse) psoriasis
- Erythrodermic psoriasis
- Sebopsoriasis
- Napkin psoriasis
- Linear psoriasis

Psoriasis is associated with several comorbidities, including increased incidence of myocardial infarction, stroke, and death, particularly in patients with moderate-to-severe psoriasis.[20–23] Psoriasis has been shown to be an independent risk factor for cardiovascular disease,[24,25] and it is important to screen patients for other cardiovascular risk factors in their social and medical histories, because modification of these can help offset their increased risk. Cardiovascular risk factors include smoking status, diet, and any previous diagnoses of hypertension, diabetes, dyslipidemia, or obesity.

Treatment history should also be recorded. Although the ability to predict treatment responses to a given agent are still very limited, patients that have been on previous biologics and failed generally respond less well to other biologic agents, even when these are in a different class. The nature of this decreased therapeutic response is still unclear. There is a broad differential diagnosis for psoriasis that physicians should consider (Table 1.1), and treatment failures may prompt a reconsideration of the diagnosis.

CUTANEOUS LESIONS

Psoriasis Vulgaris

Psoriasis vulgaris, or chronic plaque psoriasis, is the most common clinical manifestation of psoriasis, affecting approximately 90% of psoriasis patients. Psoriasis vulgaris is characterized by well-demarcated, erythematous, raised plaques with white micaceous scale. Lesions vary in size from pinpoint papules to large plaques and tend to be symmetrically distributed on the scalp, postauricular skin, elbows, gluteal cleft, and knees. These lesions produce significant amounts of scale and removing the scale produces pinpoint bleeding (the Auspitz sign), which is a sign of the dilated

TABLE 1.1
Differential diagnosis of psoriasis

Psoriasis Vulgaris	Guttate	Erythrodermic	Pustular
Common			
• Discoid/nummular eczema • Cutaneous T-cell lymphoma (CTCL) • Tinea corporis	• Pityriasis rosea • Pityriasis lichenoides chronica • Lichen planus	• Drug-induced erythroderma • Eczema • CTCL/Sézary syndrome • Pityriasis rubra pilaris	• Impetigo • Superficial candidiasis • Reactive arthritis syndrome • Superficial folliculitis
Consider			
• Pityriasis rubra pilaris • Seborrheic dermatitis • Subacute cutaneous lupus erythematosus • Erythrkeratoderma (either erythrokeratoderma variabilis and/or progressive symmetric erythrokeratoderma) • Hypertrophic lichen planus • Lichen simplex chronicus • Contact dermatitis • Chronic cutaneous lupus erythematosus/discoid lupus erythematosus • Hailey-Hailey disease (more flexural) • Intertrigo (flexures) • *Candida* infection (flexures) • Bowen disease/squamous cell carcinoma in situ • Extramammary Paget disease	• Small plaque parapsoriasis • Pityriasis lichenoides et varioliformis acuta (PLEVA) • Lichen planus • Drug eruption • Secondary syphilis		• Pemphigus foliaceus • Immunoglobulin A pemphigus • Sneddon-Wilkinson disease (subcorneal pustular dermatosis) • Migratory necrolytic erythema • Transient neonatal pustular melanosis • Acropustulosis of infancy • Acute generalized exanthematous pustulosis

capillaries below the epidermis and thinned suprapapillary plate. Disease presentation is impressively variable among patients, and the clinical findings can change quickly even within the same patient.

Psoriatic lesions can be induced by trauma, and this is known as Koebnerization or the isomorphic response. This phenomenon is more likely to occur when the disease is flaring and is an all-or-nothing response (meaning if psoriasis appears at one site of injury then it will appear at all sites of injury). The isomorphic response typically appears 7 to 14 days after injury, and the lifetime prevalence of the phenomenon is estimated to be 25% to 75%.[26] The isomorphic response is not specific to psoriasis.

Historically, psoriasis vulgaris has been subclassified by the shape and scale of the plaques. Today, the terms have little significance clinically, but they connect the modern disease to its long history. *Psoriasis geographica* describes plaques that resemble a land map. *Psoriasis gyrata* consists of confluent, connected plaques with a circinate appearance. *Rupioid* lesions present in the shape of a cone or limpet. *Ostraceous* plaques have a circular, hyperkeratotic concave lesion resembling an oyster shell. *Elephantine psoriasis* refers to large, thick, scaly plaques on the lower extremities. *Annular* lesions have partial central clearing, giving a ring-shaped appearance, and are associated with a good prognosis because the annular shape suggests clearing (Fig. 1.1). Finally, a hypopigmented ring on the periphery of an individual plaque, or Woronoff ring, may be seen after treatment with UV radiation or topical steroids. Woronoff rings are thought to be caused by inhibition of prostaglandin synthesis and are associated with lesional clearing and a good prognosis.[27]

Guttate Psoriasis

Derived from the Latin *gutta*, "a drop," guttate psoriasis is distinguished by the eruption of small psoriatic papules across the upper trunk and proximal extremities (Fig. 1.2). Guttate psoriasis typically presents in children, adolescents, and young adults. It is often preceded by a streptococcal throat infection, and less commonly, perianal strep infections, and more than half of patients will have molecular evidence of a recent streptococcal infection, such as an elevated antistreptolysin O, anti-DNase B, or streptozyme titer. Despite this association, antibiotics are not helpful in the treatment of guttate psoriasis and do not alter the course of the disease.[28] One-third to one-half of patients who develop guttate psoriasis will later develop chronic plaque psoriasis. As mentioned above, guttate psoriasis shows the strongest association with HLA-Cw6.[29]

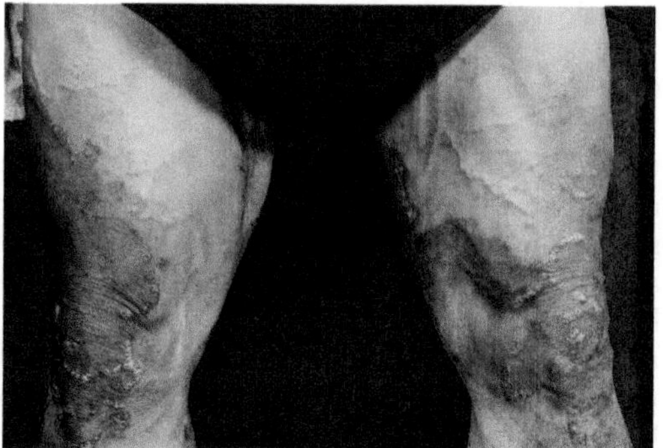

Fig. 1.1 Annular plaque psoriasis. There are well-defined erythematous plaques with thick micaceous scale on the periphery.

Inverse Psoriasis (Flexural Psoriasis)

Inverse, or flexural, psoriasis is distinguished by psoriatic lesions appearing in the major skin folds, such as in the axillae, inguinal creases, intergluteal cleft, umbilicus, and inframammary folds. Lesions are erythematous and sharply demarcated, with a glossy appearance and little to no scale. The lesion may contain a central fissure. The sharp demarcation and glossy appearance help distinguish the lesions from other diseases of the skin folds. Sweating is decreased in affected areas and localized fungal or bacterial infections may be a trigger.

Erythrodermic Psoriasis

Erythrodermic psoriasis is the generalized form of disease and affects all body sites: face, trunk, extremities, hands, and feet. Erythema is more prominent and the scaling is finer, more superficial and diffuse, as compared with psoriasis vulgaris. Patients lose their autonomic control of body temperature and may present with systemic symptoms. They lose excessive heat from generalized vasodilation and so may shiver to try to compensate. In warm climates, there is a risk for hyperthermia because patients do not sweat from their psoriatic lesions.[30] The generalized vasodilatation also puts patients at risk for high-output cardiac failure, impaired hepatic and renal function, and lower extremity edema. Erythrodermic psoriasis is thought to have 2 general presentations: first, as a chronic form that is thought to be a slow progression of psoriasis vulgaris (Fig. 1.3). A second form is distinguished by its sudden onset and may be a generalized Koebner reaction to treatments such as phototherapy or anthralin. Finally, other generalized forms of psoriasis may give an appearance of erythrodermic psoriasis as they heal, such as generalized pustular psoriasis.

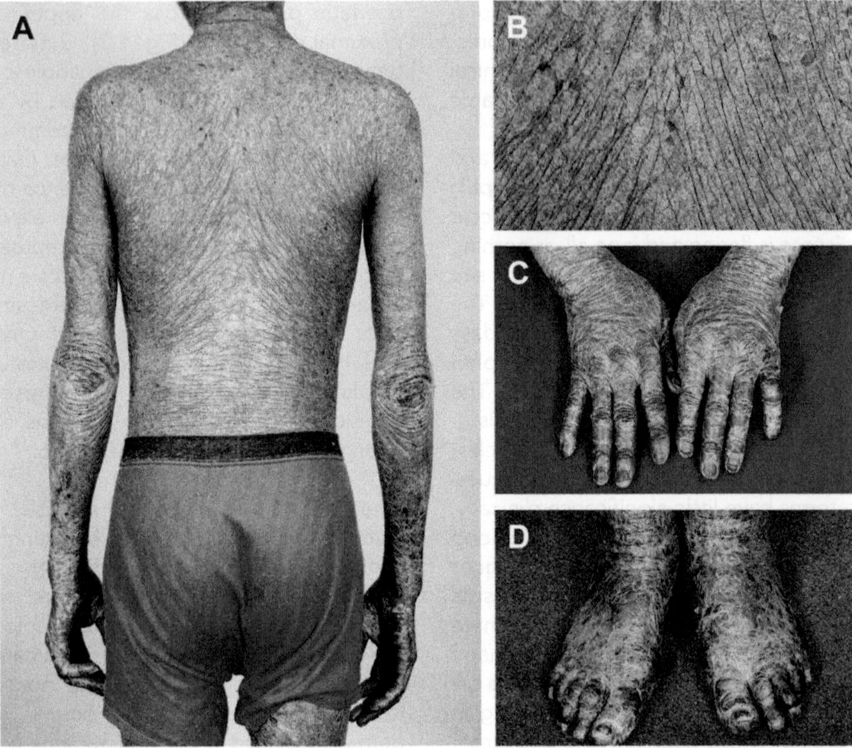

Fig. 1.2 Erythrodermic psoriasis associated with HIV. (*A*) Cutaneous disease often worsens as a patient's CD4 count drops. (*B*) Thick micaceous scale. (*C*) There was confluent erythema and scale on the hands. Note the prominent oil spots below the fingernails and swelling of the left fifth PIP joint. (*D*) There is confluent scale on the feet with subtle erythema. Note the left third toe dactylitis, also known as a "sausage digit," a manifestation of psoriatic arthritis.

Pustular Psoriasis

Clinically, pustular psoriasis is distinguished by the appearance of 2- to 3-mm sterile pustules that show infiltrated subcorneal neutrophils on histopathologic examination (Fig. 1.4). There are 4 main clinical categories of pustular psoriasis: generalized pustular psoriasis (von Zumbusch type), annular pustular psoriasis, impetigo herpetiformis, and localized forms (including pustulosis palmaris et plantaris [PPP] and acrodermatitis continua of Hallopeau) (Box 1.2). Finally, SAPHO syndrome (synovitis, acne, pustulosis, hyperostosis, osteitis) is a genetic syndrome that typically presents in children and young adults, and palmoplantar pustulosis is a main feature.

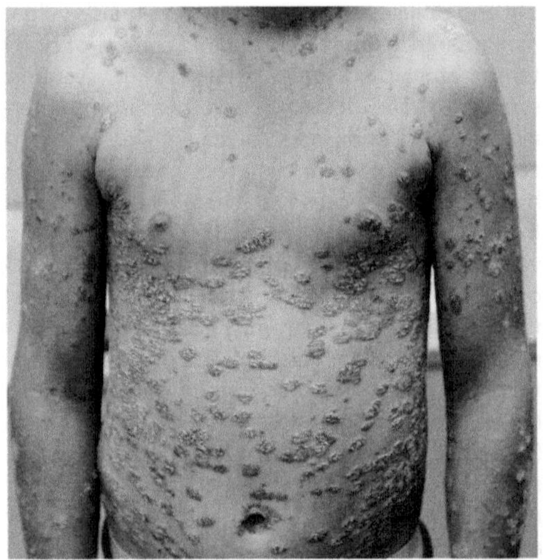

Fig. 1.3 Guttate psoriasis, involving the upper extremities and torso. Clinically, the micaceous scale helps differentiate this disorder.

Generalized Pustular Psoriasis (von Zumbusch)

Generalized pustular psoriasis (von Zumbusch) is an acute variant of pustular psoriasis typified by several days of fever preceding the sudden generalized eruption of sterile pustules across the body—face, trunk, extremities, nail beds, palms, and soles. The attacks may occur in waves, and the skin is painful. On examination, there is a background of erythematous skin that initially starts as patches but spreads to become confluent, leading to erythroderma. With chronic disease, there may be atrophy of the fingertips.

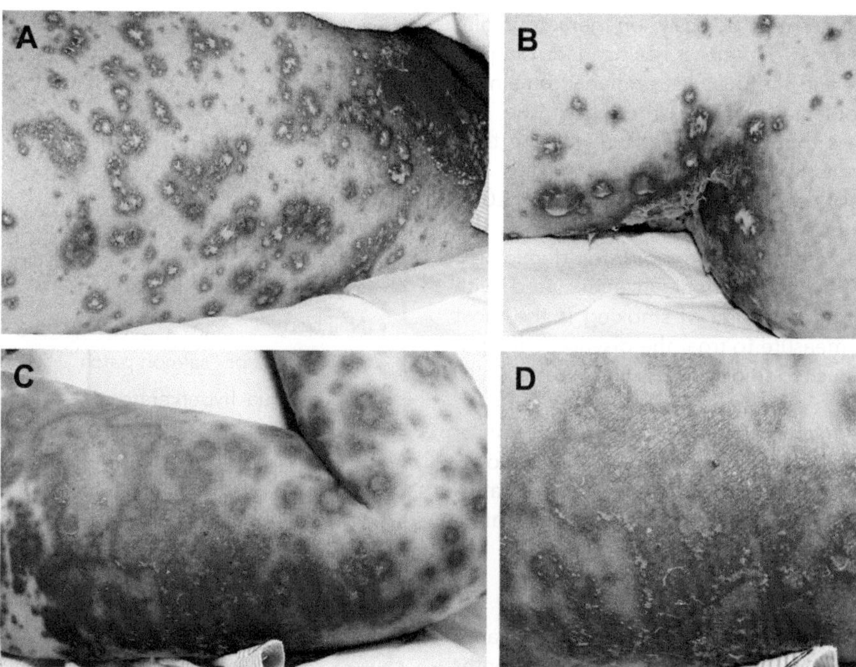

Fig. 1.4 Pustular psoriasis. The patient shown in (*A*) and (*B*) demonstrates flaccid subcorneal pustules on an erythematous base. Note the pus accumulating in the dependent half of the pustules. The patient shown in (*C*) and (*D*) had pustules form an annular or circinate pattern with an erythematous center. This may resemble erythema annulare centrifugum or impetigo herpetiformis.

The cause of attacks is unknown but possible triggering factors include infections, irritating topical treatments (provoking a Koebner phenomenon), and withdrawal of systemic corticosteroids.

Generalized pustular psoriasis may have life-threatening complications, including hypocalcemia, acute respiratory distress syndrome, bacterial superinfection leading to sepsis, and dehydration.[31,32] The severity of the disease makes rapid control important, and therefore, medications with a rapid onset of action should be chosen. Drugs that have been used successfully include methotrexate, cyclosporine, infliximab,[33] and systemic corticosteroids.[34]

Loss-of-function mutations in the *IL36RN* gene, encoding IL-36 receptor antagonist (IL-36ra), have been found in patients with generalized pustular psoriasis. IL-36ra is an anti-inflammatory cytokine that inhibits signaling of proinflammatory IL-36 proteins (α, β, and γ).[35]

BOX 1.2
Clinical subtypes of pustular psoriasis

- Generalized pustular psoriasis (von Zumbusch)
- Annular pustular psoriasis
- Impetigo herpetiformis
- Localized pustular psoriasis
  - Pustulosis palmaris et plantaris
  - Acrodermatitis continua (of Hallopeau)
  - SAPHO (synovitis, acne, pustulosis, hyperostosis, osteitis)

Annular Pustular Psoriasis and Impetigo Herpetiformis

Annular pustular psoriasis is a rare form of pustular psoriasis that presents with pustules on an erythematous ring. It may initially resemble gyrate erythemas, such as erythema annulare centrifugum. It can present during pregnancy, typically in the early third trimester, and is called impetigo herpetiformis. There is significant risk for hypocalcemia, and while the disease typically improves after delivery, it may recur during subsequent pregnancies.[31,36] There is often no personal or family history of psoriasis.

Localized Pustular Psoriasis Variants

There are 2 main forms of localized pustular psoriasis: PPP and acrodermatitis continua (of Hallopeau). PPP is characterized by sterile pustules on the palmoplantar surfaces with yellow-brown macules. There may be scaly, erythematous plaques. A minority of patients has psoriatic plaques elsewhere, and the pustules primarily remain on the palmoplantar surfaces throughout the disease. PPP is thought to affect femalemore than male patients, with a ratio of approximately 3:1, and typically presents between the ages of 20 to 60. In contrast to plaque psoriasis, PPP is not associated with any HLA type. In epidemiologic surveys, PPP has been highly associated with smoking, and cessation of smoking is the most important measure to treat the disease.[37] If a patient continues to smoke, PPP is highly resistant to treatment.

Acrodermatitis continua is a rare eruption of sterile pustules on the fingers or toes that slowly extends proximally. Chronic disease leads to atrophy of the digit and destruction of the nail matrix. It is difficult to treat.

Napkin Psoriasis

Napkin psoriasis typically presents in the diaper (napkin) areas between the ages of 3 and 6 months with a red, confluent patch. Scattered small, red, papules with psoriatic white scale may appear a few days later on the rest of the body. It typically responds readily to topical steroids and usually resolves by 1 year of age.

Linear Psoriasis

Linear psoriasis is a rare form of the disease that typically presents as a linear plaque on an extremity or dermatome of the trunk. There may be an underlying nevus, such as an inflammatory linear verrucous epidermal nevus (ILVEN). Separating linear psoriasis and ILVEN into distinct diseases is controversial.[38]

RELATED PHYSICAL FINDINGS

Nail Findings

Nail involvement is common in psoriasis and is seen in up to 40% of psoriasis patients.[18] It increases with age, extent of disease, duration of disease, and presence of psoriatic arthritis. Findings are classified as either evidence of nail matrix or nail bed disease (Box 1.3). Nail matrix disease leads to pitting, onychorrhexis, Beau lines, leukonychia, and thinning of the nail plate. Nail bed disease leads to findings of oil drops (or "salmon patches"), subungual hyperkeratosis, and splinter hemorrhages. Fingernails are more often affected than toenails, and nail involvement may cause pain and restrictions on activities of daily life.

Nail pitting is one of the most common nail findings with psoriasis. Typically, there are single or multiple 0.5- to 2.0-mm pits irregularly arranged on the dorsal nail plate. Nail pitting is caused by foci of parakeratosis at the proximal nail matrix, which forms the dorsal nail plate, causing poor keratinization. Nail pitting is not unique to psoriasis and can also be seen in alopecia areata and other disorders. The nail pitting of alopecia areata is typically thought to be more linear than in psoriasis, although this is not always the case. Other findings of nail matrix disease include leukonychia, a result of disease in the midportion of the nail matrix, and widespread disease leads to crumbling of the nail plate.

Oil drops are translucent red-yellow discolorations on the nail bed, below the nail plate. They are a result of psoriasiform hyperplasia, parakeratosis, and microvascular changes of the nail bed and trapping of neutrophils under the nail plate.[39] Unlike nail pits, oil drops on the nail bed are a unique finding of psoriasis. Other nail bed findings with psoriasis include splinter hemorrhages, from capillary bleeding at thinned suprapapillary plates, onycholysis, and subungual hyperkeratosis. These findings are not as specific to psoriasis. Anonychia, complete loss of nails, is common in acrodermatitis continua, but nail findings are not typically seen in other localized variants of pustular psoriasis. Nail changes are important to note clinically because they have been associated with increased risk for psoriatic arthritis.

BOX 1.3
Nail findings in psoriasis

- Nail matrix
  - Nail plate pits
  - Onychorrhexis
  - Beau lines
  - Nail plate thinning
  - Erythema of the lunula
- Nail bed
  - Oil drops or "salmon patch"
  - Subungual hyperkeratosis
  - Onycholysis
  - Splinter hemorrhages
- Proximal and lateral nail folds
  - Cutaneous psoriasis

PSORIATIC ARTHRITIS

Psoriatic arthritis occurs in 5% to 30% of patients with cutaneous psoriasis, and its prevalence may be underestimated.[40] Cutaneous disease typically precedes the joint disease by about 10 to 12 years, but about 10% to 15% of patients with psoriatic arthritis present without skin findings. Diagnosis is difficult to establish because there is no serologic marker, and the radiographic hallmark, erosive changes, may occur years after the initial periarticular inflammation. Classic findings include asymmetric involvement of both the distal (DIP) and proximal (PIP) interphalangeal joints, seen in about 40% of patients.[41] In contrast to rheumatoid arthritis, involvement of the metacarpophalangeal joints is rare. Prolonged disease in the PIP and DIP of a single digit can lead to swelling (dactylitis) and the appearance of a "sausage" digit. Enthesitis, or inflammation at the insertion site of tendons into bones, is also a common finding in psoriatic arthritis and is seen in approximately 20% of patients with psoriatic arthritis.[42] Arthritis mutilans is the most severe form of psoriatic arthritis with extensive joint damage and bone resorption and is seen in 5% of patients.[41] Early diagnosis of psoriatic arthritis alters the treatment approach for a patient, as the physician should consider systemic or biologic medications to prevent life-changing morbidity from arthritic changes, even when cutaneous disease is limited.

LABORATORY TESTS

Most patients can be diagnosed based on their clinical history and features alone. However, histopathologic examination can be helpful to establish the diagnosis in difficult cases. The typical histopathologic features of chronic plaque psoriasis and guttate psoriasis have been discussed previously (see "Development of Lesions").

Pustular psoriasis is distinguished on histopathology by the presence of neutrophils migrating from dilated vessels and pooling in the upper epidermis, within the upper Malpighian layer below the stratum corneum. In newer lesions, there may be mild acanthosis, whereas older lesions have more typical psoriasiform hyperplasia.

There are no serum markers that are specific for psoriasis and regularly used to establish a diagnosis. Laboratory workup is typically aimed at ruling out other disease processes in the differential diagnosis, such as checking an antinuclear antibody to test for connective tissue disease. Nonetheless, it can be important to check serum markers in patients with severe disease to assess for systemic complications. Patients may have a decreased serum albumin, secondary to the negative nitrogen balance from the turnover of their skin, or elevated uric acid, increasing their risk for developing gouty arthritis.

Many patients with psoriasis manifest altered lipid profiles with elevated levels of high-density lipoproteins, altered cholesterol-triglyceride ratios in very low-density lipoprotein particles, and elevated plasma apolipoprotein-A1 concentrations.[43] These alterations in lipids may contribute to the increased cardiovascular risk for psoriasis patients. Other risk factors of cardiovascular disease should be considered and appropriate laboratory tests ordered, because patients with psoriasis are predisposed to cardiovascular disease (see later discussion). General markers of systemic inflammation, such as C-reactive protein and erythrocyte sedimentation rate, are elevated in a minority of patients with chronic plaque psoriasis and may suggest the presence of psoriatic arthritis.

COMPLICATIONS

Psoriatic patients have increased morbidity and mortality from cardiovascular disease, which correlates with the severity and length of disease.[44] Younger patients with psoriasis are at particular risk, because a large population-based cohort study using the UK General Practice Research Database found that 30-year-olds with severe psoriasis had a relative risk of myocardial infarction of 3.10 as compared with healthy controls.[21] Other large epidemiology studies have shown that patients with psoriasis are 2.9-fold more likely to have a diagnosis of metabolic syndrome—which is defined by having 3 of 5 risk factors for cardiovascular disease, including obesity, hypertriglyceridemia, low high-density lipoprotein, hypertension, or diabetes. Psoriasis patients had increased rates of hypertension (35.6% in psoriatic patients vs 20.6% in controls), and hyperlipidemia (29% vs 17.1%).[45] Psoriasis is thought to be an independent risk factor for the development of metabolic syndrome because psoriasis patients have increased odds of having hypertension even after controlling for age, sex, smoking status, and other variables.[46] There is an increased prevalence of rheumatoid arthritis (prevalence ratio [PR] 3.8), Crohn disease (PR 2.1), and ulcerative colitis (PR 2.0) in patients with psoriasis.[45] There is an increased risk of both Hodgkin lymphoma and cutaneous T-cell lymphoma in psoriasis, particularly in patients with severe disease.[47]

The psychological impact of psoriasis on patients is profound. Cutaneous disease leads to concerns about appearance, lowered self-esteem, social rejection, guilt, embarrassment, emptiness, sexual problems, and impairment of professional ability (Fig. 1.5). These stressors lead to higher rates of anxiety, depression, and suicidal ideation in psoriasis patients than in the

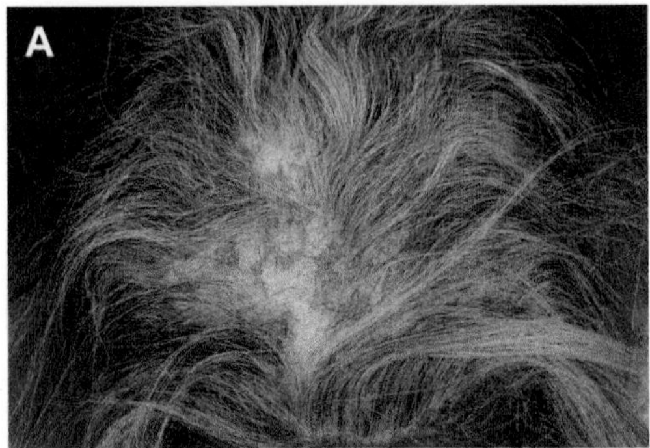

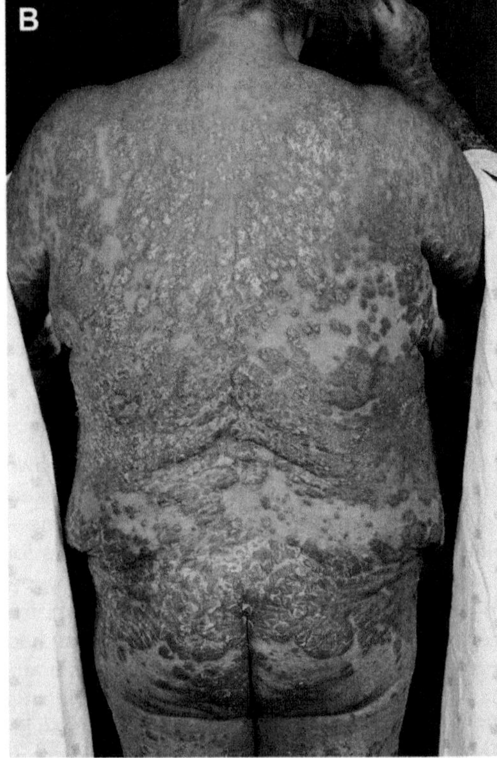

Fig. 1.5 Psoriatic alopecia and plaque psoriasis. (*A*) Chronic inflammation and scale from psoriasis have led to alopecia. This is typically a nonscarring alopecia but the inflammation may be so severe that there is permanent destruction of hair follicles. (*B*) The same patient demonstrated widespread erythematous plaques with micaceous scale in a symmetric distribution.

general population.[48] Pruritus and pain may exacerbate these psychosocial stressors. These issues impact a large number of psoriatic patients with one survey finding 79% of respondents reporting their psoriasis caused a negative impact on their life.[49]

MODIFYING FACTORS

Obesity and smoking have both been associated with more severe presentations of psoriasis.[50] Smoking also seems to play a role in the onset of psoriasis. Neither characteristic affects treatment strategies, although all patients should be encouraged to quit and follow a healthy diet. Quitting tobacco is particularly important for patients with palmoplantar pustulosis because tobacco use may drive the process and is associated with recalcitrant disease.

Bacterial and viral infections have also been associated with psoriasis flares or the onset of disease. There is a clear association between streptococcal throat infection and guttate psoriasis, but streptococcal infections may exacerbate chronic plaque psoriasis, too.[51,52] HIV infection can present as a severe psoriasis exacerbation and, paradoxically, a patient's psoriasis may become more severe as the immunodeficiency progresses.[53] This helps to explain why treatment of a patient's underlying HIV with highly active antiretroviral therapy improves the patient's psoriasis.[54]

Finally, medications may help either induce disease or aggravate a patient's psoriasis. Medications that have been reported to aggravate psoriasis include lithium, β-blockers, TNF-α inhibitors, antimalarials, nonsteroidal anti-inflammatory drugs, type I and type II IFNs, imiquimod, angiotensin-converting enzyme inhibitors, and gemfibrozil. The mechanism and clinical presentation of drug-exacerbated psoriasis vary. For example, lithium is thought to decrease levels of inositol, an important component of the intracellular second messenger system, altering calcium homeostasis and keratinocyte differentiation. β-Blockers decrease cellular AMP, an important intracellular signaling protein, altering calcium homeostasis, driving keratinocyte proliferation and inhibiting keratinocyte differentiation.[55] Counterintuitively, TNF-α inhibitors may cause a psoriasiform dermatitis in patients with rheumatoid arthritis or inflammatory bowel disease.[56] Most patients reported developed palmoplantar pustulosis, but about one-third developed chronic plaque psoriasis.[57] Psoriasis patients traveling to countries where antimalarial prophylaxis is needed should be warned that their disease may flare and plan accordingly.

TREATMENT

Psoriasis is an exciting field because the number of medications available for treating patients is broad and growing quickly. Most, but not all, of these agents are immunomodulatory medications. Despite the high efficacy of these medications, older and more traditional therapies still have an important role as adjunctive treatment. This chapter provides a general introduction to the major categories of treatment: topical therapies, phototherapy, oral medications, and biologic medications (Table 1.2). This chapter covers topical treatments at depth but leaves the other modalities for the remainder of this book.

In formulating a treatment regimen, the clinician must balance the patient's goals with the measurable severity of the disease, patient-specific factors (such as psoriatic arthritis, pregnancy, or a history of malignancy), and limits set by payors. There is no cure for psoriasis, and treatment can be frustrating, with many patients reporting their treatment regimens being ineffective. With the advent of highly effective biologics and the high level of treatment responses achieved with these drugs, patient's expectations have grown. Therefore, these feelings are only likely to grow.

As patients will use these medications for years, safety is also a major concern and deserves a frank discussion with patients. New treatments, which can be highly efficacious, often have the shortest safety record. Furthermore, although some treatments are safe for continuous use, others have cumulative toxicity that limits their use. Treatments may lose efficacy over time either through a process called tachyphylaxis, which is mostly limited to topical treatments, through the development of neutralizing antibodies to a particular biologic agent, or possibly through the changing nature of inflammatory responses in psoriatic skin, requiring the change or the addition of other modalities. Physicians must individualize a treatment regimen to the patient and, if there is disease progression, progression of disease will likely have to use treatments in combination to achieve long-term control.

TOPICAL THERAPIES

Most patients with psoriasis are treated initially with topical treatments, and these medications can be used safely with nearly every other treatment available (Box 1.4). Topical treatments are often inexpensive and efficacious and have an excellent safety profile. Despite these benefits, 40% of patients report being noncompliant with their topical treatments because they feel these treatments are time-consuming and cosmetically unacceptable.[58] Cosmetic considerations are particularly important, and physicians should prescribe a medication as both a cream, to be used during the day, and a more potent ointment, to be used at night. It is important to give a sufficient volume of medication for the patient to treat their skin lesions appropriately, and 400 g of a topical agent is required to entirely cover an average sized adult twice daily for 1 week.

CORTICOSTEROIDS

Topical corticosteroids are commonly first-line therapy in mild-to-moderate psoriasis and on sensitive skin, such as the flexures and genitalia. These medications work by causing nuclear translocation of glucocorticoid receptors, leading to a wide variety of effects. Patients typically see improvement with 2 to 4 weeks of daily treatment and then can taper to a maintenance phase of applying the creams only 2 to 3 days per week. Long-term daily use of topical corticosteroids may cause skin atrophy, telangiectasias, stretch marks, and adrenal suppression (from systemic absorption). With long-term use, these agents lose their efficacy, and patients should be switched to an alternative formulation. Upon discontinuation of a topical steroid, a patient's disease may rebound.[59] Topical corticosteroids are inexpensive, effective, and safe, when used appropriately; therefore, they should be a part of every patient's treatment plan.

VITAMIN D_3 AND ANALOGUES

The topical vitamin D preparations that are commercially available for the treatment of skin

TABLE 1.2
Treatments for psoriasis

Topical	Phototherapy	Systemic	Biologics
• Corticosteroids • Vitamin D analogues • Tazarotene • Salicylic acid • Calcineurin inhibitors (for inverse psoriasis)	• Narrowband UVB (310–331 NM) • Broadband UVB • PUVA • Excimer laser (308 NM)	• Cyclosporine • Methotrexate • Acitretin • Fumaric acid esters (available in Germany but not the US or UK) • Apremilast	TNF-α inhibitors • Etanercept • Humira • Infliximab IL-12/IL-23 inhibitor • Ustekinumab IL-17 inhibitor • Secukinumab • Ixekizumab

BOX 1.4
Topical therapies

- Topical steroids
- Vitamin D analogues
- Tazarotene
- Calcineurin inhibitors
  - Tacrolimus
  - Pimecrolimus
- Dithranol
- Coal tar
- Salicylic acid

disease include calcipotriene (or calcipotriol), calcitriol, tacalcitol, and maxacalcitol (tacalcitol and maxacalcitol are not currently available in the United States). Topical calcipotriene is commonly thought of as being about as potent as a mild topical steroid. These medications are more effective if applied twice daily rather than once daily and do not lose their efficacy with long-term use.[60] Irritation to the skin is a common side effect, so patients should be instructed not to apply vitamin D preparations to sensitive skin. There are almost no systemic side effects when these medications are used appropriately. However, hypercalcemia can occur if a patient applies more than 100 g per week of calcipotriene or 200 g per week of calcitriol. Treatment with calcipotriene can complement the use of potent topical corticosteroids, with patients applying topical calcipotriene 5 times per week when they taper their topical steroid to 2 times per week, minimizing the risk for steroid-induced atrophy.

TAZAROTENE

Tazarotene is a third-generation retinoid available in 0.05% and 0.1% gels and a cream formulation. It is used primarily to reduce plaque thickness and scaling. It is not as effective for plaque erythema. The drug's specific molecular targets are unknown, but it is thought to act by binding to retinoic acid receptors. Local irritation is a significant side effect and is dose related. Therefore, this medication is best used in combination with topical corticosteroids or phototherapy. By decreasing thickness and causing irritation, tazarotene lowers the minimal erythema dose for both UVB and UVA. Therefore, if tazarotene is started in the middle of a phototherapy course, it is recommended that the UV dose be reduced by at least one-third.[61]

TOPICAL CALCINEURIN INHIBITORS

Tacrolimus and pimecrolimus are topical calcineurin inhibitors, blocking both T-lymphocyte function and IL-2 production. In clinical trials, neither agent proved efficacious for chronic plaque psoriasis. However, there is evidence that tacrolimus is effective for the treatment of inverse psoriasis.[62,63] Clinically, these agents are limited by their main side effect, which is a burning sensation at the application site. The US Food and Drug Administration has placed a "black-box warning" on these medications after anecdotal reports of malignancy were published. The American Academy of Dermatology and the American Academy of Allergy, Asthma, and Immunology have protested these warnings. Furthermore, large after-marketing surveillance databases of the topical formulations have not detected any increased risk of lymphoma or cutaneous malignancies.[64]

SALICYLIC ACID

Salicylic acid is a topical keratolytic that lowers the pH of the stratum corneum and reduces keratinocyte adhesion. This helps to soften plaques and reduce their scale, which enhances the penetration of other therapies. Like tazarotene, it is often best used in combination with a topical corticosteroid. Unlike tazarotene, salicylic acid decreases the efficacy of UVB phototherapy.[59] Systemic absorption can occur if applied to more than 20% of the body surface area, particularly in patients with renal or hepatic dysfunction. There are no placebo-controlled studies using salicylic acid as monotherapy.

BLAND EMOLLIENTS

Patients should be encouraged to apply bland emollients regularly between medical treatments. Emollients can limit dryness, scale, and pruritus. They should be applied immediately after bathing or showering for maximum effect. They can also be applied over a thin layer of a topical medication to improve hydration of the skin. By smoothing the skin and preventing epidermal scatter, emollients may increase the efficacy of phototherapy.

PHOTOTHERAPY

Goeckerman first started using artificial light sources to treat psoriasis in the 1920s—using a combination of topical crude coal tar and subsequent UV irradiation. In the 1970s, photochemotherapy with psoralen and UVA light (PUVA) was developed, but has now been mostly discontinued given increased incidence of skin cancer,

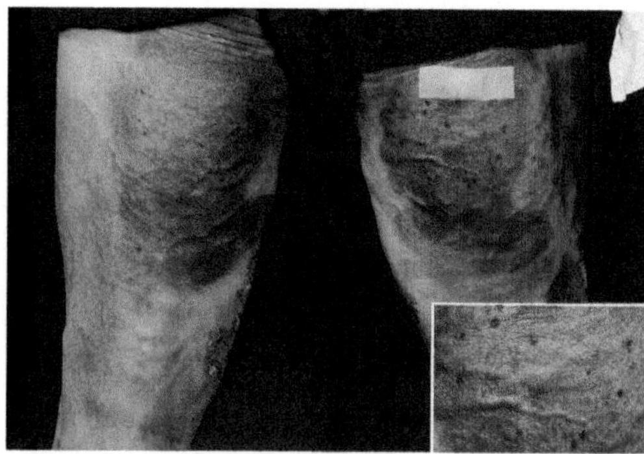

Fig. 1.6 Lentigines from ultraviolet treatment of psoriasis. Chronic damage from the ultraviolet treatment of these psoriatic patches has led to the formation of lentigines bilaterally. There is also epidermal atrophy, likely from chronic use of topical steroids. A closer view of the lentigines and epidermal atrophy (inset).

particularly squamous cell carcinoma (Fig. 1.6).[65] In the 1980s, narrow band UVB (311–313 nm) was developed and shown to be efficacious. Since that time, phototherapy has proven to be a safe, effective treatment for psoriasis that does not cause immunosuppression.

ORAL AGENTS

Methotrexate, acitretin, and cyclosporine have been available for years and were the cornerstones of psoriasis treatment before biologic therapies (Box 1.5). These agents have been overshadowed by newer biologic agents, but they remain effective and inexpensive. They have side effects that make them inappropriate for certain patients but are largely well tolerated. Apremilast and tofacitinib (currently approved for rheumatoid arthritis) are new additions to this class.

BIOLOGIC THERAPY

Since 1998, with the release of etanercept, there has been an explosion in the development of new biologic agents (Box 1.6). These agents have piggy-backed on the increased understanding of the genetics and immunology that drive psoriasis. These molecules are targeted and potent, and after-marketing surveillance shows that they have an excellent safety profile. This is an exciting time for the treatment of psoriasis with multiple classes of biologics available: TNF-α inhibitors, anti-p40 (IL-12/IL-23 antagonists), IL-17 inhibitors, and the promise of new anti-p19 inhibitors (selective for IL-23) on the horizon. These medications are changing the treatment of patients with psoriasis and improving clinical outcomes.

BOX 1.5
Oral therapies

- Cyclosporine
- Methotrexate
- Acitretin
- Apremilast

BOX 1.6
Biologic therapies

- TNF-α inhibitors
  - Etanercept
  - Adalimumab
  - Infliximab
- IL-12/IL-23 p40 subunit inhibitor
  - Ustekinumab
- IL-17 inhibitor
  - Secukinumab
  - Ixekizumab

REFERENCES

1. Henseler T, Christophers E. Psoriasis of early and late onset: characterization of two types of psoriasis vulgaris. J Am Acad Dermatol 1985;13(3):450–6.
2. Sagoo GS, Cork MJ, Patel R, et al. Genome-wide studies of psoriasis susceptibility loci: a review. J Dermatol Sci 2004;35(3):171–9.
3. Elder JT, Nair RP, Guo SW, et al. The genetics of psoriasis. Arch Dermatol 1994;130(2):216–24.
4. Trembath RC, Clough RL, Rosbotham JL, et al. Identification of a major susceptibility locus on chromosome 6p and evidence for further disease loci revealed by a two stage genome-wide search in psoriasis. Hum Mol Genet 1997;6(5):813–20.
5. Cox AJ, Watson W. Histological variations in lesions of psoriasis. Arch Dermatol 1972;106(4):503–6.
6. Baker BS, Swain AF, Fry L, et al. Epidermal T lymphocytes and HLA-DR expression in psoriasis. Br J Dermatol 1984;110(5):555–64.
7. Baker BS, Swain AF, Griffiths CE, et al. Epidermal T lymphocytes and dendritic cells in chronic plaque psoriasis: the effects of PUVA treatment. Clin Exp Immunol 1985;61(3):526–34.
8. Ellis CN, Gorsulowsky DC, Hamilton TA, et al. Cyclosporine improves psoriasis in a double-blind study. JAMA 1986;256(22):3110–6.
9. Wrone-Smith T, Nickoloff BJ. Dermal injection of immunocytes induces psoriasis. J Clin Invest 1996;98(8):1878–87.

10. Uyemura K, Yamamura M, Fivenson DF, et al. The cytokine network in lesional and lesion-free psoriatic skin is characterized by a T-helper type 1 cell-mediated response. J Invest Dermatol 1993;101(5):701–5.
11. Zaba LC, Cardinale I, Gilleaudeau P, et al. Amelioration of epidermal hyperplasia by TNF inhibition is associated with reduced Th17 responses. J Exp Med 2007;204(13):3183–94.
12. Eyerich S, Eyerich K, Pennino D, et al. Th22 cells represent a distinct human T cell subset involved in epidermal immunity and remodeling. J Clin Invest 2009;119(12):3573–85.
13. Fuentes-Duculan J, Suarez-Farinas M, Zaba LC, et al. A subpopulation of CD163-positive macrophages is classically activated in psoriasis. J Invest Dermatol 2010;130(10):2412–22.
14. Wang H, Peters T, Kess D, et al. Activated macrophages are essential in a murine model for T cell-mediated chronic psoriasiform skin inflammation. J Clin Invest 2006;116(8):2105–14.
15. Stratis A, Pasparakis M, Rupec RA, et al. Pathogenic role for skin macrophages in a mouse model of keratinocyte-induced psoriasis-like skin inflammation. J Clin Invest 2006;116(8):2094–104.
16. Zaba LC, Fuentes-Duculan J, Eungdamrong NJ, et al. Psoriasis is characterized by accumulation of immunostimulatory and Th1/Th17 cell-polarizing myeloid dendritic cells. J Invest Dermatol 2009;129(1):79–88.
17. Zaba LC, Krueger JG, Lowes MA. Resident and "inflammatory" dendritic cells in human skin. J Invest Dermatol 2009;129(2):302–8.
18. Gudjonsson JE, Karason A, Runarsdottir EH, et al. Distinct clinical differences between HLA-Cw*0602 positive and negative psoriasis patients–an analysis of 1019 HLA-C- and HLA-B-typed patients. J Invest Dermatol 2006;126(4):740–5.
19. Christophers E. Psoriasis–epidemiology and clinical spectrum. Clin Exp Dermatol 2001;26(4):314–20.
20. Wu JJ, Choi YM, Bebchuk JD. Risk of myocardial infarction in psoriasis patients: a retrospective cohort study. J Dermatolog Treat 2015;26(3):230–4.
21. Gelfand JM, Neimann AL, Shin DB, et al. Risk of myocardial infarction in patients with psoriasis. JAMA 2006;296(14):1735–41.
22. Gelfand JM, Troxel AB, Lewis JD, et al. The risk of mortality in patients with psoriasis: results from a population-based study. Arch Dermatol 2007;143(12):1493–9.
23. Gelfand JM, Dommasch ED, Shin DB, et al. The risk of stroke in patients with psoriasis. J Invest Dermatol 2009;129(10):2411–8.
24. Hjuler KF, Bottcher M, Vestergaard C, et al. Increased prevalence of coronary artery disease in severe psoriasis and severe atopic dermatitis. Am J Med 2015;128(12):1325–34.e2.
25. Mehta NN, Yu Y, Pinnelas R, et al. Attributable risk estimate of severe psoriasis on major cardiovascular events. Am J Med 2011;124(8):775.e1-6.
26. Weiss G, Shemer A, Trau H. The Koebner phenomenon: review of the literature. J Eur Acad Dermatol Venereol 2002;16(3):241–8.
27. van de Kerkhof PC. The Woronoff zone surrounding the psoriatic plaque. Br J Dermatol 1998;139(1):167–8.
28. Chalmers RJ, O'Sullivan T, Owen CM, et al. A systematic review of treatments for guttate psoriasis. Br J Dermatol 2001;145(6):891–4.
29. Mallon E, Bunce M, Savoie H, et al. HLA-C and guttate psoriasis. Br J Dermatol 2000;143(6):1177–82.
30. Johnson C, Shuster S. Eccrine sweating in psoriasis. Br J Dermatol 1969;81(2):119–24.
31. Zelickson BD, Muller SA. Generalized pustular psoriasis. A review of 63 cases. Arch Dermatol 1991;127(9):1339–45.
32. Abou-Samra T, Constantin JM, Amarger S, et al. Generalized pustular psoriasis complicated by acute respiratory distress syndrome. Br J Dermatol 2004;150(2):353–6.
33. Varma R, Cantrell W, Elmets C, et al. Infliximab for the treatment of severe pustular psoriasis: 6 years later. J Eur Acad Dermatol Venereol 2008;22(10):1253–4.
34. Umezawa Y, Ozawa A, Kawasima T, et al. Therapeutic guidelines for the treatment of generalized pustular psoriasis (GPP) based on a proposed classification of disease severity. Arch Dermatol Res 2003;295(Suppl 1):S43–54.
35. Marrakchi S, Guigue P, Renshaw BR, et al. Interleukin-36-receptor antagonist deficiency and generalized pustular psoriasis. N Engl J Med 2011;365(7):620–8.
36. Oumeish OY, Parish JL. Impetigo herpetiformis. Clin Dermatol 2006;24(2):101–4.
37. Michaelsson G, Gustafsson K, Hagforsen E. The psoriasis variant palmoplantar pustulosis can be improved after cessation of smoking. J Am Acad Dermatol 2006;54(4):737–8.
38. Happle R. Linear psoriasis and ILVEN: is lumping or splitting appropriate? Dermatology 2006;212(2):101–2.
39. Kvedar JC, Baden HP. Nail changes in cutaneous disease. Semin Dermatol 1991;10(1):65–70.
40. Nestle FO, Kaplan DH, Barker J. Psoriasis. N Engl J Med 2009;361(5):496–509.
41. Reich K, Kruger K, Mossner R, et al. Epidemiology and clinical pattern of psoriatic arthritis in Germany: a prospective interdisciplinary epidemiological study of 1511 patients with plaque-type psoriasis. Br J Dermatol 2009;160(5):1040–7.

42. Radtke MA, Reich K, Blome C, et al. Prevalence and clinical features of psoriatic arthritis and joint complaints in 2009 patients with psoriasis: results of a German national survey. J Eur Acad Dermatol Venereol 2009;23(6):683–91.
43. Mallbris L, Granath F, Hamsten A, et al. Psoriasis is associated with lipid abnormalities at the onset of skin disease. J Am Acad Dermatol 2006;54(4):614–21.
44. Mallbris L, Akre O, Granath F, et al. Increased risk for cardiovascular mortality in psoriasis inpatients but not in outpatients. Eur J Epidemiol 2004;19(3):225–30.
45. Augustin M, Reich K, Glaeske G, et al. Co-morbidity and age-related prevalence of psoriasis: analysis of health insurance data in Germany. Acta Derm Venereol 2010;90(2):147–51.
46. Cohen AD, Weitzman D, Dreiher J. Psoriasis and hypertension: a case-control study. Acta Derm Venereol 2010;90(1):23–6.
47. Gelfand JM, Shin DB, Neimann AL, et al. The risk of lymphoma in patients with psoriasis. J Invest Dermatol 2006;126(10):2194–201.
48. Gupta MA, Gupta AK, Watteel GN. Early onset (< 40 years age) psoriasis is comorbid with greater psychopathology than late onset psoriasis: a study of 137 patients. Acta Derm Venereol 1996;76(6):464–6.
49. Krueger G, Koo J, Lebwohl M, et al. The impact of psoriasis on quality of life: results of a 1998 National Psoriasis Foundation patient-membership survey. Arch Dermatol 2001;137(3):280–4.
50. Herron MD, Hinckley M, Hoffman MS, et al. Impact of obesity and smoking on psoriasis presentation and management. Arch Dermatol 2005;141(12):1527–34.
51. Telfer NR, Chalmers RJ, Whale K, et al. The role of streptococcal infection in the initiation of guttate psoriasis. Arch Dermatol 1992;128(1):39–42.
52. Gudjonsson JE, Thorarinsson AM, Sigurgeirsson B, et al. Streptococcal throat infections and exacerbation of chronic plaque psoriasis: a prospective study. Br J Dermatol 2003;149(3):530–4.
53. Obuch ML, Maurer TA, Becker B, et al. Psoriasis and human immunodeficiency virus infection. J Am Acad Dermatol 1992;27(5 Pt 1):667–73.
54. Vittorio Luigi De Socio G, Simonetti S, Stagni G. Clinical improvement of psoriasis in an AIDS patient effectively treated with combination antiretroviral therapy. Scand J Infect Dis 2006;38(1):74–5.
55. O'Brien M, Koo J. The mechanism of lithium and beta-blocking agents in inducing and exacerbating psoriasis. J Drugs Dermatol 2006;5(5):426–32.
56. Famenini S, Wu JJ. Infliximab-induced psoriasis in treatment of Crohn's disease-associated ankylosing spondylitis: case report and review of 142 cases. J Drugs Dermatol 2013;12(8):939–43.
57. Ko JM, Gottlieb AB, Kerbleski JF. Induction and exacerbation of psoriasis with TNF-blockade therapy: a review and analysis of 127 cases. J Dermatolog Treat 2009;20(2):100–8.
58. Richards HL, Fortune DG, O'Sullivan TM, et al. Patients with psoriasis and their compliance with medication. J Am Acad Dermatol 1999;41(4):581–3.
59. Menter A, Korman NJ, Elmets CA, et al. Guidelines of care for the management of psoriasis and psoriatic arthritis. Section 3. Guidelines of care for the management and treatment of psoriasis with topical therapies. J Am Acad Dermatol 2009;60(4):643–59.
60. Ramsay CA. Management of psoriasis with calcipotriol used as monotherapy. J Am Acad Dermatol 1997;37(3 Pt 2):S53–4.
61. Hecker D, Worsley J, Yueh G, et al. Interactions between tazarotene and ultraviolet light. J Am Acad Dermatol 1999;41(6):927–30.
62. Zonneveld IM, Rubins A, Jablonska S, et al. Topical tacrolimus is not effective in chronic plaque psoriasis. A pilot study. Arch Dermatol 1998;134(9):1101–2.
63. Gribetz C, Ling M, Lebwohl M, et al. Pimecrolimus cream 1% in the treatment of intertriginous psoriasis: a double-blind, randomized study. J Am Acad Dermatol 2004;51(5):731–8.
64. Margolis DJ, Abuabara K, Hoffstad OJ, et al. Association between malignancy and topical use of pimecrolimus. JAMA Dermatol 2015;151(6):594–9.
65. Chuang TY, Heinrich LA, Schultz MD, et al. PUVA and skin cancer. A historical cohort study on 492 patients. J Am Acad Dermatol 1992;26(2 Pt 1):173–7.

CHAPTER 2

Ultraviolet B Phototherapy

Sandra Pena, BS, Dane Hill, MD, Steven R. Feldman, MD, PhD

KEYWORDS

• Phototherapy • Narrowband UV-B • UV therapy • Psoriasis • Excimer laser

KEY POINTS

- Phototherapy with UV light can be used in the treatment of several cutaneous disorders.
- Phototherapy is an efficacious treatment option in the management of psoriasis and should be a first therapy considered in patients with moderate-to-severe plaque psoriasis.
- Narrowband UV-B is used as the first-line phototherapy treatment option for moderate-to-severe psoriasis due to its clinical efficacy and mild side-effect profile.
- Targeted UV-B therapy phototherapy and employment of excimer lasers are excellent options for patients with more limited disease, although there are now reports of use for extensive disease.

INTRODUCTION

Definition

Phototherapy refers to the use of nonionizing radiation, from the UV range, in the treatment of skin disorders (Table 2.1).[1] It represents an efficacious, cost-effective, and generally nonimmunosuppressive staple in the management of psoriasis.[2]

History

The use of sunlight in the treatment of cutaneous diseases can be traced back to ancient times. Evidence dating thousands of years demonstrates the use of plant extracts, including those from the *Ammi majus* plant (psoralens), followed by sun exposure to treat vitiligo in Egypt and India.[3] However, it was not until the late nineteenth century that heralded major advances in the development and use of phototherapy.[4] In 1901, Niels Ryberg Finsen published the results of the treatment of lupus vulgaris with a carbon arc lamp, which marked a breakthrough in the treatment of skin diseases. For this, Finsen received a Nobel Prize in medicine, the first and only one ever awarded in the field of dermatology.[5]

Shortly after in 1925, William Goeckerman combined the use of UV radiation with coal tar in the treatment of psoriasis.[6] The Goeckerman regimen as it came to be known would remain a mainstay in phototherapy treatment of psoriasis for several decades.[7] A major shortcoming of the Goeckerman regimen was the low output of the lamps. However, in 1978, Wiskemann introduced broadband UV-B radiation in a closed chamber to treat psoriasis, which mitigated this drawback.[8] Despite these advances, broadband UV-B radiation was less efficacious than psoralens followed by UV-A radiation, also known as PUVA therapy, and as a result, did not gain widespread popularity.[5] It was not until the late 1970s when Parrish and Jaenicke determined the action spectrum of psoriasis with a peak response at 313 nm that gave impetus to narrowband (NB) UV-B as a new phototherapeutic modality.[9] In 1988, both Van Weelden and colleagues[10] and Green and colleagues[11] demonstrated the superior clinical efficacy of NB UV-B and subsequently marked the decline of broadband-UV-B (BB-UV-B) use for psoriasis.

Types

This chapter provides an overview of UVB phototherapy in the management of psoriasis.

Broadband ultraviolet B (290–320 nm)

Broadband (BB) UV-B phototherapy was initially described in the Goeckerman regimen in 1925. For many decades, BB-UV-B remained an option in the psoriasis treatment arsenal despite being less efficacious than other treatment modalities. Presently, however, BB-UV-B has largely been replaced by NB-UV-B radiation, which has demonstrated superior efficacy in clearing psoriatic lesions.[12]

TABLE 2.1
Ultraviolet radiation spectrum

UV Spectrum (10–400 nm)	
Abbreviation	**Wavelength (nm)**
UV-A	320–400
UV-B	290–320
UV-C	200–290

Narrowband ultraviolet B (311–313 nm)

First defined in 1976, NB-UV-B has taken the place of BB-UV-B in the treatment and management of psoriasis.[9] NB-UV-B has gained popularity over PUVA in the treatment of psoriasis for several reasons. First, NB-UV-B had similar efficacy rates compared with PUVA.[12] Therefore, NB-UV-B is generally favored over PUVA due to greater ease of use for the patient. Another factor is the increased risk of squamous cell cancer (SCC) associated with PUVA treatments. The risk of SCC increases as the number of PUVA treatments increases.[13] NB-UV-B phototherapy has not been shown to incur any increased risk of skin cancer.[14] Last, NB-UV-B is safe to use in children and pregnant patients and lacks psoralen-related side effects, which ultimately makes it more favorable as an initial phototherapy modality.[15]

TARGETED PHOTOTHERAPY

Targeted phototherapy is a method of phototherapy in which only affected areas of skin are treated. Various devices can be used to deliver focused UV-B radiation on skin lesions while sparing uninvolved skin. These devices include high fluence devices, like the excimer laser and flash lamp, and lower output devices, like UV-B light-emitting diodes.[16] Introduced in 1997, the 308-nm excimer laser contains an unstable mixture of xenon and chloride, which form "excited dimmers." It is the dissociation of these dimers that produces the monochromatic wavelength, which is transmitted via a fiber-optic cable to the lesion.[17] The excimer laser allows for targeted therapy that spares uninvolved skin, especially in areas that are otherwise difficult to treat, like the scalp, hands, and feet.[17] In addition, it can generate high fluencies of UV-B, resulting in faster clearing and fewer exposures.[18] Although the excimer laser is not suitable for large body surface areas because the treatment may be considerably resource intensive and lengthy, the availability of more powerful UV emitting devices (and aggressive treatment protocol) is extending the range of area that can be treated.[7,19] Although targeted treatment has generally been used for mild, localized psoriasis, it can also be used for severe psoriasis of the palms/soles or even for extensive disease.

TANNING BEDS

The use of commercial tanning beds may be a viable alternative for patients in which in-office and home phototherapy are either unaccessible or impractical. Although evidence to support the routine use of tanning beds may be sparse, approximately 36% to 52% of patients have used tanning beds in the treatment of their psoriasis.[20,21] However, given the increased risk of skin cancer and full-body UV exposure, tanning bed use remains controversial, and not all dermatologists agree that they should be used.

INDICATIONS

Indications for UV-B radiation include psoriasis, atopic dermatitis, vitiligo, and mycosis fungoides, among several others (Table 2.2).[22]

MECHANISM OF ACTION

The epidermal layer of human skin, composed primarily of keratinocytes, absorbs most UV radiation, with only the longer wavelengths having the ability to penetrate the dermis. It was thought that UV-B's antiproliferative properties were a

TABLE 2.2
Ultraviolet B phototherapy indications

Common	Less Common
Psoriasis	Acquired perforating dermatosis
Vitiligo	Chronic urticaria
Atopic dermatitis	Cutaneous graft-versus-host disease
Mycosis fungoides	Polymorphous light eruption
Pruritus (associated with renal disease, polycythemia vera)	Cutaneous mastocytosis
	Granuloma annulare
	Lichen planus
	Lichen simplex chronicus
	Lymphomatoid papulosis
	Parapsoriasis
	Pityriasis lichenoides
	Pityriasis rosea
	Pityriasis rubra pilaris
	Seborrheic dermatitis

From Walker D, Jacobe H. Phototherapy in the age of biologics. Semin Cutan Med Surg 2011;30(4):196; with permission.

result of direct DNA damage; however, recent evidence suggests that phototherapy also exerts immunomodulatory effects.[23] Specifically, UV-B radiation diminishes type-1 T-cell predominance by altering cytokine profiles, induces apoptosis of keratinocytes and T cells, and depletes Langerhan cell numbers.[24–26]

Human T helper (Th) lymphocytes can be separated into T effector cells, which protect the body from pathogens, and regulatory T cells, which dampen immune responses when they become dangerous to the host. Different subsets of effector T helper cells are distinguished based on their cytokine production profiles in addition to transcription factors and homing receptor expression.[27] The main T helper subsets include Th1, Th2, and Th17. In psoriasis, it is the Th1/Th17 T cells that overexpress Th1 and Th17 cytokines, which, in turn, influence the hyperproliferation of keratinocytes and the resultant inflammation.[28]

UV-B radiation shifts the dysregulated predominance of Th1/Th17-mediated immune response in psoriasis to more of a Th2 response. Specifically, UV-B phototherapy induces interleukin-10 (IL-10) production in human keratinocytes, which is a major regulatory cytokine in the Th2 pathway.[29] In addition, phototherapy downregulates Th1/Th17 proinflammatory pathways by decreasing pathogenic cytokine (IL-23, IL-20, interferon-γ, IL-17, IL-22) production.[30]

Furthermore, UV-B exerts its therapeutic effects by inducing apoptosis. Apoptosis is a process of programmed cell death in response to noxious stimuli. Evidence indicates that one mechanism in which UV-B clears psoriatic lesions is through the induction of apoptosis in keratinocytes, epidermal T cells, and to a lesser extent, Langerhans cells.[26,31,32]

Last, UV-B is involved in promoting localized immunosuppression. In addition to apoptosis, UV-B radiation influences the migration of Langerhans cells from the epidermis as well as decreases dendritic cell expression of B7 costimulatory signals, which is necessary for the stimulation and activation of T cells.[32,33]

EFFICACY

Efficacy can be evaluated with regards to fluency, clearance, remission times, and number of treatments.[16] The Psoriasis Area and Severity Index (PASI) score was developed as a tool to measure the severity of psoriasis. A variant of that score, the PASI-75, determines the percentage of patients that achieved 75% reduction in the baseline PASI score and is a common measure of treatment efficacy.

Broadband Ultraviolet B

UV-B radiation is efficacious in the treatment and management of psoriasis. By virtue of being discovered first, BB-UV-B has a longer safety record than NB-UV-B but is less efficacious in the treatment of psoriasis. Only selective BB-UV-B (305–325 nm) has shown evidence of being as effective as NB-UV-B in clearing chronic plaque psoriasis.[12]

Narrowband Ultraviolet B

NB-UV-B phototherapy is an effective therapeutic option in the treatment of plaque psoriasis. In a systematic review of 41 randomized control trials, 68% of patients receiving NB-UV-B monotherapy achieved plaque clearance, whereas 62% achieved PASI-75.[34] When compared with oral PUVA, NB-UV-B may be less efficacious in clearing lesions but favored overall because of less risk of adverse events and increased ease of use.[12,35]

If NB-UV-B phototherapy alone is insufficient to manage a patient's disease, then a combination of NB-UV-B plus topical or systemic adjuncts may be considered.[4] Emollients, including petroleum jelly, mineral oil, and coal tar, may result in improved plaque clearance.[35] In addition, calcipotriol and maxacalcitol (vitamin D analogues) and psoralens at higher concentrations may also facilitate lesion resolution.[35] Regarding systemic adjuncts to NB-UV-B phototherapy, the addition of methotrexate to NB-UV-B renders the treatment more efficacious than NB-UV-B alone.[35] Combining phototherapy with retinoids or cyclosporine decreases the cumulative NB-UV-B dose needed to clear psoriasis. Combination therapy using biologics may potentiate their efficacy, but sufficient data are lacking.[35]

Data in children and pregnant women have also been promising, because 51% of pediatric patients achieved complete clearance and an additional 41% had a 75% reduction in their PASI score.[36]

TARGETED PHOTOTHERAPY

Recent meta-analyses using a PASI clearance of 75% evaluated the efficacy of targeted NB-UV-B in the treatment of plaque psoriasis and demonstrated efficacy rates for the excimer (308-nm) laser to be 70%, 59% for excimer (308-nm) light, and 49% for localized NB-UV-B (311–313-nm) light.[37]

In addition, the excimer laser can clear psoriasis, with about 70% of patients having a 75% or greater reduction in their psoriatic lesions.[37,38] Although partial clearance is possible in as few as one session, usually higher frequency treatments (2 to 3 per week) are considered to be more effective, with higher rates of complete clearance.[37,39] In one multicenter trial for mild-to-moderate plaque-type psoriasis, 84% and 35% of subjects demonstrated PASI score improvement of at least 75% and 90%, respectively, after 10 or fewer treatments.[40] In addition, the 308-nm excimer laser required fewer visits while remaining relatively effective when compared with whole-body phototherapy.[40]

Similarly to NB-UV-B, combination therapies that use the excimer laser with topical adjuncts resulted in higher efficacy rates compared with monotherapy alone.[41]

TANNING BEDS

Efficacy of commercial tanning is difficult to assess due to the lack of standardization of tanning bed devices and lamps as well as by the poor compliance of tanning regimens.[42,43]

Although tanning beds primarily emit UVA radiation, approximately 0.5% to 5.0% of the total light output is within the UV-B spectrum.[42] One controlled trial compared low UV-B output (0.7%) lamps to higher UV-B output (4.6%) lamps in the treatment of psoriasis and determined that when equal erythema doses were given, there was a similar significant improvement in PASI scores.[44] In addition, higher output lamps achieved mean reductions in PASI scores of 35.4% $\pm$ 24.1% in 80% of patients.[45]

SAFETY

UV-B is generally well tolerated and safe in almost all patients, including children and pregnant women.[35,36,46] The most common acute side effect is "sunburn," which is a red phototoxic reaction that occurs about 24 hours after treatment.[47] Erythema is usually dose-dependent and has comparable rates between NB-UV-B versus BB-UV-B therapy.[9,47] Pruritus has occasionally been described in psoriatic lesions following UV-B therapy. However, this may be due more to the underlying disease process rather than secondary to phototherapy.[17] Hyperpigmentation is another common side effect of UV-B phototherapy that can interfere with treatment compliance depending on the patient's tolerance of skin color changes.[48] Pregnant patients should be informed of the possible increased risk of melasma secondary to UV-B phototherapy.[49]

Other less common acute effects include blistering, cataract formation, and reactivation of herpes simplex virus infection. Blistering and painful erythema have been seen in approximately 16% of patients and may be caused by a quick reduction in acanthosis and desquamation before defensive mechanism, that is, pigmentation and increases in stratum corneum, take place.[37,50] There have been a few cases reporting the reactivation of herpes simplex virus infection following phototherapy; therefore, precautionary measures should be taken in those prone to frequent relapses.[51] UV-B phototherapy has not been associated with an increased risk of fetal abnormalities or prematurity and seems to be the safest therapy in extensive disease. However, overheating should be avoided due to the increased risk of neural tube defects.[46]

The most common long-term effect is photoaging, which may present as wrinkling, lentigines, and telangiectasias.[49] The most concerning long-term outcome is photocarcinogenesis. NB-UV-B probably confers less of a cancer risk compared with PUVA but may be 2 to 3 times more carcinogenic than BB-UV-B at similar doses.[52,53] However, the risk of skin cancer in psoriasis patients treated with NB-UV-B correlated with the number of treatments, yet the overall risk of malignancy in the NB-UV-B-treated patients was not greater than in the general population.[54] In addition, although NB-UV-B treatment has not been linked to any skin cancers, long-term follow-up data are lacking.[15] Therefore, providers should continue counseling patients regarding skin cancer risk with NB-UV-B treatment. In addition, ongoing skin cancer monitoring of patients, in addition to genital and facial shielding, is recommended.

TARGETED PHOTOTHERAPY

Evidence suggests that targeted phototherapy is safer than whole-body phototherapy by reducing the amount of unnecessary radiation.[16] Adverse events are associated with higher cumulative UV-B doses and increased number of treatments.[16]

Given its targeted nature, the adverse effects of the excimer laser are limited to the area that was targeted and are similar to those of NB-UV-B. Short-term effects include erythema, blistering, and hyperpigmentation.[40] Blisters are noted more often with the use of higher doses.[38] Hyperpigmentation may be psychologically distressful for patient; however, it tends to resolve with the discontinuation of treatment.[40] Long-term safety data in patients treated with the excimer laser, including children and pregnant women, are lacking but generally considered to be safe.[49]

TANNING BEDS

Unsupervised use of commercial tanning beds is problematic and increases the likelihood of acute side effects that include phototoxic reactions, blisters, and itching.[43,45] Long term, there is an increased risk of developing melanoma, SCC, and basal cell carcinoma in patients who have ever used a recreational tanning bed compared with those who have not.[43] In addition to history of use, younger age at first use and increased frequency of sessions incur greater risk of skin cancers in recreational tanners.[43]

PRECAUTIONS

Although normally safe in most patients, UV-B phototherapy is absolutely contraindicated in patients with xeroderma pigmentosum or lupus erythematosus (Table 2.3).

MONITORING

Prior to initiating treatment, patients should be classified according to their disease severity. Patients whose lesions are localized (<10% body surface area) are typically considered to have mild-to-moderate disease. Those who have generalized lesions (>10% of body surface area involvement) are categorized as having severe disease. However, patients with less than 10% BSA involvement can also be considered as having severe disease when debilitating symptoms that interfere with activities of daily living are present. Those with mild disease can be treated with topical treatments or targeted phototherapy, whereas severe disease usually warrants phototherapy or systemic therapies.[2]

TABLE 2.3
Contraindications to ultraviolet B phototherapy

Absolute	Relative
Xeroderma pigmentosum Lupus erythematosus	Photosensitivity disorder Taking photosensitizing medications History of melanoma History of atypical nevi Multiple risk factors for melanoma History of multiple nonmelanoma skin cancers Immunosuppressed secondarily to organ transplant

Data from Menter A, Korman NJ, Elmets CA, et al. Guidelines of care for the management of psoriasis and psoriatic arthritis: section 5. Guidelines of care for the treatment of psoriasis with phototherapy and photochemotherapy. J Am Acad Dermatol 2010;62(1):120.

When proceeding with phototherapy, patients should be educated about the use of goggles and genital shields, and treatment regimens should be standardized (Tables 2.4 and 2.5).[49] In addition, the starting dose of UV-B radiation should be determined based on the patient's skin sensitivity. Patient's skin sensitivity can be estimated based on the patient's Fitzpatrick skin phototype (Table 2.6) or through determination of a minimal erythema dose (MED), which is the amount of UV radiation required to produce minimal erythema. The initial dose should be between 50% and 70% of MED, which has been found to have maximum efficacy and safety in both dark- and light-skinned patients.[7]

To determine the MED, adjacent areas of skin are exposed to increasing doses of UV radiation, and after 24 to 48 hours, graded based on their degree of erythema. The erythematous skin exposed to the shortest duration of UV radiation is defined as the MED.[55] The degree of erythema can be

TABLE 2.4
Dosing broadband ultraviolet B

According to Skin Type		
Skin Type	**Initial UV-B Dose (mJ/cm²)**	**UV-B Increase After Each Treatment (mJ/cm²)**
I	20	5
II	25	10
III	30	15
IV	40	20
V	50	25
VI	60	30
According to MED		
Initial UV-B		50% of MED
Treatments 1–10		Increase by 25% of initial MED
Treatments 11–20		Increase by 10% of initial MED
Treatments ≥21		As ordered by physician
If Subsequent Treatments are Missed for		
4–7 d		Keep dose the same
1–2 wk		Decrease dose by 50%
2–3 wk		Decrease dose by 75%
3–4 wk		Start over

Administered 3-5×wk.

Data from Zanolli MD, Feldman SR. Phototherapy treatment protocols for psoriasis and other phototherapy responsive dermatoses. 2nd ed. New York: Informa Healthcare; 2004. p. 2.

TABLE 2.5
Dosing narrowband ultraviolet B

According to Skin Type			
Skin Type	Initial UV-B Dose (mJ/cm²)	UV-B Increase After Each Treatment (mJ/cm²)	Maximum Dose (mJ/cm²)
I	130	15	2000
II	220	25	2000
III	260	40	3000
IV	330	45	3000
V	350	60	5000
VI	400	65	5000
According to MED			
Initial UV-B		50% of MED	
Treatments 1–20		Increase by 10% of initial MED	
Treatments ≥21		Increase as ordered by physician	
If Subsequent Treatments are Missed for			
4–7 d		Keep dose the same	
1–2 wk		Decrease dose by 25%	
2–3 wk		Decrease dose by 50% or start over	
3–4 wk		Start over	
Maintenance Therapy for NB-UV-B After >95% Clearance			
1×/wk	NB-UV-B for 4 wk	Keep dose the same	
1×/2 wk	NB-UV-B for 4 wk	Decrease dose by 25%	
1×/4 wk	NB-UV-B	50% of highest dose	

Administered 3–5×/wk.

From Menter A, Korman NJ, Elmets CA, et al. Guidelines of care for the management of psoriasis and psoriatic arthritis: section 5. Guidelines of care for the treatment of psoriasis with phototherapy and photochemotherapy. J Am Acad Dermatol 2010;62(1):118; with permission.

assessed either subjectively, which may have more intraobserver variability, or objectively, using a chroma meter. However, one study looking at objective versus subjective measures of erythema found both to be in good agreement.[56]

MED is considered safe and allows for a higher starting dose compared with a skin type–based regimen resulting in quicker results and fewer treatment sessions.[57] In addition, MED can vary among skin type, and therefore, testing is recommended. However, an MED-based regimen may be more labor intensive and time consuming,

TABLE 2.6
Fitzpatrick skin phototype

SPT	Reaction to Sun Exposure
I	Always burns, never tans. White skin
II	Always burns, sometimes tans. White skin
III	Sometimes burns, gradually tans. White skin
IV	Sometimes burns, tans well. Light brown skin
V	Rarely burns, always tans. Brown skin
VI	Never burns, always tans. Dark brown/black skin

From Roberts WE. Skin type classification systems old and new. Dermatol Clin 2009;27(4):531; with permission.

and therefore, many physicians may choose to tailor treatment based on skin type due to greater convenience.[58]

Typically, treatment sessions 3 times per week are recommended for NB-UV-B (up to 5 times per week for BB-UV-B and daily for tanning beds). However, barring any extenuating circumstances, treatment 3 times per week may be more favorable to minimize radiation exposure as well as toxicities.[59] Dose increments, on the other hand, depend on the individual patient with the goal being to maintain a mild perceptible erythema throughout treatment.[58] Typically, it takes 20 to 36 treatments to see significant improvement for moderate-to-severe psoriasis treatment with NB-UV-B.[35]

There are no agreed-upon guidelines for the use of maintenance phototherapy. As a result, treatment should continue until total clearance is achieved or treatment fails to result in further improvement.[58] Some patients achieve clearing and long-term remission, and treatment can be stopped. For those whose disease tends to recur, a maintenance regimen can be used in which the frequency of treatments is gradually reduced to once a week or every other week. The decision to continue with maintenance therapy is left to the discretion of the practitioner and patient.[7]

TARGETED PHOTOTHERAPY

For patients with limited disease, targeted phototherapy using an excimer laser is a worthwhile treatment option. Currently, there is limited evidence for dosing protocols using the excimer laser (Table 2.7). The initial dose is determined by the patient's skin type and the thickness of the plaque, while further doses are adjusted

TABLE 2.7
Dosing for excimer laser

Initial Dose for Psoriasis				
Plaque Thickness	**Induration Score**	**Fitzpatrick Skin Type I–III (Dose in mJ/cm²)**	**Fitzpatrick Skin Type IV–VI (Dose in mJ/cm²)**	
None 0	0	—	—	—
Mild	1	500	400	—
Moderate	2	500	600	—
Severe	3	700	900	—
Dose for Subsequent Treatments				
No Effect	**Minimal Effect**	**Good Effect**	**Considerable Improvement**	**Moderate/Severe Erythema (with or Without Blistering)**
No erythema at 12–24 h and no plaque improvement	Slight erythema at 12–24 h but no significant improvement	Mild to moderate erythema response 12–24 h	Significant improvement with plaque thinning or reduced scaliness or pigmentation occurred	
Typical Dosing Change from Prior Treatment Dose				
Increase dose by 25%	Increase dose by 15%	Maintain dose	Maintain dose or reduce dose by 15%	Reduce dose by 25% (treat around blistered area, do not treat blistered area until it heals or crust disappears)

From Menter A, Korman NJ, Elmets CA, et al. Guidelines of care for the management of psoriasis and psoriatic arthritis: section 5. Guidelines of care for the treatment of psoriasis with phototherapy and photochemotherapy. J Am Acad Dermatol 2010;62(1):124; with permission.

according to response to prior treatment.[49] Treatment sessions are usually 2 to 3 times per week with a minimum of 48 hours between sessions and are continued for 3 to 6 weeks.[49]

VACCINATIONS

There are no limitations on vaccinations.

SUMMARY

Phototherapy is an efficacious treatment option in the management of psoriasis and should be the first therapy considered in patients with moderate-to-severe plaque psoriasis. A common barrier to this therapy is the inconvenience of patients needing to come to the office 2 to 3 times per week for treatment.

- NB-UV-B phototherapy is first-line treatment for psoriasis because of less risk of adverse events and increased ease of use when compared with oral PUVA.
- Combination therapies with topical adjuncts may help improve clearance rates in patients compared with limited response to monotherapy alone. Thick emollient creams should be avoided because they can prevent penetration of UV-B radiation.[60]
- Targeted therapy is an important alternative for patients with photoresponsive, localized disease.
- Home phototherapy can be an effective alternative to office-based phototherapy while increasing patient satisfaction with treatment.[61] Compliant and motivated patients could be considered appropriate candidates for home UV-B therapy, under dermatologist supervision.
- Although the recreational use of tanning beds is discouraged, therapeutic use of tanning beds may be recommended by some dermatologists for patients for whom in-office or home phototherapy is not feasible.
- Patients should be continued on phototherapy for 25 to 40 sessions at a frequency of at least 2 to 3 times per week and a dose of 6 to 10 times the baseline MED for

BB-UV-B and 4 to 6 times the baseline MED for NB-UV-B before considering discontinuation due to treatment failure.[62]

REFERENCES

1. Pathak M, Fitzpatrick T. The evolution of photochemotherapy with psoralens and UVA (PUVA): 2000 BC to 1992 AD. J Photochem Photobiol B 1992; 14(1–2):3–22.
2. Feldman S, Garton R, Averett W, et al. Strategy to manage the treatment of severe psoriasis: considerations of efficacy, safety and cost. Expert Opin Pharmacother 2003;4(9):1525–33.
3. Hönigsmann H. History of phototherapy in dermatology. Photochem Photobiol Sci 2013;12(1): 16–21.
4. Lim H, Silpa-archa N, Amadi U, et al. Phototherapy in dermatology: a call for action. J Am Acad Dermatol 2015;72(6):1078–80.
5. Roelandts R. The history of phototherapy: something new under the sun? J Am Acad Dermatol 2002;46(6):926–30.
6. Goeckerman W. Treatment of psoriasis. Northwest Med 1925;24:229–31.
7. Totonchy M, Chiu M. UV-based therapy. Dermatol Clin 2014;32(3):399–413.
8. Wiskemann A. Recent developments in light therapy. Dermatol Wochenschr 1963;20(147):377–83.
9. Parrish J, Jaenicke K. Action spectrum for phototherapy of psoriasis. J Invest Dermatol 1981;76(5): 359–62.
10. Van Weelden H, Baart De La Faille H, Young E, et al. A new development in UVB phototherapy of psoriasis. Br J Dermatol 1988;119(1):11–9.
11. Green C, Ferguson J, Lakshmipathi T, et al. 311 nm UVB phototherapy—an effective treatment for psoriasis. Br J Dermatol 1988;119(6):691–6.
12. Chen X, Yang M, Cheng Y, et al. Narrow-band ultraviolet B phototherapy versus broad-band ultraviolet B or psoralen-ultraviolet A photochemotherapy for psoriasis. Cochrane Database Syst Rev 2013;(10):CD009481.
13. Stern R. The risk of squamous cell and basal cell cancer associated with psoralen and ultraviolet therapy: a 30-year prospective study. J Am Acad Dermatol 2012;66(4):553–62.
14. Hearn R, Kerr A, Rahim K, et al. Incidence of skin cancers in 3867 patients treated with narrow-band ultraviolet B phototherapy. Br J Dermatol 2008; 159(4):931–5.
15. Dogra S, De D. Narrowband ultraviolet B in the treatment of psoriasis: the journey so far! Indian J Dermatol Venereol Leprol 2010;76:652–61.
16. Mudigonda T, Dabade T, Feldman S. A review of targeted ultraviolet B phototherapy for psoriasis. J Am Acad Dermatol 2012;66(4):664–72.
17. Beggs S, Short J, Rengifo-Pardo M, et al. Applications of the excimer laser. Dermatol Surg 2015; 41(11):1201–11.
18. He Y, Zhang X, Dong J, et al. Clinical efficacy of a 308 nm excimer laser for treatment of psoriasis vulgaris. Photodermatol Photoimmunol Photomed 2007;23(6):238–41.
19. Debbaneh M, Levin E, Sanchez Rodriguez R, et al. Plaque-based sub-blistering dosimetry: reaching PASI-75 after two treatments with 308-nm excimer laser in a generalized psoriasis patient. J Dermatolog Treat 2015;26(1):45–8.
20. Fleischer A, Feldman S, Rapp S, et al. Alternative therapies commonly used within a population of patients with psoriasis. Cutis 1996;58(3):216–20.
21. Turner R, Farr P, Walshaw D. Many patients with psoriasis use sunbeds. BMJ 1998;317(7155):412.
22. Walker D, Jacobe H. Phototherapy in the age of biologics. Semin Cutan Med Surg 2011;30(4): 190–8.
23. Krutmann J, Morita A. Mechanisms of ultraviolet (UV) B and UVA phototherapy. J Investig Dermatol Symp Proc 1999;4(1):70–2.
24. DeSilva B, McKenzie R, Hunter J, et al. Local effects of TL01 phototherapy in psoriasis. Photodermatol Photoimmunol Photomed 2008;24(5):268–9.
25. Krueger J. Successful ultraviolet B treatment of psoriasis is accompanied by a reversal of keratinocyte pathology and by selective depletion of intraepidermal T cells. J Exp Med 1995;182(6):2057–68.
26. Piskin G, Tursen U, Sylva-Steenland R, et al. Clinical improvement in chronic plaque-type psoriasis lesions after narrow-band UVB therapy is accompanied by a decrease in the expression of IFN-gamma inducers—IL-12, IL-18 and IL-23. Exp Dermatol 2004;13(12):764–72.
27. Jadali Z, Eslami M. T cell immune responses in psoriasis. Iran J Allergy Asthma Immunol 2014;13(4): 220–30.
28. Wong T, Hsu L, Liao W. Phototherapy in psoriasis: a review of mechanisms of action. J Cutan Med Surg 2013;17(1):6–12.
29. Enk C, Sredni D, Blauvelt A, et al. Induction of IL-10 gene expression in human keratinocytes by UVB exposure in vivo and in vitro. J Immunol 1995;154: 4851–6.
30. Johnson-Huang L, Suarez-Fariatas M, Sullivan-Whalen M, et al. Effective narrow-band UVB radiation therapy suppresses the IL-23/IL-17 axis in normalized psoriasis plaques. J Invest Dermatol 2010;130(11):2654–63.
31. Weatherhead S, Farr P, Jamieson D, et al. Keratinocyte apoptosis in epidermal remodeling and clearance of psoriasis induced by UV radiation. J Invest Dermatol 2011;131(9):1916–26.
32. Kolgen W, Both H, van Weelden H, et al. Epidermal langerhans cell depletion after artificial ultraviolet B

irradiation of human skin in vivo: apoptosis versus migration. J Invest Dermatol 2002;118(5):812–7.

33. Weiss J, Renkl A, Denfeld R, et al. Low-dose UVB radiation perturbs the functional expression of B7.1 and B7.2 co-stimulatory molecules on human Langerhans cells. Eur J Immunol 1995;25(10): 2858–62.
34. Almutawa F, Alnomair N, Wang Y, et al. Systematic review of UV-based therapy for psoriasis. Am J Clin Dermatol 2013;14(2):87–109.
35. Sokolova A, Lee A, D Smith S. The safety and efficacy of narrow band ultraviolet B treatment in dermatology: a review. Am J Clin Dermatol 2015; 16(6):501–31.
36. Pavlovsky M, Baum S, Shpiro D, et al. Narrow band UVB: is it effective and safe for paediatric psoriasis and atopic dermatitis? J Eur Acad Dermatol Venereol 2010;25(6):727–9.
37. Almutawa F, Thalib L, Hekman D, et al. Efficacy of localized phototherapy and photodynamic therapy for psoriasis: a systematic review and meta-analysis. Photodermatol Photoimmunol Photomed 2013; 31(1):5–14.
38. Gerber W, Arheilger B, Ha T, et al. 308-nm excimer laser treatment of psoriasis: a new phototherapeutic approach. Br J Dermatol 2003;149(6):1250–8.
39. Asawanonda P, Anderson R, Chang Y, et al. 308-nm excimer laser for the treatment of psoriasis. Arch Dermatol 2000;136(5):619–24.
40. Feldman S, Mellen B, Housman T, et al. Efficacy of the 308-nm excimer laser for treatment of psoriasis: results of a multicenter study. J Am Acad Dermatol 2002;46(6):900–6.
41. Mehraban S, Feily A. 308nm excimer laser in dermatology. J Lasers Med Sci 2013;5(1):8–12.
42. Fleischer A, Lee W, Adams D, et al. Tanning facility compliance with state and federal regulations in North Carolina: a poor performance. J Am Acad Dermatol 1993;28(2):212–7.
43. Radack K, Farhangian M, Anderson K, et al. A review of the use of tanning beds as a dermatological treatment. Dermatol Ther (Heidelb) 2015; 5(1):37–51.
44. Das S, Lloyd J, Walshaw D, et al. Response of psoriasis to sunbed treatment: comparison of conventional ultraviolet A lamps with new higher ultraviolet B-emitting lamps. Br J Dermatol 2002;147(5):966–72.
45. Fleischer A, Clark A, Rapp S, et al. Commercial tanning bed treatment is an effective psoriasis treatment: results from an uncontrolled clinical trial. J Invest Dermatol 1997;109(2):170–4.
46. Kurizky P, Ferreira C, Nogueira L, et al. Treatment of psoriasis and psoriatic arthritis during pregnancy and breastfeeding. An Bras Dermatol 2015;90(3): 367–75.
47. Vangipuram R, Feldman S. Ultraviolet phototherapy for cutaneous diseases: a concise review. Oral Dis 2016;22(4):253–9.
48. Jo S, Yoon H, Woo S, et al. Time course of tanning induced by narrow-band UVB phototherapy in Korean psoriasis patients. Photodermatol Photoimmunol Photomed 2006;22(4):193–9.
49. Menter A, Korman N, Elmets C, et al. Guidelines of care for the management of psoriasis and psoriatic arthritis. J Am Acad Dermatol 2010;62(1):114–35.
50. Calzavara-Pinton P, Zane C, Candiago E, et al. Blisters on psoriatic lesions treated with TL-01 lamps. Dermatology 2000;200(2):115–9.
51. Perna J, Mannix M, Rooney J, et al. Reactivation of latent herpes simplex virus infection by ultraviolet light: a human model. J Am Acad Dermatol 1987; 17(3):473–8.
52. Young A. Carcinogenicity of UVB phototherapy assessed. Lancet 1995;345(8962):1431–2.
53. Man I, Crombie I, Dawe R, et al. The photocarcinogenic risk of narrowband UVB (TL-01) phototherapy: early follow-up data. Br J Dermatol 2005; 152(4):755–7.
54. Osmancevic A, Gillstedt M, Wennberg A, et al. The risk of skin cancer in psoriasis patients treated with UVB therapy. Acta Derm Venereol 2014;94(4): 425–30.
55. Heckman C, Chandler R, Kloss J, et al. Minimal erythema dose (MED) testing. J Vis Exp 2013;(75): e50175.
56. Bodekaer M, Philipsen P, Karlsmark T, et al. Good agreement between minimal erythema dose test reactions and objective measurements: an in vivo study of human skin. Photodermatol Photoimmunol Photomed 2013;29(4):190–5.
57. Baron E, Suggs A. Introduction to photobiology. Dermatol Clin 2014;32(3):255–66.
58. Lapolla W, Yentzer B, Bagel J, et al. A review of phototherapy protocols for psoriasis treatment. J Am Acad Dermatol 2011;64(5):936–49.
59. Dawe RS, Wainwright NJ, Cameron H, et al. Narrow-band (TL-01) ultraviolet B phototherapy for chronic plaque psoriasis: three times or five times weekly treatment? Br J Dermatol 1998;138(5):833–9.
60. Lebwohl M, Martinez J, Weber P, et al. Effects of topical preparations on the erythemogenicity of UVB: implications for psoriasis phototherapy. J Am Acad Dermatol 1995;32(3):469–71.
61. Koek M, Buskens E, van Weelden H, et al. Home versus outpatient ultraviolet B phototherapy for mild to severe psoriasis: pragmatic multicentre randomised controlled non-inferiority trial (PLUTO study). BMJ 2009;338:b1542.
62. Lui H. Phototherapy of psoriasis: update with practical pearls. J Cutan Med Surg 2002;6(0):17–21.

CHAPTER 3

Psoralen-Ultraviolet Light A Therapy

Lauren M. Madigan, MD, Henry W. Lim, MD

KEYWORDS

• Psoralen-UV-A • PUVA • Photochemotherapy • Psoriasis

KEY POINTS

- Psoralen-UV-A (PUVA) photochemotherapy involves use of either an oral or topical psoralen followed by exposure to long-wave UV-A radiation. This combination leads to a clinically beneficial phototoxic response, which has been used therapeutically for a wide array of dermatoses.
- PUVA is an effective form of therapy for chronic plaque-type psoriasis with the potential for induction of long-term remission.
- Use of PUVA photochemotherapy has become limited secondary to cumbersome administration, acute toxicity, the availability of alternative modalities, and, most notably, the risk of carcinogenesis.
- Although caution must be exercised when administering PUVA, it remains a viable treatment option for individuals with recalcitrant disease, darker skin types, and localized, refractory forms of psoriasis, such as palmoplantar pustulosis.

INTRODUCTION

Photochemotherapy broadly refers to a treatment method that uses a photosensitizing compound and ultraviolet radiation. Psoralen-UV-A (PUVA) therapy more specifically involves use of either an oral or a topical psoralen followed by exposure to long-wave UV-A radiation (320–400 nm). This combination leads to a clinically beneficial phototoxic response, which has been used therapeutically for a wide array of dermatoses. The use of psoralen photochemotherapy dates back thousands of years to ancient Egypt and India, where the pigment-inducing qualities of naturally occurring plants were anecdotally described and applied to pigmentary disorders such as vitiligo. The period ranging from the 1930s to 1960s saw the chemical and structural identification of psoralens with extraction and synthesis.[1] PUVA, in its modern form, was established by 1947 for the treatment of vitiligo and was subsequently adapted for use in psoriasis by Pinkus in 1951.[2] The development of a high-intensity UV-A light source in 1974 firmly established the use of this modality as a highly effective treatment of psoriasis.[3] Over time, treatment options for psoriasis have expanded and regular use of PUVA therapy has declined because of its photocarcinogenic potential. This chapter discusses the mechanism of PUVA as well as efficacy, dosing, safety, and precautions.

MECHANISM OF ACTION

Psoralens are furocoumarins that are either naturally derived or synthetically produced.[4] Currently, in North America, 8-methoxypsoralen (8-MOP) is the only available oral and topical formulation, whereas in Europe, 5-methoxypsoralen (5-MOP) is used due to its lower potential for phototoxicity and reduced gastrointestinal side effects. Trimethylpsoralen (TMP) has been traditionally used for bath PUVA, a practice that has been chiefly used in Scandinavian countries.[5,6] The lower phototoxic potential of TMP has also led to its use, primarily in South Asia, in combination with sunlight exposure.

Following oral ingestion or topical application, the psoralen intercalates between DNA base pairs but remains quiescent in the absence of ultraviolet radiation. Upon initial exposure to UV-A, cyclobutane monoadducts are formed with pyrimidine bases. When a second photon of energy is absorbed, psoralen-DNA cross-linking occurs, which inhibits DNA replication and causes cell cycle arrest (Fig. 3.1).[4]

In addition to direct effects on cellular DNA, numerous changes in the cutaneous microenvironment have been observed following PUVA treatment. Psoralen photosensitization leads to altered cytokine secretion, including an increase in the expression of interleukins-1, -6, and -10 as well as immunosuppressive prostaglandins. Adhesion molecules and growth factor receptors are similarly modulated as is demonstrated by intercellular adhesion molecule-1, whose upregulation—a hallmark of inflammatory skin conditions—is effectively mitigated by photochemotherapy.[7] Alteration in these mediators leads to transformation from a T helper 1 (Th1) and Th17 profile to a Th2 phenotype.[5] Activated psoralens also interact with molecular oxygen, leading to the formation of reactive oxygen species.

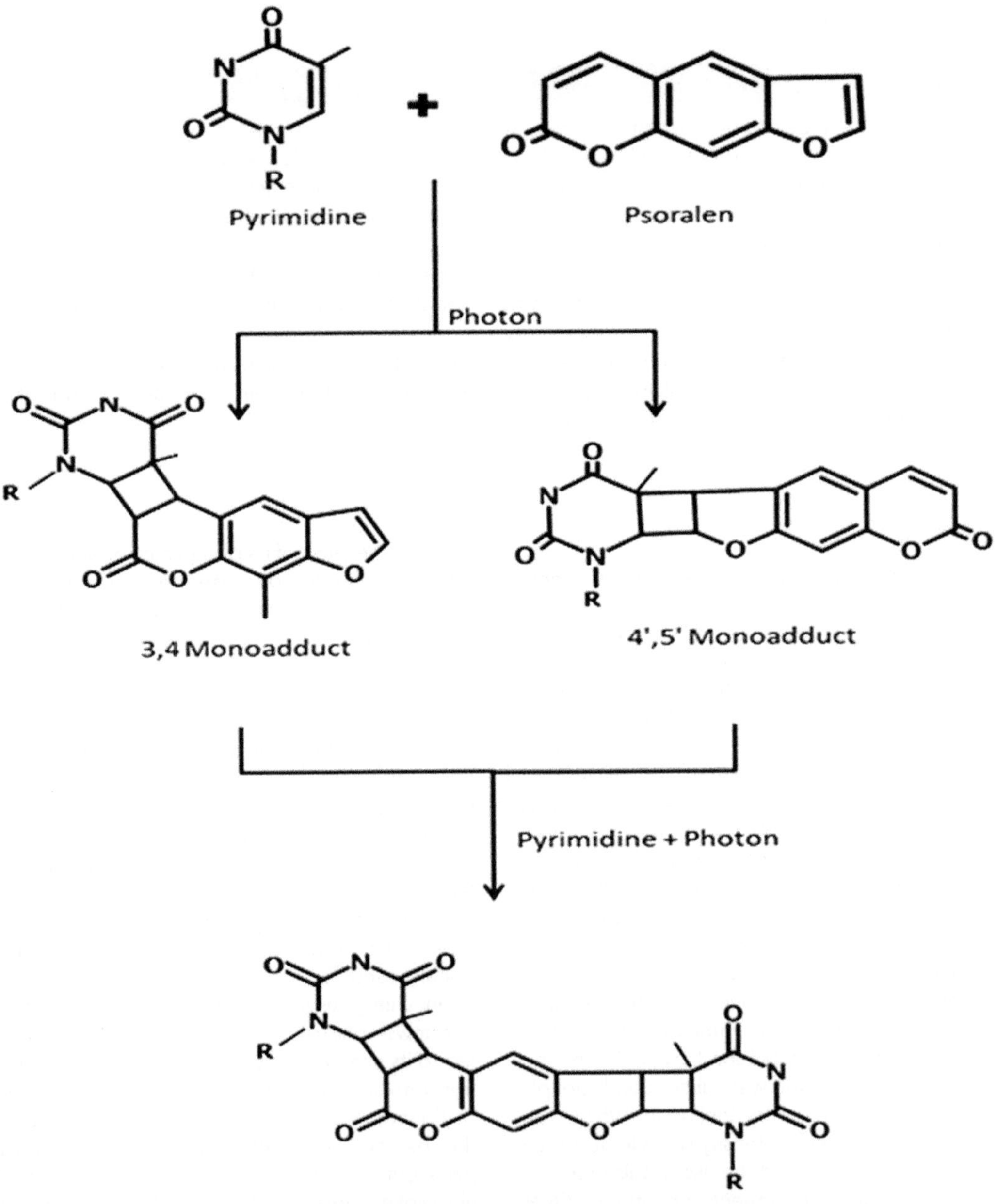

Fig. 3.1 Psoralen biochemical pathway.

These reactive molecules and free radicals result in cell membrane damage by lipid peroxidation, disruption of mitochondria, and activation of eicosanoid pathways.[4]

Following successful PUVA therapy, there is a decline in proliferating epidermal cells and a significant reduction in the epidermal thickness of psoriatic lesions. Current evidence suggests that this is mediated, in part, by induction of p53 and Fas pathways with subsequent keratinocyte apoptosis. There is evidence that differential expression of microRNAs plays a large role in p53-dependant apoptosis with significant upregulation of miR-4516 and increased Retinoic Acid Inducible Gene-1 signaling, leading to induction of autophagy and reduced cell migration.[8,9]

Although effective at reducing epidermal keratinocyte proliferation, PUVA is far more potent at inducing apoptosis in lymphocytes, which may be related to suppression of Bcl-2 expression.[4,8] In one in vitro study, there was virtual elimination of CD3 expression following bathwater treatment with either TMP or 8-MOP.[10] The degree of lymphocyte depletion has been reported to correlate with clinical response.[6]

A major advantage of PUVA over UV-B phototherapy is that UV-A penetrates deeper into the skin. As a result, cellular effects can be detected throughout the epidermis, papillary dermis, and superficial vascular plexus, leading to alterations in dermal dendritic cells, mast cells, endothelial cells, and infiltrating immune cell function.[5]

EFFICACY

Numerous studies have demonstrated the efficacy of PUVA in treating psoriasis. These studies include 2 early and integral investigations—one in the United States in 1977 and one in Europe in 1981—that firmly established PUVA as an effective therapeutic option. The American study used oral 8-MOP and high-intensity UV-A radiation. Of the 1139 patients included in the final analysis, clearance was noted in 88% and was reached at a mean of 23.6 treatments. Of note, clearance was defined as having macular erythema, hyperpigmentation, or normal-appearing skin.[11] Initial dosing was based on skin phototype, and a fixed dose was used for escalation of therapy in the absence of erythema.[11] In the European study, data from 18 separate institutions were pooled and evaluated. In agreement with the US cohort, 88.8% of the 3175 patients treated with PUVA achieved a response better than "marked improvement" over an average of 20 exposures. Dosing in this study was determined by the minimal phototoxicity dose, and subsequent adjustment was individualized to each patient.[12] These findings were of paramount importance when considering that patients with severe, generalized involvement previously required inpatient hospitalization to achieve comparable results. Similarly, impressive response rates were noted in 2 comparative studies that evaluated the efficacy of PUVA in relation to narrowband (NB) UV-B. The PUVA-associated clearance rates reported in these studies were 70% and 84%, which, in both instances, were superior to NB-UV-B therapy. Clearance in these trials was defined as either 95% to 100% improvement or total clearance of psoriatic plaques above the knees, respectively.[13,14] Of note, long-term remission (>6 months) was also achieved by a larger proportion of the subjects treated with PUVA (35% vs 12% in the NB-UV-B cohort).[14]

A *Cochrane Review* formally comparing PUVA and NB-UV-B for the treatment of psoriasis was reported in 2013. As with most phototherapeutic interventions, the analyzed studies were confounded by disparate dosing strategies, frequency of use, and outcome measures.[5] Of the 3 studies included, one revealed that NB-UV-B was as effective as oral PUVA, whereas the other 2 found PUVA to be superior to NB-UV-B.[15] A European review similarly concluded that PUVA had superior efficacy, when compared with NB-UV-B, as well as a higher probability of remission at 6 months (odds ratio = 2.73; 95% confidence interval [CI] 1.19–6.27).[16] The duration of remission has been correlated with Psoriasis Area and Severity Index scores at the end of treatment.[17] In clinical practice, this difference in response and remission period must be weighed against the potential for carcinogenesis (to be discussed later in detail). Several studies have demonstrated that bath PUVA is not only as effective as orally administered PUVA but also requires a lower cumulative dose of UV-A and has fewer associated adverse effects.[5,18–21] This treatment option, however, requires preparation of psoralen-containing bath water, immersion of the patient in the bathtub, and irradiation with UV-A immediately after completion of bathing. In light of the resources needed to properly administer bath PUVA, its use has been limited worldwide.

Combination Therapy

Effective combination regimens have been sought in an effort to reduce the cumulative dose of UV-A and potentially mitigate the associated risks. Topical corticosteroids, calcipotriol, and tazarotene are all considered synergistic with PUVA and carry minimal additional side effects.[5] Concomitant exposure to NB-UV-B has also been investigated for use in recalcitrant cases. In a bilateral comparison study, patients were noted to reach clearance in an average of only 11.3 treatments with a mean cumulative UV-A dose that was less than half of what was given with PUVA monotherapy.[22] Despite these findings, UV-B-PUVA combination therapy is not used due to concerns for increased photocarcinogenicity.

The combination of PUVA and oral retinoids has been well studied. In a randomized, placebo-controlled trial, 96% of subjects who received adjunctive acitretin therapy attained marked or complete clearance in comparison to 80% of subjects who received PUVA phototherapy alone. Significantly, the cumulative UV-A dose for patients in the acitretin/PUVA arm was 42% less than those who did not receive combination therapy.[23] These findings are supported by another placebo-controlled trial, which found the combination of oral retinoids and PUVA to be superior in many regards, including a decrease in lesional scores, number of sessions, and total cumulative dose of UV-A required before clearance. On average, the patients in this study experience a decrease in treatment duration of 18 days when treated with concurrent PUVA and acitretin.[24] The combination of these 2 therapies may also help to reduce the potential side effects. Not only is a lower cumulative dose of UV-A required but acitretin may also provide protection with regard to cutaneous malignancy.[25] Because of the potential for increased carcinogenesis, concurrent treatment with cyclosporine is generally not recommended. The safety of combination therapy with methotrexate has also been challenged, although to a lesser degree.[5]

DOSING

8-MOP is available orally in a variety of preparations, including crystals, micronized crystals, and a liquid, which has a higher, earlier, and more reproducible peak concentration. The liquid formulation enclosed in a soft gel capsule is currently the most widely available.[4] Following ingestion, oral psoralens are metabolized in the liver and ultimately renally excreted after 12 to 24 hours. Psoralens are subject to a first-pass effect that can lead to drastic variability in plasma concentration following slight alterations in administration.[4] The initial dose of psoralen is based on the patient's weight, as outlined in Table 3.1. UV-A should be delivered 1 hour following ingestion, with the initial UV-A dose dependent on the patient's phototype. Table 3.2 lists dosing guidelines. Ideally, patients should refrain from eating 1 hour before and 1 hour after dosing because food impairs the absorption of methoxypsoralen. Strict adherence to fasting is not usually feasible, however, as ingestion of psoralens on an empty stomach can lead to gastrointestinal side effects such as nausea, and less commonly, vomiting. In practice, most practitioners recommend that the psoralen be taken with a small meal. Care must be taken to ensure that the type of food, amount of food, and the time interval between the meal and psoralen dosing are held constant to minimize variations in the serum levels. For topical PUVA therapy, 0.1% 8-MOP in an emollient base is recommended and should be applied 30 minutes before exposure to UV-A starting at a dose of 0.25 to 0.5 J/cm^2 and increasing by 0.25 to 0.5 J/cm^2 as tolerated.[5]

TABLE 3.1
Weight-based dosing of oral 8-methoxypsoralen for oral psoralen plus ultraviolet light A therapy

Patient's Weight		
lb	**kg**	**Dose (mg)**
<66	<30	10
66–143	30–65	20
144–200	66–91	30
>200	>91	40

Adapted from Menter A, Korman NJ, Elmets CA, et al. Guidelines of care for the management of psoriasis and psoriatic arthritis. Section 5. Guidelines of care for the treatment of psoriasis with phototherapy and photochemotherapy. J Am Acad Dermatol 2010;62(1):126; with permission.

TABLE 3.2
Dosing of ultraviolet light A for psoralen plus ultraviolet light A photochemotherapy

Skin Type	Initial Dose (J/cm^2)	Increments (J/cm^2)	Maximum Dose (J/cm^2)
I	0.5	0.5	8
II	1.0	0.5	8
III	1.5	1.0	12
IV	2.0	1.0	12
V	2.5	1.5	20
VI	3.0	1.5	20

Adapted from Menter A, Korman NJ, Elmets CA, et al. Guidelines of care for the management of psoriasis and psoriatic arthritis. Section 5. Guidelines of care for the treatment of psoriasis with phototherapy and photochemotherapy. J Am Acad Dermatol 2010;62(1):126; with permission.

SAFETY

Acute toxicities are well recognized and are among the most common adverse effects related to PUVA. Within the initial large American and European studies, erythema (with associated pruritus, tingling, and pigmentation) and gastrointestinal symptoms (such as nausea and vomiting) were most common.[11,12] As noted previously, some of the gastrointestinal complaints can be mitigated with coingestion of a small meal or use of an alternative psoralen (5-MOP). Unlike UV-B, PUVA-induced erythema peaks at 48 to 72 hours and persists for longer periods of time—up to 1 week or more.[26] When large areas are affected by phototoxicity, systemic symptoms such as fever and malaise may be present due to significant cytokine release.[4]

Other acute toxicities, including headache, blistering, dizziness, melanonychia, and photo-onycholysis, have been reported (Fig. 3.2).[5,11,12] Induction or worsening of certain cutaneous diseases, such as blistering disorders, has been well described as has phototoxicity from other medications that the patient might be taking. Hepatic toxicity is also of concern because of observed liver damage in rodents receiving excessive doses, although the clinical relevance of these findings and the incidence of true hepatitis are likely negligible in patients without severe underlying liver dysfunction.[5] Ocular complications, on the other hand, do occur in individuals who resist use of eye protection. In one study of 82 patients who refused UV-A blocking sunglasses following treatment, 20 patients developed conjunctival hyperemia and 21 patients demonstrated decreased lacrimation.[27] No patients within this study developed lens opacities despite the ability of psoralens to bind proteins within the lens. In a 25-year prospective study of a large US cohort, there was no increase in the incidence of either visual impairment or cataract formation, findings which may reflect the careful use of eye protection among investigators.[28]

With long-term use of PUVA, photoaging is an expected side effect because of changes in dermal collagen, loss of elasticity, and pigmentary changes. In addition, chronic exposure to PUVA had been associated with PUVA lentiginosis (the formation of diffuse, stellate lentigines; Fig. 3.3), cutaneous amyloid deposition, hypertrichosis, and chromonychia (Fig. 3.4).[5,29,30] Although these adverse reactions may be cosmetically disturbing, the greatest risk attributed to prolonged use is the potential for the development of skin cancer.

Nonmelanoma Skin Cancer

As PUVA has mutagenic effects on cellular DNA and immunosuppressive activity, it is not surprising that there have been concerns regarding the risk of cutaneous malignancy since its inception. In a 30-year prospective study involving a large American cohort (the PUVA Follow-Up study), 3000 squamous cell carcinomas (SCC) developed—a value that is approximately 30 times higher than would be expected based on population incidence data. These SCC were also noted to be distributed in anatomic sites that are not as commonly affected, such as the extremities and genitals. The correlation was not as strong for basal cell carcinomas (BCC), which demonstrated a 5-fold greater incidence with more than half of the detected tumors occurring in areas where there was some degree of shielding during therapy. Overall, the greatest determinate of risk for the development of skin cancer was the total number of treatments administered. Although patients who had received less than 150 treatments did not demonstrate a clinically important increase in SCC, those subjects who had received between 350 and 450 treatments

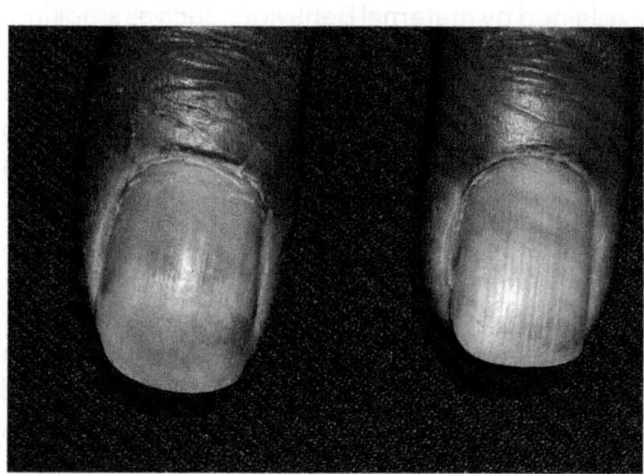

Fig. 3.2 PUVA-associated photo-onycholysis.

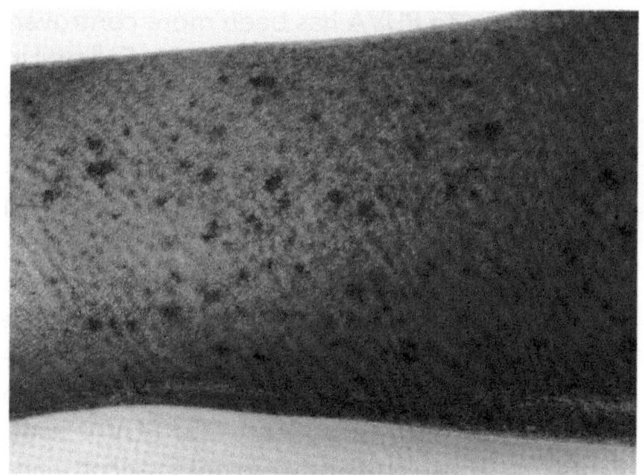

Fig. 3.3 PUVA lentiginosis.

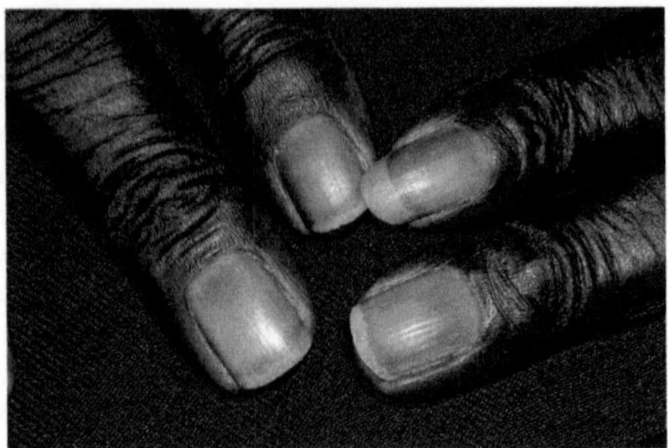

Fig. 3.4 Blue discoloration of the lunulae secondary to PUVA therapy.

were noted to have an incidence rate ratio of 6.01 (95% CI 4.41–8.20).[31] A recent, large systematic review also revealed an increased incidence of cutaneous tumors in PUVA-treated patients with a disproportionate elevation in SCC. The risk in European studies was found to be lower than the US cohort described above. This finding was attributed to a higher average UV-A dose as well as an overall high incidence of lighter phototypes receiving therapy in the American study.[32] As alluded to previously, the risk in many of the trials analyzed was particularly elevated with regard to SCC of the male genitalia. In a prospective cohort of 892 PUVA-treated men, the incidence of an invasive penile or scrotal SCC was elevated 52.6-fold (95% CI 19.3–114.6) compared with the general Caucasian population. The highest risk was appreciated among men receiving high-dose PUVA as well as exposure to both PUVA and topical tar/UV-B radiation.[33] It is important to note that an increased risk of skin cancer has not been demonstrated in patients of darker skin types receiving oral psoralen or in patients who only receive PUVA bath therapy.[34,35]

Malignant Melanoma

The relationship between malignant melanoma and exposure to PUVA has been more controversial. Long-term data from the PUVA Follow-Up study revealed an increased risk that first emerged approximately 15 years after the time of first treatment. From year 15 to year 21, the incidence relative risk of all melanomas increased to 5.4 (95% CI 2.2–11.2) with a further increase to 9.3 (95% CI 3.2–26.6) over the following 27 months. A dose response relationship was appreciated with more than a 4-fold increase in the incidence of melanoma after 15 years of latency in patients who had been exposed to at least 200 PUVA treatments.[36,37] These findings were not in accordance with 3 retrospective European studies and 2 other US cohorts, which did not find any increase in the incidence of melanoma.[32,38,39]

PRECAUTIONS

Contraindications

Absolute contraindications to PUVA include known systemic lupus erythematosus, porphyria, xeroderma pigmentosum, and photosensitivity with a known action spectrum in the UV-A range (eg, solar urticaria). Caution is also advised in any individual with a predisposition to cutaneous malignancy, including patients with lightly pigmented skin that burns easily, those with a history of multiple nonmelanoma skin cancers or malignant melanoma, those who are significantly immunosuppressed, and patients with a history of exposure to either arsenic or ionizing radiation. Care must be taken in patients with severe hepatic disease because toxicity is more of a true concern in this population. In addition, PUVA should not be administered to patients with limited ability to stand within the booth or to those who are claustrophobic.[5]

Special Populations

Pregnancy and lactation

Although UV-A therapy alone can lead to unique ramifications for pregnant patients (ie, induction or worsening of melasma), much attention has been directed toward the potential risk of psoralen ingestion at the time of conception or during pregnancy. Three separate investigations—a prospective analysis of pregnant women included in the Follow-Up study, a prospective follow-up analysis conducted by the European Network of Teratology Information Services, and a retrospective review of women treated with PUVA in Sweden—found an absence of significant congenital anomalies within the treatment groups.[40–42] The Swedish study did, however, identify a marked increase in low-birth-weight infants when pregnancy occurred following treatment. Although not fully explained by maternal behaviors, such as smoking, the investigators could not exclude the possibility that the underlying disease process itself was responsible for this outcome.[42] It is important to consider that the cohorts included in these studies were relatively small. At the current time, oral psoralens are considered to be pregnancy category C, and it is prudent to avoid administering oral PUVA therapy to pregnant women.[43] Similar risks may not pertain to topical psoralen because plasma levels are not significantly increased unless applied to a large body surface area. As psoralen is excreted in human milk, PUVA should not be administered to nursing mothers.[5]

Children

Because of the concern for photocarcinogenicity and premature photoaging, oral PUVA is rarely used in the pediatric population. Among patients enrolled in the initial PUVA Follow-up study in 1975 and 1976, a total of 26 subjects were aged 15 years or younger at the time of their first treatment. Within that small cohort, one male patient developed 2 BCC before the age of 21.[44] Although the power of the study is limited, this finding raises concern, especially because further phototherapy or immunomodulatory agents may be required later in life. In general, significant caution should be taken in this population, and alternative modalities—such as NB-UV-B—are preferred. Based on the data obtained from adult subjects, topical PUVA may be a viable alternative for children with palmar and plantar disease due to lower systemic absorption.[45]

MONITORING

Because of the risk of associated cutaneous malignancy and ocular damage—among many other potential adverse events—a careful full skin examination and a complete ocular evaluation should be performed at baseline. As directed by history, specific laboratory parameters including liver enzymes and autoimmune serologies (ANA, anti-Ro/La antibodies) may also be prudent. In a study that evaluated 27,840 person-years of data, no significant decrease in the skin cancer risk was noted during the first 15 years after cessation of PUVA therapy.[46] This persistence of risk highlights the need for ongoing, full-body skin examinations for any patient with a prior exposure, especially those with a high total cumulative dose. This recommendation is likely of less importance in individuals with darkly pigmented skin. Although the literature has yet to find a significant long-term risk of cataracts in patients who received PUVA, yearly ophthalmologic evaluations are recommended.[5]

Monitoring is most important in patients with a higher inherent risk for skin cancer and those in whom maintenance therapy has been used. PUVA maintenance therapy is almost never done currently because of limited available data regarding safety and the assumption of further risk without clear benefit. In one right-to-left side prospective, comparison study, the mean interval between therapy and relapse was nearly identical for areas that had received short-term maintenance therapy in comparison to those that did not. The investigators of this study concluded that this practice should be avoided.[47]

VACCINATION

As this form of therapy does not result in systemic immune suppression, there are no concerns regarding vaccination before—or during—PUVA therapy.

SUMMARY

PUVA is an effective form of therapy for psoriasis with the potential for induction of long-term remission. Its use has, in many ways, fallen out of favor due to cumbersome administration, acute toxicity, the availability of alternative modalities (such as NB-UV-B) and—most notably—the concern for photocarcinogenesis. For patients with moderate-to-severe psoriasis, it is appropriate to consider NB-UV-B and targeted phototherapy with excimer laser as the first therapeutic options (in addition to topical treatments). In those who show an inadequate response to 20 to 30 treatments of NB-UV-B, the options then would be considerably broader and include PUVA, traditional systemic medications (eg, methotrexate, cyclosporine), biologics, and phosphodiesterase 4 inhibitors. PUVA can be considered as the first-line UV-based therapy in patients with darker skin and those with thick lesions because UV-A penetrates deeper into the skin when compared with NB-UV-B. Topical PUVA is also an excellent treatment option for palmoplantar pustulosis.

As the landscape of pharmacology continues to change dramatically with regard to psoriasis, PUVA will remain an important component of the dermatologist's armamentarium for approaching an often complicated and challenging disease.

REFERENCES

1. Pathak MA, Fitzpatrick TB. The evolution of photochemotherapy with psoralens and UVA (PUVA): 2000 BC to 1992 AD. J Photochem Photobiol B 1992;14(1–2):3–22.
2. Lapolla W, Yentzer BA, Bagel J, et al. A review of phototherapy protocols for psoriasis treatment. J Am Acad Dermatol 2011;64(5):936–49.
3. Parrish JA, Fitzpatrick TB, Tanenbaum L, et al. Photochemotherapy of psoriasis with oral methoxsalen and longwave ultraviolet light. N Engl J Med 1974; 291(23):1207–11.
4. Honigsmann H. Phototherapy for psoriasis. Clin Exp Dermatol 2001;26(4):343–50.
5. Menter A, Korman NJ, Elmets CA, et al. Guidelines of care for the management of psoriasis and psoriatic arthritis. Section 5. Guidelines of care for the treatment of psoriasis with phototherapy and

photochemotherapy. J Am Acad Dermatol 2010; 62(1):114–35.
6. Zanolli M. Phototherapy treatment of psoriasis today. J Am Acad Dermatol 2003;49(2 Suppl): S78–86.
7. Krutmann J, Morita A. Mechanisms of ultraviolet (UV) B and UVA phototherapy. J Investig Dermatol Symp Proc 1999;4(1):70–2.
8. El-Domyati M, Moftah NH, Nasif GA, et al. Evaluation of apoptosis regulatory proteins in response to PUVA therapy for psoriasis. Photodermatol Photoimmunol Photomed 2013;29(1):18–26.
9. Chowdhari S, Saini N. Gene expression profiling reveals the role of RIG1 like receptor signaling in p53 dependent apoptosis induced by PUVA in keratinocytes. Cell Signal 2016;28(1):25–33.
10. Coven TR, Walters IB, Cardinale I, et al. PUVA induced lymphocyte apoptosis: mechanism of action in psoriasis. Photodermatol Photoimmunol Photomed 1999;15(1):22–7.
11. Melski JW, Tanenbaum L, Parrish JA, et al. Oral methoxsalen photochemotherapy for the treatment of psoriasis: a cooperative clinical trial. J Invest Dermatol 1977;68(6):328–35.
12. Henseler T, Wolff K, Honigsmann H, et al. Oral 8-methoxypsoralen photochemotherapy of psoriasis. The European PUVA Study: a cooperative study among 18 European centres. Lancet 1981;1(8225): 853–7.
13. Spuls PI, Witkamp L, Bossuyt M, et al. A systematic review of five systemic treatments for severe psoriasis. Br J Dermatol 1997;137(6):943–9.
14. Gordon PM, Diffey BL, Matthews JN, et al. A randomized comparison of narrow-band TL-01 phototherapy and PUVA photochemotherapy for psoriasis. J Am Acad Dermatol 1999;41(5 Pt 1): 728–32.
15. Chen X, Yang M, Cheng Y, et al. Narrow-band ultraviolet B phototherapy versus broad-band ultraviolet B or psoralen-ultraviolet A photochemotherapy for psoriasis. Cochrane Database Syst Rev 2013;(10):CD009481.
16. Archier E, Devaux S, Castela E, et al. Efficacy of psoralen UV-A therapy vs. narrowband UV-B therapy in chronic plaque psoriasis: a systematic literature review. J Eur Acad Dermatol Venereol 2012; 26(Suppl 3):11–21.
17. Racz E, Prens EP. Phototherapy and photochemotherapy for psoriasis. Dermatol Clin 2015;33(1):79–89.
18. Cooper EJ, Herd RM, Priestley GC, et al. A comparison of bathwater and oral delivery of 8-methoxypsoralen in PUVA therapy for plaque psoriasis. Clin Exp Dermatol 2000;25(2):111–4.
19. Collins P, Rogers S. Bath-water compared with oral delivery of 8-methoxypsoralen PUVA therapy for chronic plaque psoriasis. Br J Dermatol 1992; 127(4):392–5.
20. Lowe NJ, Weingarten D, Bourget T, et al. PUVA therapy for psoriasis: comparison of oral and bathwater delivery of 8-methoxypsoralen. J Am Acad Dermatol 1986;14(5 Pt 1):754–60.
21. Turjanmaa K, Salo H, Reunala T. Comparison of trioxsalen bath and oral methoxsalen PUVA in psoriasis. Acta Derm Venereol 1985;65(1):86–8.
22. Momtaz TK, Parrish JA. Combination of psoralens and ultraviolet A and ultraviolet B in the treatment of psoriasis vulgaris: a bilateral comparison study. J Am Acad Dermatol 1984;10(3):481–6.
23. Tanew A, Guggenbichler A, Hönigsmann H, et al. Photochemotherapy for severe psoriasis without or in combination with acitretin: a randomized, double-blind comparison study. J Am Acad Dermatol 1991;25(4):682–4.
24. Saurat JH, Geiger JM, Amblard P, et al. Randomized double-blind multicenter study comparing acitretin-PUVA, etretinate-PUVA and placebo PUVA in the treatment of severe psoriasis. Dermatologica 1988;177(4):218–24.
25. Lebwohl M, Drake L, Menter A, et al. Consensus conference: acitretin in combination with UVB or PUVA in the treatment of psoriasis. J Am Acad Dermatol 2001;45(4):544–53.
26. Ibbotson SH, Dawe RS, Farr PM. The effect of methoxsalen dose on ultraviolet-A-induced erythema. J Invest Dermatol 2001;116(5):813–5.
27. Calzavara-Pinton PG, Carlino A, Manfredi E, et al. Ocular side effects of PUVA-treated patients refusing eye sun protection. Acta Derm Venereol Suppl (Stockh) 1994;186:164–5.
28. Malanos D, Stern RS. Psoralen plus ultraviolet A does not increase the risk of cataracts: a 25-year prospective study. J Am Acad Dermatol 2007; 57(2):231–7.
29. Greene I, Cox AJ. Amyloid deposition after psoriasis therapy with psoralen and long-wave ultraviolet light. Arch Dermatol 1979;115(10):1200–2.
30. Hashimoto K, Masanobu K. Colloid-amyloid bodies in PUVA-treated human psoriatic patients. J Invest Dermatol 1979;72(2):70–80.
31. Stern RS, Study PFU. The risk of squamous cell can basal cell cancer associated with psoralen and ultraviolet A therapy: a 30-year prospective study. J Am Acad Dermatol 2012;66(4):553–62.
32. Archier E, Devaux S, Catela E, et al. Carcinogenic risks of Psoralen UV-A therapy and narrowband UV-B therapy in chronic plaque psoriasis: a systematic literature review. J Eur Acad Dermatol Venereol 2012;26(Suppl 3):22–31.
33. Stern RS, Bagheri S, Nichols K, et al. The persistent risk of genital tumors among men treated with psoralen plus ultraviolet A (PUVA) for psoriasis. J Am Acad Dermatol 2002;47(1):33–9.
34. Murase JE, Lee EE, Koo J. Effect of ethnicity on the risk of developing nonmelanoma skin cancer

following long-term PUVA therapy. Int J Dermatol 2005;44(12):1016–21.
35. Hannuksela-Svahn A, Sigurgeirsson B, Pukkala E, et al. Trioxsalen bath PUVA did not increase the risk of squamous cell skin carcinoma and cutaneous malignant melanoma in a joint analysis of 944 Swedish and Finnish patients with psoriasis. Br J Dermatol 1999;141(3):497–501.
36. Stern RS, Nichols KT, Vakeva LH. Malignant melanoma in patients treated for psoriasis with methoxsalen (psoralen) and ultraviolet A radiation (PUVA). The PUVA Follow-Up Study. N Engl J Med 1997; 336(15):1041–5.
37. Stern RS, Study PFU. The risk of melanoma in association with long-term exposure to PUVA. J Am Acad Dermatol 2001;44(5):755–61.
38. Forman AB, Roenigk HH Jr, Caro WA, et al. Long-term follow-up of skin cancer in the PUVA-48 cooperative study. Arch Dermatol 1989;125(4):515–9.
39. Chuang TY, Heinrich LA, Schultz MD, et al. PUVA and skin cancer: a historical cohort study on 492 patients. J Am Acad Dermatol 1992;26(2 Pt 1):173–7.
40. Stern RS, Lange R. Outcomes of pregnancies among women and partners of men with a history of exposure to methoxsalen photochemotherapy (PUVA) for the treatment of psoriasis. Arch Dermatol 1991;127(3):347–50.
41. Garbis H, Elefant E, Bertolotti E, et al. Pregnancy outcome after periconceptional and first trimester exposure to methoxsalen photochemotherapy. Arch Dermatol 1995;131(4):492–3.
42. Gunnarskog JG, Kallen AJ, Lindelof BG, et al. Psoralen photochemotherapy (PUVA) and pregnancy. Arch Dermatol 1993;129(3):320–3.
43. Neild VS, Scott LV. Plasma levels of 8-methoxypsoralen in psoriatic patients receiving topical 8-methoxypsoralen. Br J Dermatol 1982;106(2):199–203.
44. Stern RS, Nichols KT. Therapy with orally administered methoxsalen and ultraviolet A radiation during childhood increases the risk of basal cell carcinoma. The PUVA follow-up study. J Pediatr 1996;129(6):915–7.
45. Pasic A, Ceovic R, Lipozencic J, et al. Phototherapy in pediatric patients. Pediatr Dermatol 2003;20(1):71–7.
46. Nijsten TEC, Stern RS. The increased risk of skin cancer is persistent after discontinuation of psoralen + ultraviolet A: a cohort study. J Invest Dermatol 2003;121(2):252–8.
47. Radakovic S, Seeber A, Honigsmann H, et al. Failure of short-term psoralen and ultraviolet A light maintenance treatment to prevent early relapse in patients with chronic recurring plaque-type psoriasis. Photodermatol Photoimmunol Photomed 2009; 25(2):90–3.

CHAPTER 4

Methotrexate

Vidhi V. Shah, BA, Elaine J. Lin, MD, Shivani P. Reddy, BS,
Jashin J. Wu, MD

KEYWORDS

• Methotrexate • MTX • Folate antagonist • CHAMPION • RESTORE1

KEY POINTS

- Methotrexate (MTX) remains a safe and effective modality for the treatment of severe, recalcitrant psoriasis when used appropriately.
- The exact mechanism of action of MTX in psoriasis is unknown, but it is thought to involve an immune modulatory effect on the T-cell–mediated inflammation in psoriasis.
- Studies demonstrate improvement of psoriatic lesions using 10 to 25 mg per week MTX as a single oral, intramuscular, or intravenous dose.
- Adverse effects reported after MTX therapy include nausea, loss of appetite, vomiting, diarrhea, bone marrow toxicity, pulmonary toxicity, and hepatotoxicity.
- Close monitoring of hematologic, liver, and renal function tests are indicated before and during MTX treatment.

INTRODUCTION

Methotrexate (MTX) is a well-established systemic treatment for moderate-to-severe psoriasis and psoriatic arthritis (PsA).[1] The US Food and Drug Administration (FDA) first approved the use of MTX for the treatment of severe, recalcitrant, disabling psoriasis in 1972.[2–4] Today, approximately 20,000 to 30,000 psoriatic patients in the United States receive MTX treatment yearly.[5]

MTX is the mainstay of treatment in rheumatoid arthritis (RA), and the rheumatologic literature thoroughly describes its safety profiles, which include the common side effects of nausea, loss of appetite, vomiting, and diarrhea, and more severe adverse effects (AEs) of bone marrow, pulmonary, and hepatic toxicity.[5] Greater knowledge of MTX and its effect on patients with RA has promoted conscientious use of this medication in patients battling with moderate-to-severe plaque psoriasis. Dermatologists have expanded indications for prescribing MTX to other forms of severe psoriasis, including PsA, erythrodermic psoriasis, acute and localized forms of pustular psoriasis, nail psoriasis, psoriasis that is recalcitrant to alternative treatments, and/or psoriasis that significantly impacts a patient's economic or psychological well-being and does not respond appropriately to retinoid, phototherapy, or psoralen and UV-A therapy.[3,5,6] There are many off-label uses of MTX, such as scleroderma, dermatomyositis, alopecia areata, and others.[7–9] In addition to psoriasis and RA, MTX is FDA approved for use in malignant neoplastic diseases, including gestational choriocarcinoma, chorioadenoma destruens, hydatidiform mole, acute lymphocytic leukemia, meningeal leukemia, mycosis fungoides, non-Hodgkin lymphomas as well as cancers of the head and neck, breast, and lung, but doses for malignancies are much higher than those used for dermatologic indications.[10]

Physicians caring for patients with psoriasis taking MTX are faced with the challenge of identifying optimal therapeutic doses, while managing adverse side effects. Appropriate use of MTX requires a gradual increasing of dosages paired with careful patient management.[11] Several guidelines on MTX dosing regimens have been published and are largely based on expert opinions, although administration strategies vary widely.[4,11]

MTX is manufactured as oral tablets or intramuscular, intravenous, or intra-arterial injections. The tablet form is 2.5 mg MTX disodium, whereas the injection is 25 mg/mL MTX sodium. The recommended starting dose schedule for psoriasis is a once-weekly, low-dose schedule of either a single oral, intramuscular, or intravenous 7.5- to

15-mg per week dose until adequate response is achieved or a divided oral dose schedule 2.5 mg at 12-hour intervals for a total of 3 doses (Fig. 4.1).[3] Some physicians recommend a test dose as low as 5 mg for the first week of treatment.[12] Dosages should be adjusted to the individual patient (ie, reduced doses for decreased renal function, the elderly patient, or persons with low body mass index vs greater doses for those with extensive, intractable disease), while avoiding higher doses. MTX can be used for long-term management of plaque psoriasis and should be continued until optimal clinical responses are achieved. There is not an established maximum dose, although many use 25 to 30 mg as a maximum. Following improvement of lesions, dosages are typically tapered to the lowest effective dose and may be continued long term with adequate monitoring owing to the risk of toxicity. MTX should be kept in an area that is not readily accessible to children. Tablets and injection vials should be stored in areas with little heat or moisture, adequate light protection, and room temperatures 59°F to 86°F (15°C to 30°C). Special care should be taken not to freeze injection vials.[10]

MECHANISM OF ACTION

MTX is a folate antagonist that interferes with de novo purine synthesis by inhibiting the enzyme dihydrofolate reductase. This critical enzyme is responsible for converting dihydrofolate to tetrahydrofolate, and its inhibition lowers the synthesis of DNAs, particularly purines and thymidylate. For this reason, MTX effectively hinders cellular replication (Fig. 4.2).[3,5]

The exact mechanism of action of MTX in the treatment of moderate-to-severe plaque psoriasis is not fully understood. Traditionally, the antiproliferative role of MTX was assumed to be most effective against the rapidly proliferating psoriatic epidermis. Inhibition of DNA synthesis during the S phase of the cell cycle would theoretically decrease epithelial cell production and parallel keratinization rates of normal skin.[13]

However, this long-standing theory has been disproven.[3,13] Novel concepts emphasize this drug's immune modulatory properties that downgrade the psoriasis inflammatory cascade by promoting apoptosis and suppressing intracellular adhesion molecule expression of T cells involved in the pathogenesis of psoriasis. In addition, MTX inhibits neutrophil chemotaxis and reduces levels of tumor necrosis factor-α (TNF-α) and interleukin-1 (IL-1).[3,14,15] These ideas represent fundamental advances in the understanding of the pathogenesis and treatment of psoriasis in the last decade, and further studies are needed to better elucidate its immune activity.[16]

EFFICACY

There is a scant amount of evidence regarding the efficacy of MTX in plaque psoriasis, despite its former widespread usage. Much of the existing drug data is primarily derived from trials involving patients with RA.[5] To date, large randomized, controlled trials, such as the CHAMPION, RESTORE, M10-255, and a few smaller trials, have been conducted to evaluate the efficacy and safety of MTX for the treatment of plaque psoriasis.[17] Table 4.1 provides a summary of these trials, including their comparative interventions, primary endpoints, and outcomes.

CHAMPION

The CHAMPION trial was a phase 3, placebo-controlled study that was the first to compare oral MTX to adalimumab and placebo for the treatment of psoriasis.[17] The study enrolled 271 patients from 28 different sites across Europe and Canada and randomized them in a 2:2:1 ratio to receive MTX, adalimumab, or placebo for 16 weeks. Oral MTX was dosed at 7.5 mg at week 0, increased to 10 mg/wk at week 2, and finally 15 mg/wk at week 4. Patients who achieved Psoriasis Area and Severity Index (PASI) 50 by week 8 were maintained on the 15-mg/wk dose, and those who did not were increased to 20 mg/wk. Any patient not achieving PASI-50 by week 12 was increased to a maximum study

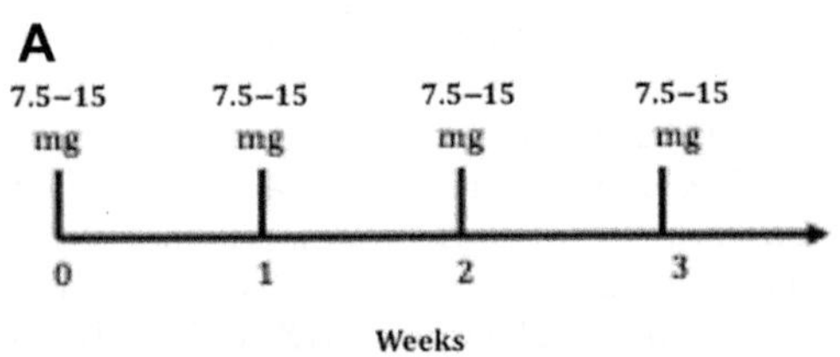

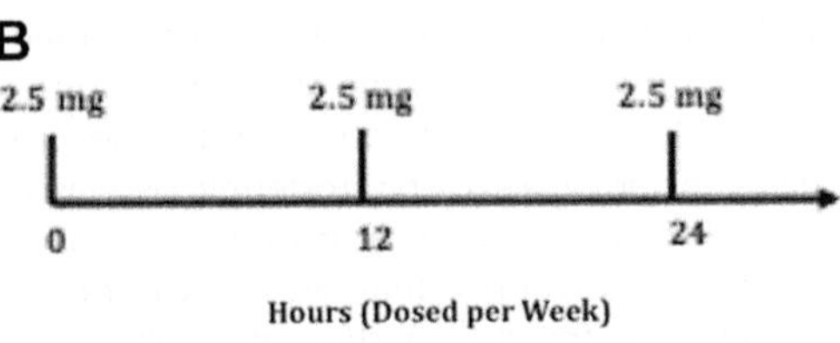

Fig. 4.1 MTX dosing regimen for psoriasis. (*From* Czarnecka-Operacz M, Sadowska-Przytocka A. The possibilities and principles of methotrexate treatment of psoriasis—the updated knowledge. Postepy Dermatol Alergol 2014;31:392–400.)

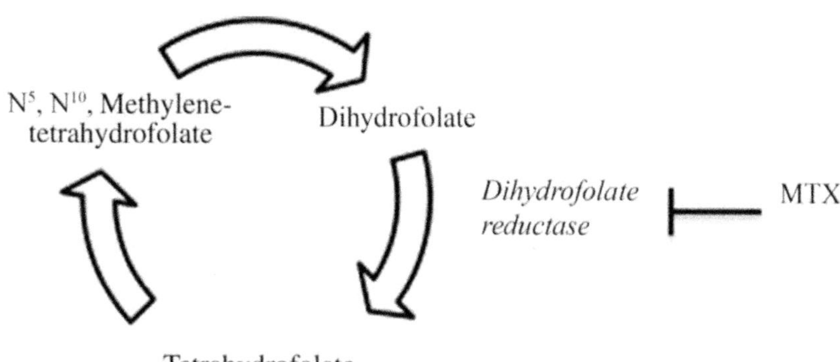

Fig. 4.2 MTX mechanism of action.

dose of 25 mg/wk. Efficacy was defined as achieving a PASI 75 response after 16 weeks of treatment. Patients with prior exposure to TNF antagonists were excluded.[17] The trial demonstrated greater PASI-75 scores for adalimumab (79.6%) to oral MTX (35.5%) and placebo (18.9%) for the treatment of plaque psoriasis.[17] Further analysis of the CHAMPION trial suggests that week 12 may be a crucial time period to decide whether a patient should continue MTX treatment or change to a different medication.[27] Fig. 4.3 demonstrates the efficacy data of the CHAMPION trial.[27]

RESTORE1

The RESTORE1 trial was a phase 3, open-label, randomized, controlled trial that compared the efficacy and safety of oral MTX to infliximab in adults with moderate-to-severe plaque psoriasis.[18] The study enrolled 868 patients, who were randomized in a 3:1 ratio to receive infliximab 5 mg/kg (infusions at weeks 0, 2, 6, 14, and 22) or MTX 2.5-mg tablets (15 mg/wk for the first 6 weeks, which could be increased to 20 mg/wk if patients failed to achieve PASI-25 from baseline by week 6). Patients who were intolerant to the treatment or had not achieved PASI-50 from baseline by week 16 were able to switch treatment groups. Patients who switched from MTX to infliximab therapy were administered infliximab infusions at weeks 16, 18, and 22. Patients who switched from infliximab to MTX received 15 mg MTX weekly until week 22. Last treatments were administered at week 22, and final follow-up occurred at week 26. Folic acid supplementation was recommended, but not required. The primary efficacy endpoint was defined as a PASI-75 at week 16, whereas additional major endpoints included PASI-75 at week 26 and a Physician Global Assessment (PGA) score of cleared or minimal (0 or 1, respectively) at weeks 16 and 26. Patients with previous exposure to MTX were excluded from the study. MTX was found to be less efficacious than infliximab in patients with moderate-to-severe plaque psoriasis, and by week 16, 63 of 215 (29%) patients taking MTX switched to infliximab. Only 9 of 653 (1%) infliximab patients switched to MTX. At week 16, 78% of infliximab patients attained PASI-75 in comparison to 42% on MTX therapy (P<.001). This score was consistent at week 26 when 77% of infliximab achieved PASI-75, whereas only 31% of MTX patients achieved PASI-75 (P<.001). In general, higher percentage of infliximab patients achieved PASI-50 and PASI-75 than MTX patients at all visits.[18]

M10-255

The M10-255 trial was a phase 3, randomized, double-blinded, clinical study comparing oral MTX with folic acid to briakinumab, a human monoclonal antibody targeting IL-12 and IL-23.[19] The study enrolled 317 patients randomized to receive either briakinumab or MTX. Baseline MTX dosage was 5 mg/wk at week 0 to 15 mg/wk and escalated by 5 mg at weeks 10 and 16 if patients did not achieve a PASI-75 or PGA 0 to 1. The primary endpoint consisted of PASI-75 or PGA 0 to 1 at 24 and 52 weeks. Results demonstrated greater percentage of patients achieving clearance with briakinumab (81.8%) than MTX (39.9%) at week 24 and 66.2% versus 23.9% at week 52, respectively (P<.001).[19]

SMALLER STUDIES

Smaller studies have also demonstrated efficacy of MTX in psoriasis. Flystrom and colleagues[20] compared the short-term effectiveness of MTX to cyclosporine (CsA) in a randomized, controlled trial. A total of 37 patients with plaque psoriasis were treated with MTX using an initial dose of 7.5 mg/wk, maximum dose of 15 mg/wk, and 5 mg/d of folic acid supplementation. The primary

TABLE 4.1
Efficacy data of methotrexate studies

Study, Year (n = Subjects)	Comparator (mg)	MTX Dosing mg (no. wk)	MTX a. PASI-75 b. PASI-50 c. PASI-90 Outcome (%)	Comparator a. PASI-75 b. PASI-50 c. PASI-90 Outcome (%)
CHAMPION,[17] 2008 (n = 271)	Adalimumab, placebo	7.5 (0–1) 10.0 (2–3) 15.0 (4–7) 20.0 (8–12)[a] 25.0 (2–16)[a]	a. 35.5 b. NR c. 13.6	a. 79.6, 18.9 b. NR c. 51.3, 11.3
RESTORE1,[18] (n = 868)	Infliximab	15.0 (1–5) 20.0 (6–16)[a]	a. 42 b. 61 c. 19	a. 78 b. 87 c. 55
M10–255,[19] (n = 317)	Briakinumab	5.0 (0) 10.0 (1) 15.0 (2–9) 20.0 (10–15)[a] 25.0 (16–24)	a. 39.9 b. 23.9 c. NR[a]	a. 81.8 b. 66.2 c. NR[a]
Flystrom et al,[20] 2008 (n = 84)	CsA	7.5 (0–12) 15.0 (0–12)[a]	a. 24 b. 65 c. 11	a. 58 b. 87 c. 29
Heydendael et al,[21] 2003 (n = 88)	CsA	15.0 (1–4) 22.5 (5–16)	a. 60 b. NR c. 40	a. 71 b. NR c. 33
Akhyani et al,[22] 2010 (n = 38)	MMF	7.5 (0–1) 15 (2–4) 20 (5–12)	a. 73.3 b. 100 c. 26.7	a. 58.8 b. 82.4 c. 11.8
Dogra et al,[23] 2012	MTX (25 mg vs 10 mg)	N/A	a. 72 b. NR c. NR	a. 92 b. NR c. NR
Ho et al,[24] 2010	TCM	2.5–5 (0–1) 10 (1–2)[a]	a. 63 b. 79 c. NR	a. 0 b. 14 c. NR
Fallah Arani et al,[25] 2011	Fumaric acid	5 (0–1) 15 (2–12) 12.5 (13) 10 (14) 5 (15) 2.5 (16)	a. 24 b. 60 c. 8	a. 19 b. 42 c. 4
Revicki et al,[26] 2008	Adalimumab	7.5–25 (0–15)[a]	a. 80 b. 88 c. 51	a. 36 b. 62 c. 14

Abbreviations: CsA, cyclosporine; NR, not reported; TCM, traditional Chinese medicine.
[a] Step up therapy if response was inadequate and no AEs were noted, the dosage was increased.
Data from Refs.[17–26]

endpoint was PASI-75 response at 12 weeks, which was achieved in 58% using MTX. There was a statistically significant difference in efficacy that was greater in the CsA treatment group.[20] Heydendael and colleagues[21] conducted a randomized, controlled trial also comparing MTX to CsA. A total of 43 patients were treated with MTX using an initial dose of 15 mg/wk, maximum dose of 22.25 mg/wk, and no folic acid supplementation. Fourteen MTX patients experienced elevated liver enzymes and were excluded from the study. At 16 weeks, approximately 60% of these patients achieved a PASI-75; however, no significant difference in efficacy was found between MTX and CsA treatment groups. Akhyani and colleagues[22] compared the efficacy and safety of mycophenolate mofetil (MMF) and MTX in the treatment of chronic plaque psoriasis.

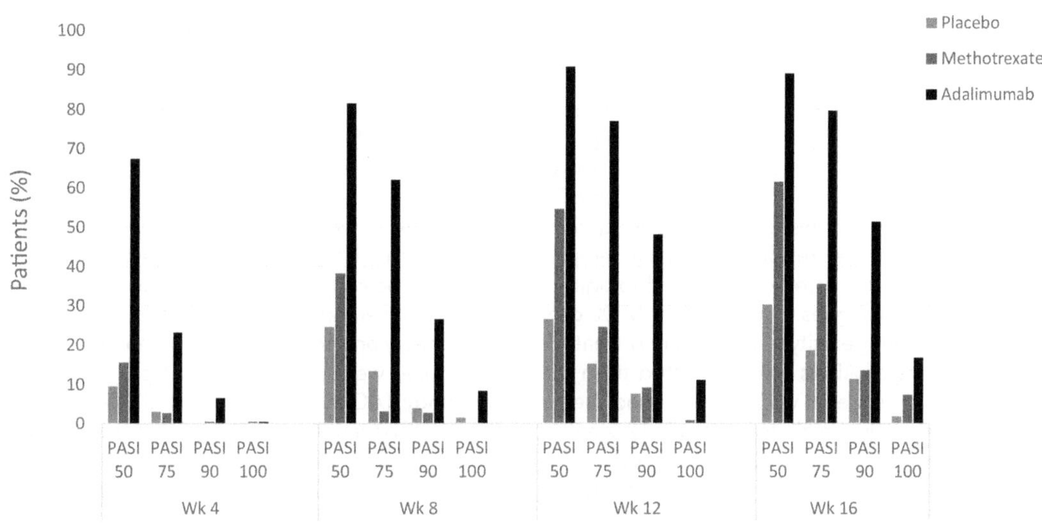

Fig. 4.3 Efficacy data of CHAMPION trial.

Eighteen patients were administered MTX using an initial dose of 7.5 mg/wk. Following 12 weeks of treatment, patients in the MTX group achieved a PASI-75 of 53.3%. No significant differences in efficacy were found between MTX and MMF.[22] Ranjan and colleagues[28] compared the therapeutic efficacy of MTX at 15 to 20 mg/wk versus hydroxycarbamide at 3 to 4.5 g/wk. The primary endpoint was percentage reduction of baseline PASI scores over 12 weeks. The mean percentage reduction in the MTX group was 77.28 $\pm$ 28 and 48.47 $\pm$ 26.53 in the hydroxycarbamide group. A greater percentage of patients in the MTX group demonstrated greater than 75% reduction in the PASI scores than hydroxycarbamide (66.66% and 13.33%, respectively).[28] A systematic review investigated MTX for psoriasis in 7 different trials and found that MTX 7.5 mg was less efficacious that CsA 3 mg, and MTX 15 mg was equally as efficacious as CsA 2.5 mg and fumaric acid ester. MTX 7.5–25 mg was less efficacious than both adalimumab and infliximab.

The data from these clinical trials and small studies suggest that MTX therapy for psoriasis is generally effective if the side effects are tolerable. Week 12 may represent an appropriate time for dermatologists to decide whether MTX is improving psoriasis or should be discontinued for alternative options. Additional randomized, controlled clinical studies in patients with psoriasis are needed to explore the efficacy profile of MTX and to validate the current prescribing guidelines.

EFFICACY IN REDUCTION OF IMMUNOGENICITY

Immunogenicity refers to the ability of therapeutic protein products to stimulate an immune response, specifically, the development of anti-drug antibodies (ADAs). These antibodies act by neutralizing or binding to therapeutic protein products, and their presence is often concerning for impending biologic failure. Moreover, ADAs can trigger potentially dangerous immune-complex AEs, such as serum sickness, bronchospasm, thromboembolic events, and Arthus and infusion reactions.[29] Emerging evidence suggests that concomitant administration of disease-modifying anti-rheumatic drugs (DMARDs) such as MTX with biologic therapy can reduce the effects of biologic-associated immunogenicity. Administration of MTX in the context of biologic therapy may decrease ADAs' formation in a dose-dependent manner, thus improving drug survival, protecting drug efficacy, and promoting better patient outcomes.[29]

The data for MTX for the reduction of immunogenicity are promising, yet are largely established in patients with RA. Biologics indicated for the treatment of moderate-to-severe plaque psoriasis, etanercept, infliximab, adalimumab, ustekinumab, secukinumab, and ixekizumab, all pose the risk of immunogenicity, but few studies exist that investigate the value of the MTX-biologic combination in this population.[29–31] Lecluse and colleagues[30] conducted a prospective observational cohort study assessing ADAs in 29 patients receiving adalimumab for plaque psoriasis over 24 weeks. Thirteen of 29 patients (45%) developed ADAs; interestingly, none of their 3 patients who received concomitant MTX therapy developed ADAs. In a follow-up study, Menting and colleagues[32] extended this cohort to 80 patients, including the original 29 patients. The long-term consequences of ADA after 24 weeks of adalimumab treatment were assessed and ADA concentrations were collected at baseline and at 12, 24, and 52 weeks. Overall, 39 of 90 (49%) patients developed ADAs. Three of 8 (37.5%) patients receiving concomitant MTX (2.5–20 mg/wk) at the start of therapy developed low titers of ADA. Thus, concomitant treatment with MTX did not significantly reduce ADAs in this study. The investigators possibly attribute their results to the small sample size of patients administered MTX with biologics.

Chiu and colleagues[33] found that MTX can decrease immunogenicity in adalimumab-treated patients. Titers of ADAs were collected from 53 patients with psoriasis vulgaris who had been treated with adalimumab for at least 12 weeks. Fifty-five percent of patients initiated MTX 10 ± 3.2 mg weekly (range 5–15 mg weekly) at the start of adalimumab therapy, whereas 45% of patients started MTX 5 ± 9.2 months after biologic treatment. Lower titers of ADAs were found in patients administered MTX in comparison to adalimumab monotherapy ($P<.05$). Interestingly, no difference in ADAs was found between patients treated with greater than 7.5 mg MTX versus less than 7.5 mg MTX. Investigators concluded that early initiation of MTX during biologic therapy might reduce the risk of developing ADAs later on, although this difference was marginally significant.

The addition of MTX, even after the development of ADA, could provide a safe and effective strategy to maintain biologic efficacy. Present literature suggests that MTX is potentially efficacious in reducing ADAs; however, the number of patients studied is limited, and this data should be interpreted with caution. The efficacy of concomitant MTX therapy with biologics needs further research and larger prospective trials with greater sample sizes necessary to validate coadministration of MTX with biologics.[29]

EFFICACY IN PSORIATIC ARTHRITIS

Various therapies, including corticosteroids, DMARDs, and biologic DMARDs, exist to target the pain, inflammation, joint destruction, and ensuing debilities affiliated with PsA. After nonsteroidal anti-inflammatory drugs (NSAIDs), MTX is one of the most widely used DMARDs. Despite its widespread use for the management of PsA, there are very few placebo-controlled studies that have investigated its effectiveness. Furthermore, the existing clinical trials provide insufficient or conflicting evidence regarding its value in the synovitis and inflammation associated with PsA.[34]

Recent evidence from controlled clinical trials suggests that MTX is not efficacious for PsA; however, the significant limitations of these studies hamper conclusive results. The Methotrexate in Psoriatic Arthritis study, a multicenter placebo-controlled trial involving 221 subjects with PsA, reported that MTX therapy has little to no disease-modifying effect. Subjects were randomized to receive either MTX or placebo for 6 months. MTX was initiated at 7.5 mg/wk, increased to 10 mg/wk at week 4, and 15 mg/wk at week 8. Sixty-seven of the 109 MTX subjects and 61 of 112 placebo subjects completed the study. Investigators observed no statistical improvement with the primary endpoint, Psoriatic Arthritis Response Criteria, as well as the American College of Rheumatology (ACR20) and 28-joint disease activity score.[35] Conversely, the Tight Control of Psoriatic Arthritis study, a multicenter, open-label, randomized, controlled trial involving 206 subjects with PsA reported the beneficial effects of MTX in PsA. Patients received MTX either as tight control protocol or as standard care, with 104 subjects receiving a mean dose of greater than 15 mg/wk. At 12 weeks, improvements in multiple clinical outcomes were demonstrated. A higher proportion of patients receiving greater than 15 mg/wk achieved ACR20, ACR50, and PASI75.[36]

In addition, large-scale registries, including the NOR-DMARD Norwegian registry and the University of Toronto PsA registry, and several observational studies report substantial improvements with MTX in joint disease in isolated and combination therapy. The paucity of clinical trial information and confounding results among different studies that evaluate the efficacy of MTX in PsA largely contributes to the lack of understanding.[37]

SAFETY

MTX has higher chance of serious side effects owing to its systemic drug distribution and drug action. Patients should be well informed of the signs and symptoms of these AEs before beginning MTX therapy. The most important side effects are hepatotoxicity, myelosuppression, and pulmonary fibrosis. Systematic review of data receiving long-term low-dose MTX indicated that 33% progress to liver disease.[38] The safety data from certain randomized, controlled clinical trials have provided important information regarding MTX use in psoriasis.

CHAMPION

Safety and AE assessments in the CHAMPION trial were continued up until 70 days after the last treatment. Eighty-nine (80.9%) patients in the MTX-treated group, 79 (73.8%) patients in the adalimumab-treated group, and 49 (79.2%) patients in the placebo group reported adverse events. There were no serious infections reported during this study, and no significant differences were seen in infection rates between the groups. Serious AEs varied between groups. In the MTX-treated group, there was 1 case of hepatitis secondary to MTX use. In the adalimumab-treated patients, there was 1 case of pancreatitis and 1 case of an ovarian cyst enlargement. There was 1 case of calculus of the right uteropelvic junction in the placebo-treated group. Overall, 8 patients discontinued the study due to AEs: 6 MTX patients (due to upper abdominal pain, retrobulbar optic neuritis, hepatitis) and 3 cases of abnormal liver function tests (LFTs) and 1 adalimumab and 1 placebo patient due to elevated aspartate aminotransferase (AST) and alanine aminotransferase (ALT) concentrations. There were no reported cases of tuberculosis or deaths during this study.

RESTORE1

Safety assessments in the RESTORE1 trial demonstrated similar instances of AE in both MTX and infliximab groups. Up until week 16, AE experienced by MTX patients included nasopharyngitis (5%), fatigue (8%), headache (7%), and nausea (7%). AE common to the infliximab group included infusion-related reactions (9%), nasopharyngitis (6%), and headache (5%). Numerical data indicated that the incidence of serious and severe AEs was greater in the infliximab group than MTX group, although no statistical analysis for significance was performed.

Toxicity

Most drug safety information has been extrapolated from rheumatologic studies for safe administration of MTX to patients with moderate-to-severe plaque psoriasis.[16] There are few evidence-based studies on plaque psoriasis patients, and data chiefly rely on case studies, clinical experience, and retrospective studies. Side effects of MTX are dose and frequency dependent, but have been appreciated at all drug levels. Table 4.1 provides an overview of the common, less common, and relatively rare AEs associated with MTX use. Decreasing or dividing the dosages, administering intramuscular or subcutaneous injections, or providing concomitant food or folic acid 1 mg supplementation can successfully reduce side effects.

Drug and Food Interactions

Special care should be taken with medications that have the potential to displace MTX from its protein binding sites (salicylates, sulfonamides, phenytoin, penicillin, and tetracycline) or decrease renal tubular secretion (NSAIDs, probenecid), thereby increasing plasma drug concentrations to toxic levels.[39] It is generally recommended to avoid prescribing other drugs with known nephrotoxic (aminoglycosides, amphotericin B, or CsA) or hepatotoxic (retinoid, azathioprine, sulfasalazine) effects in patients using MTX.[39] Antibiotics may interfere with the normal gut flora and reduce intestinal absorption of MTX. Vitamins, especially folate supplements, can decrease the effectiveness of MTX but may help relieve some AEs such as increased LFTs, nausea, vomiting, abdominal upset, alopecia, or stomatitis (Table 4.2). Use of radiotherapy and MTX increases the risk for osteonecrosis or soft tissue necrosis. The bioavailability of MTX is significantly reduced with food and milk products.[10]

PRECAUTIONS

Dermatologists should be aware of the cautions of MTX administration. Special attention should be given to patients with a history of immunodeficiency, hepatic disease, and certain other conditions. Otherwise, healthy individuals, including pregnant women, children, and elderly individuals, seeking treatment with MTX also require additional consideration.

TABLE 4.2
Side effects associated with methotrexate

Common	Less Common	Rare
Nausea	Headaches	Hepatotoxicity
Vomiting	Alopecia	Renal toxicity
Anorexia	Mood disturbances	Leukoencephalopathy
Stomatitis	Confusion	Blindness
Stomach ache/pain	Tinnitus	Gastrointestinal ulcers
Dizziness	Weight loss	Severe allergic reactions
Fever	Convulsions	Cardiac dysfunction
Chills, diarrhea	Anemia	Sudden death
Leukopenia	Thrombocytopenia	
Fatigue	Rashes	

Data from Pfizer. Methotrexate Product Monograph Pfizer Canada Inc. 2015.

Myelosuppression

MTX can potentially decrease all forms of blood cell counts, including red blood cells, white blood cells, neutrophils, and/or platelets. However, significant hematologic depression is uncommon if patients without risk factors are appropriately monitored. In 1 rheumatologic review, bone marrow toxicity occurred in 1.4% of closely studied patients.[40] The amount of bone marrow suppression is relative to the dose and duration of drug exposure as well as risk factors, including older age, drug-to-drug interactions, alcohol abuse, decreased renal function, absence of folic acid supplementation, hypoalbuminemia, and dosing inaccuracies. Depending on the level of hematologic irregularity, MTX is contraindicated in many patients with pre-existing bone marrow disorders and malignancies (Box 4.1). Patients who proceed with therapy and experience a significant decline in blood cell counts should immediately terminate treatment.

BOX 4.1
Absolute and relative contraindications for methotrexate

Relative contraindications

Abnormal LFTs

Alcoholism or alcoholic liver disease

Obesity

Diabetes mellitus

Abnormal renal function tests

Active infections including HIV, TB, and so forth

Recent or active hepatitis B or C

Mild-to-moderate bone marrow hypoplasia, leukopenia, thrombocytopenia, and anemia

Absolute contraindications

Pregnant or breastfeeding

Men or women seeking childbirth

Severe infections

Acute or chronic renal failure

Severe hepatic disease

Respiratory failure

Immunodeficiency syndromes

Severe bone marrow hypoplasia, leukopenia, thrombocytopenia, anemia

Active peptic ulcer

Hypersensitivity to MTX

Data from Pfizer. Methotrexate Product Monograph Pfizer Canada Inc. 2015.

Hepatotoxicity

MTX is notorious for increasing hepatic enzyme levels (approximately 15%–50% of patients) and inducing troublesome effects on the liver, including fibrosis and cirrhosis in patients taking chronic, low-dose MTX.[41] For this reason, hepatotoxicity is a major limiting factor for MTX administration in patients with psoriasis. According to the medical literature, persons with diabetes, obesity, hyperlipidemia, personal or family history of hepatic disease, exposure to hepatotoxic drugs or lack of folate supplementation, and excessive alcohol use significantly increase a patient's risk for hepatotoxicity.[11] In psoriasis patients with risk factors for hepatic fibrosis, some guidelines recommend periodic liver biopsies, although that suggestion remains controversial.[12]

Pulmonary Fibrosis

MTX has been implicated as a serious cause of pulmonary toxicity. Notably, most reported studies of MTX-induced lung disease are in patients with RA, which may be a combination of drug side effects as well as pulmonary manifestations of the autoimmune disease process. A recent meta-analysis of double-blind randomized, controlled trials of MTX versus placebo or comparative agents found no risk of adverse pulmonary events in patients with PsA, psoriasis, or inflammatory bowel disease.[42] Nevertheless, this toxicity is real, and patients should be aware of this potential AE and follow up with their physician if they experience any respiratory symptoms.

Patients with Excessive Third Space Fluids

Patients with pleural effusion, ascites, gastrointestinal tract obstruction, previous cisplatin therapy, dehydration, aciduria, and impaired renal function may be predisposed to higher than normal levels of MTX. Prolonged clearance times may result in toxicity, and increased MTX concentrations should be monitored at 24, 48, or 72 hours to determine when and for how long to administer leucovorin rescue.[10]

Teratogenicity

Use of MTX in pregnant and lactating women with psoriasis is strictly prohibited, because it is a well-established teratogen (pregnancy category X).[3] When dispensed to pregnant women, MTX can lead to abortion, death, and fetal abnormalities of the cardiac, musculoskeletal, and nervous systems.[3] Women seeking children should postpone conception for at least 1 complete ovulation cycle following suspension of MTX therapy before conception, although no optimal time period between cessation of therapy and pregnancy has been established.[3] Men should also be strongly discouraged from using MTX if seeking a pregnancy with their partner, because MTX is known to affect the process of spermatogenesis.[3]

Pediatric Use

MTX should be used with caution in children, because there are very little data on the safety and effectiveness of this drug in the pediatric population. Low dosages have proven to be beneficial in children with psoriasis as well as other rheumatologic disorders. Children less than 1 month of age should not be given MTX injection formula with benzyl alcohol. This preservative is reported to cause gasping syndrome, characterized by difficulty breathing and circulatory collapse.[10]

Geriatric Use

Not much data regarding the clinical safety of MTX are available in the elderly population. The older individual experiences age-related changes in intestinal, renal, and hepatic drug metabolism; thus, consider prescribing lower weekly dosages and monitoring for adverse events more vigilantly than in the adult population.[10]

MONITORING

The first guidelines on safety monitoring in patients receiving MTX were established in 1972. Since then, multiple updates have been published. The information presented is based on the most recently published guidelines from the American Academy of Dermatology in 2009 (Table 4.3).[43]

The potential for fatal drug toxicities mandates treatment regimens characterized by a strict dosing schedule and routine monitoring. Patients on MTX should be closely monitored for early recognition of hematopoietic, hepatic, or renal abnormalities.

Baseline Monitoring

Before initiating MTX therapy, patients should have a thorough history and physical examination, including a history of alcohol consumption, exposure to viral hepatitis, and family history of liver disease. Laboratory evaluation should include complete blood counts (CBC) with differential and platelet counts, blood urea nitrogen (BUN) and creatinine, LFTs including serum AST, ALT, alkaline phosphatase, and serum albumin and bilirubin. Patients with elevated LFTs should undergo further screening for hepatitis B virus (HBV) and hepatitis C virus. Screening for tuberculosis (TB) with a baseline purified protein derivative (PPD) test or another test for latent TB is recommended in patients who will be treated with MTX.

TABLE 4.3
Methotrexate monitoring recommendations from the American Academy of Dermatology

Monitoring	
History and physical	Routine
PPD test	Baseline
CBC (differential and platelet counts)	Baseline and every 2–4 wk until stable and then every 1–3 mo thereafter[a]
Renal function tests (serum BUN, creatinine, GFR)	Baseline and every 2–3 mo
LFTs (AST, ALT, alkaline phosphatase, albumin, bilirubin)	Baseline and every 4 wk for first 6 mo and then every 1–3 mo thereafter[a]

[a] CBC and LFT monitoring recommendations for the patient with no hematologic or hepatic abnormalities.

Data from Menter A, Korman NJ, Elmets CA, et al. Guidelines of care for the management of psoriasis and psoriatic arthritis: section 4. Guidelines of care for the management and treatment of psoriasis with traditional systemic agents. J Am Acad Dermatol 2009;61:456.

Ongoing Monitoring

Hematologic

CBC should be obtained every 2 to 4 weeks for the first few months to detect changes in leukocyte and platelet counts. Continue CBC monitoring until patient and leukocyte count are stable and then proceed to check CBC every 1 to 3 months until cessation of therapy. Patients at risk for hematologic toxicities may be affected after the first MTX dose, and CBC should be obtained before administering the second dose. It is advisable to reduce or temporarily discontinue MTX therapy should a significant reduction in platelet or leukocyte count occur and administer 10 mg/m^2 folic acid.[43]

Renal

Renal function tests including serum BUN and creatinine should be conducted at 2- to 3-month intervals. Consider calculating glomerular filtration rates (GFR) in patients with decreased renal function, such as the elderly or patients with decreased muscle mass.[43]

Liver

The issue of liver toxicity is a major concern in patients using MTX therapy. Serum AST, ALT, alkaline phosphatase, and serum albumin should be monitored monthly for the first 6 months and then 1 to 3 months thereafter. Repeat LFTs in 2 to 4 weeks if enzymes levels are elevated less than 2 times the upper limit of normal. Elevations greater than 2 times, but less than 3 times, the upper limit of normal should be closely monitored, repeated in 2 to 4 weeks, and doses decreased as necessary. Liver biopsy should be performed in patients with persistent elevations of 5 of 9 AST levels over a 1-year period or if there is a decline in serum albumin from the normal range in a patient with well-controlled disease and normal nutritional status.[43]

Patients with risk factors for hepatotoxicity from MTX (obesity, diabetes mellitus, hyperlipidemia, alcohol abuse, personal history of liver disease, family history of liver disease, elevated liver chemistry studies, or previous/concomitant exposure to other hepatotoxic drugs) require closer follow-up and evaluation. In addition, LFTs should be checked following increases in MTX dosages. If a significant abnormality in liver enzymes occurs, temporarily discontinue MTX therapy for 1 to 2 weeks and repeat LFTs. Consider liver biopsy if LFTs remain elevated for 2 to 3 months and MTX treatment is still desired.[43]

VACCINATIONS

Live and inactive vaccinations are considered to be less efficacious in a patient taking MTX. Inactivated vaccinations (injectable influenza) are not contraindicated during MTX therapy; however, live vaccines (intranasal influenza, varicella, oral typhoid, yellow fever, oral polio virus, smallpox, Bacillus Calmette-Guérin (BCG), and rotavirus) are generally not recommended. Importantly, the zoster vaccine is not contraindicated in patients taking doses of MTX less than 0.4 mg/kg/wk. In addition, measles, mumps, and rubella may be administered 6 weeks before start of MTX therapy, if indicated.

MTX has been reported to reactivate HBV, and serologic testing for viral hepatitis should be completed before starting treatment or considering vaccination. Check HBV surface antigen, HBV surface antibody, and HBV core antibody to rule out disease before starting MTX. Vaccination can be offered in patients lacking immunity to HBV, especially in patients who are at risk for exposure.[44]

SUMMARY AND RECOMMENDATIONS

MTX is a safe and effective drug for the treatment of moderate-to-severe plaque psoriasis. Consider MTX in a patient with severe, recalcitrant forms of psoriasis that have little to no risk factors for the development of dangerous side effects of MTX, and those who have failed alternative antipsoriatic medications such as topical medications and phototherapy. Based on expert experience, dermatologists should consider a starting dose of 7.5 to 15 mg/wk and escalate to a therapeutic target dose of 15 to 25 mg/wk without exceeding a total dose of 25 mg/wk. Folic acid supplementation is strongly recommended and may reduce the occurrence of side effects. Patients will typically see improvement in 6 to 8 weeks, but the authors do not consider MTX to be a failure until 12 weeks of therapy. Furthermore, a patient may have to be on 3 months of MTX before their insurance company will cover biologic therapy. Educate the patient that complete clearance of lesions is not the therapeutic goal. Since the advent of biologics, there are more available options to treat psoriasis that are more effective than MTX and have the potential for less AEs. Nevertheless, MTX may play a novel role in reducing biologic-associated immunogenicity. Additional studies are needed to validate the potential benefits of MTX and biologic coadministration. Dermatologists should carefully consider the risk-benefit ratio before beginning MTX and thoroughly include a history, physical, and laboratory evaluation of the patient, especially renal and liver function.

REFERENCES

1. Lajevardi V, Hallaji Z, Daklan S, et al. The efficacy of methotrexate plus pioglitazone vs. methotrexate alone in the management of patients with plaque-type psoriasis: a single-blinded randomized controlled trial. Int J Dermatol 2015;54:95–101.
2. Bolognia JL, Jorizzo JL, Rapini RP. Bolognia's textbook of dermatology. 3rd edition. New York: Elsevier; 2012.
3. Czarnecka-Operacz M, Sadowska-Przytocka A. The possibilities and principles of methotrexate treatment of psoriasis—the updated knowledge. Postepy Dermatol Alergol 2014;31:392–400.
4. Menting SP, Dekker PM, Limpens J, et al. Methotrexate dosing regimen for plaque-type psoriasis: a systematic review of the use of test-dose, start-dose, dosing scheme, dose adjustments, maximum dose and folic acid supplementation. Acta Derm Venereol 2016;96(1):23–8.

5. Weinstein GD, Jeffes EWB. Methotrexate. In: Koo JY, Levin EC, Leon A, et al, editors. Moderate to severe psoriasis. 4th edition. CRC Press; 2014. p. 161–6.
6. Crowley JJ, Weinberg JM, Wu JJ, et al, National Psoriasis Foundation. Treatment of nail psoriasis: best practice recommendations from the Medical Board of the National Psoriasis Foundation. JAMA Dermatol 2015;151:87–94.
7. Zulian F, Vallongo C, Patrizi A, et al. A long-term follow-up study of methotrexate in juvenile localized scleroderma (morphea). J Am Acad Dermatol 2012;67:1151–6.
8. Ruperto N, Pistorio A, Oliveira S, et al. Prednisone versus prednisone plus ciclosporin versus prednisone plus methotrexate in new-onset juvenile dermatomyositis: a randomised trial. Lancet 2016;387:671–8.
9. Anuset D, Perceau G, Bernard P, et al. Efficacy and safety of methotrexate combined with low- to moderate-dose corticosteroids for severe alopecia areata. Dermatology 2016;232:242–8.
10. Pfizer. Methotrexate Product Monograph Pfizer Canada Inc. 2015.
11. Montaudie H, Sbidian E, Paul C, et al. Methotrexate in psoriasis: a systematic review of treatment modalities, incidence, risk factors and monitoring of liver toxicity. J Eur Acad Dermatol Venereol 2011; 25(Suppl 2):12–8.
12. Kalb RE, Strober B, Weinstein G, et al. Methotrexate and psoriasis: 2009 National Psoriasis Foundation Consensus Conference. J Am Acad Dermatol 2009;60:824–37.
13. Weinstein GD, Goldfaden G, Frost P. Methotrexate. Mechanism of action on DNA synthesis in psoriasis. Arch Dermatol 1971;104:236–43.
14. Tamilselvi E, Haripriya D, Hemamalini M, et al. Association of disease severity with IL-1 levels in methotrexate-treated psoriasis patients. Scand J Immunol 2013;78:545–53.
15. Elango T, Dayalan H, Gnanaraj P, et al. Impact of methotrexate on oxidative stress and apoptosis markers in psoriatic patients. Clin Exp Med 2014; 14:431–7.
16. Ryan C, Korman NJ, Gelfand JM, et al. Research gaps in psoriasis: opportunities for future studies. J Am Acad Dermatol 2014;70:146–67.
17. Saurat JH, Stingl G, Dubertret L, et al. Efficacy and safety results from the randomized controlled comparative study of adalimumab vs. methotrexate vs. placebo in patients with psoriasis (CHAMPION). Br J Dermatol 2008;158:558–66.
18. Barker J, Hoffmann M, Wozel G, et al. Efficacy and safety of infliximab vs. methotrexate in patients with moderate-to-severe plaque psoriasis: results of an open-label, active-controlled, randomized trial (RESTORE1). Br J Dermatol 2011;165:1109–17.
19. Reich K, Langley RG, Papp KA, et al. A 52-week trial comparing briakinumab with methotrexate in patients with psoriasis. N Engl J Med 2011;365:1586–96.
20. Flytstrom I, Stenberg B, Svensson A, et al. Methotrexate vs. ciclosporin in psoriasis: effectiveness, quality of life and safety. A randomized controlled trial. Br J Dermatol 2008;158:116–21.
21. Heydendael VM, Spuls PI, Opmeer BC, et al. Methotrexate versus cyclosporine in moderate-to-severe chronic plaque psoriasis. N Engl J Med 2003;349: 658–65.
22. Akhyani M, Chams-Davatchi C, Hemami MR, et al. Efficacy and safety of mycophenolate mofetil vs. methotrexate for the treatment of chronic plaque psoriasis. J Eur Acad Dermatol Venereol 2010;24: 1447–51.
23. Dogra S, Krishna V, Kanwar AJ. Efficacy and safety of systemic methotrexate in two fixed doses of 10 mg or 25 mg orally once weekly in adult patients with severe plaque-type psoriasis: a prospective, randomized, double-blind, dose-ranging study. Clin Exp Dermatol 2012;37:729–34.
24. Ho SG, Yeung CK, Chan HH. Methotrexate versus traditional Chinese medicine in psoriasis: a randomized, placebo-controlled trial to determine efficacy, safety and quality of life. Clin Exp Dermatol 2010;35: 717–22.
25. Fallah Arani S, Neumann H, Hop WC, et al. Fumarates vs. methotrexate in moderate to severe chronic plaque psoriasis: a multicentre prospective randomized controlled clinical trial. Br J Dermatol 2011;164:855–61.
26. Revicki D, Willian MK, Saurat JH, et al. Impact of adalimumab treatment on health-related quality of life and other patient-reported outcomes: results from a 16-week randomized controlled trial in patients with moderate to severe plaque psoriasis. Br J Dermatol 2008;158:549–57.
27. Saurat JH, Langley RG, Reich K, et al. Relationship between methotrexate dosing and clinical response in patients with moderate to severe psoriasis: subanalysis of the CHAMPION study. Br J Dermatol 2011;165:399–406.
28. Ranjan N, Sharma NL, Shanker V, et al. Methotrexate versus hydroxycarbamide (hydroxyurea) as a weekly dose to treat moderate-to-severe chronic plaque psoriasis: a comparative study. J Dermatolog Treat 2007;18:295–300.
29. Jani M, Barton A, Warren RB, et al. The role of DMARDs in reducing the immunogenicity of TNF inhibitors in chronic inflammatory diseases. Rheumatology (Oxford) 2014;53:213–22.
30. Lecluse LL, Driessen RJ, Spuls PI, et al. Extent and clinical consequences of antibody formation against adalimumab in patients with plaque psoriasis. Arch Dermatol 2010;146:127–32.

31. Farhangian ME, Feldman SR. Immunogenicity of biologic treatments for psoriasis: therapeutic consequences and the potential value of concomitant methotrexate. Am J Clin Dermatol 2015;16:285–94.
32. Menting SP, van Lumig PP, de Vries AC, et al. Extent and consequences of antibody formation against adalimumab in patients with psoriasis: one-year follow-up. JAMA Dermatol 2014;150:130–6.
33. Chiu HY, Wang TS, Chan CC, et al. Risk factor analysis for the immunogenicity of adalimumab associated with decreased clinical response in Chinese patients with psoriasis. Acta Derm Venereol 2015; 95:711–6.
34. Mease PJ. Spondyloarthritis: Is methotrexate effective in psoriatic arthritis? Nat Rev Rheumatol 2012;8: 251–2.
35. Kingsley GH, Kowalczyk A, Taylor H, et al. A randomized placebo-controlled trial of methotrexate in psoriatic arthritis. Rheumatology (Oxford) 2012;51:1368–77.
36. Coates LC, Helliwell PS. Methotrexate efficacy in the tight control in psoriatic arthritis study. J Rheumatol 2016;43(2):356–61.
37. Mease P. Methotrexate in psoriatic arthritis. Bull Hosp Jt Dis 2013;71(Suppl 1):S41–5.
38. Barker J, Horn EJ, Lebwohl M, et al. Assessment and management of methotrexate hepatotoxicity in psoriasis patients: report from a consensus conference to evaluate current practice and identify key questions toward optimizing methotrexate use in the clinic. J Eur Acad Dermatol Venereol 2011; 25:758–64.
39. Nast A, Boehncke W-H, Mrowietz U, et al. S3—Guidelines on the treatment of psoriasis vulgaris (English version). Update. J Dtsch Dermatol Ges 2012;10:S1–s95.
40. Gutierrez-Urena S, Molina JF, Garcia CO, et al. Pancytopenia secondary to methotrexate therapy in rheumatoid arthritis. Arthritis Rheum 1996;39:272–6.
41. Bath RK, Brar NK, Forouhar FA, et al. A review of methotrexate-associated hepatotoxicity. J Dig Dis 2014;15:517–24.
42. Conway R, Low C, Coughlan RJ, et al. Methotrexate use and risk of lung disease in psoriasis, psoriatic arthritis, and inflammatory bowel disease: systematic literature review and meta-analysis of randomised controlled trials. BMJ 2015;350:h1269.
43. Menter A, Korman NJ, Elmets CA, et al. Guidelines of care for the management of psoriasis and psoriatic arthritis: section 4. Guidelines of care for the management and treatment of psoriasis with traditional systemic agents. J Am Acad Dermatol 2009; 61:451–85.
44. Wine-Lee L, Keller SC, Wilck MB, et al. From the Medical Board of the National Psoriasis Foundation: vaccination in adult patients on systemic therapy for psoriasis. J Am Acad Dermatol 2013;69: 1003–13.

CHAPTER 5

Acitretin

Elaine J. Lin, MD, Vidhi V. Shah, BA, Shivani P. Reddy, BS, Jashin J. Wu, MD

KEYWORDS

• Acitretin • Etretinate • Phototherapy • PUVA • Broadband UV-B • Narrowband UV-B • Teratogenic • Hyperlipidemia

KEY POINTS

- Acitretin is an effective agent for the treatment of plaque psoriasis and is often used in combination therapy (phototherapy and other systemic antipsoriatic agents).
- Acitretin is initially dosed at 10 to 25 mg/d with gradual escalation of 10 to 25 mg every 2 to 4 weeks done according disease response and patient tolerance.
- Acitretin is pregnancy category X; adequate counseling, abstinence from alcohol, birth control, and evaluation for pregnancy are required before, during, and after acitretin therapy.
- Acitretin has the added benefit of being safely used in the long term without the risk of immunosuppression.

INTRODUCTION

Acitretin has been the only oral retinoid approved by the US Food and Drug Administration (FDA) to treat psoriasis since 1997.[1] Monotherapy acitretin is a therapeutic option for the treatment of plaque psoriasis with doses up to 50 mg daily, although it is often used at lower doses in combination with systemic therapies, such as UV-B or oral psoralen plus UV-A (PUVA) phototherapy, to increase efficacy. When used in combination with phototherapy, acitretin may be often dosed at 10 to 25 mg every other day. It is also an effective monotherapy for erythrodermic and pustular forms of psoriasis as well as human immunodeficiency virus (HIV)-associated psoriasis. Acitretin is not indicated in the treatment of psoriatic arthritis.

Acitretin is the pharmacologically active metabolite of etretinate, a second-generation retinoid that was approved for psoriasis in 1986 (Fig. 5.1). Etretinate is more lipophilic and has a longer half-life than acitretin and can be detected in serum for up to 2 years after treatment discontinuation (Table 5.1).[2] Because of its more favorable pharmacokinetics, acitretin replaced etretinate in 1997. Concomitant alcohol intake indirectly increases the reverse esterification of acitretin to etretinate; a trend was found linking higher risk of etretinate formation with higher-dosage ethanol intake.[3]

Acitretin is available in 10-mg, 17.5-mg, and 25-mg gelatin capsules for oral administration.[2] For optimal absorption and bioavailability, acitretin should be taken with fatty food.[4] After oral administration, maximum plasma concentrations are reached between 0.9 and 4.6 hours; after drug cessation, elimination half-life varies from 16.5 to 111.1 hours.[5] Acitretin is extensively distributed throughout the body with approximately 95% bound to plasma proteins without tissue accumulation. After multiple doses, steady-state concentrations of acitretin are achieved within approximately 3 weeks.[2]

MECHANISM OF ACTION

Acitretin is a second-generation monoaromatic retinoid whose mechanism of action is not fully elucidated. Acitretin activates all 3 retinoic acid receptors (α, β, γ), which are nuclear receptors that are part of the steroid-thyroid hormone receptor superfamily.[6] Activation of these receptors leads to downstream gene expression, which ultimately leads to normalization of epidermal cell proliferation, differentiation, and cornification.[7] Unlike other systemic antipsoriatic medications, the effects of acitretin are not mediated through immunosuppression.

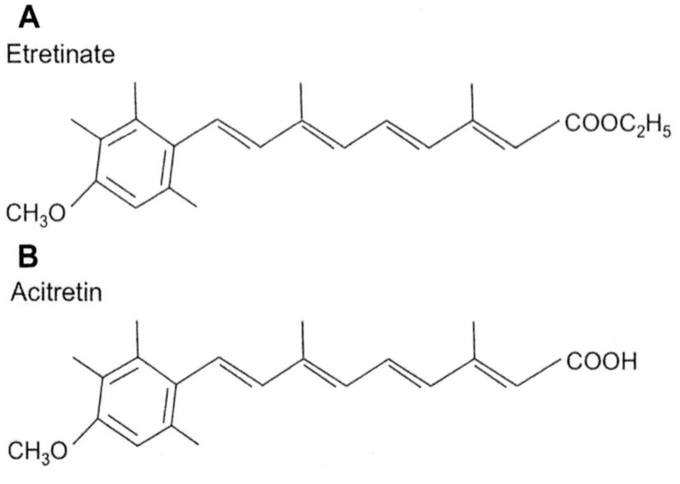

A
Etretinate

CH_3O ... $COOC_2H_5$

B
Acitretin

CH_3O ... $COOH$

Fig. 5.1 Chemical structure of etretinate (*A*) and acitretin (*B*).

EFFICACY

Monotherapy

Plaque psoriasis

Many trials have demonstrated the efficacy for acitretin monotherapy in the treatment of moderate-to-severe plaque psoriasis.[8] In an open-label multicenter study, 63 patients with severe psoriasis received acitretin at a starting dose of 50 mg daily for 4 weeks with individual dose adjustments of 10-mg increments or decrements at monthly intervals (10–70 mg) as needed thereafter.[9] The percentage of patients achieving a 75% or greater improvement in their Psoriasis Area and Severity Index score (PASI-75) after 12 weeks was 34%, and the average reduction in PASI score was 76% in comparison to baseline by the end of the 1-year follow-up period. However, only 37 patients completed 12 months of treatment, whereas the rest withdrew prematurely because of adverse effects, therapeutic failure, or concurrent illness, or were lost for administrative reasons. In a double-blinded clinical trial, 16 patients were given initial doses of 25 to 50 mg/d for 8 weeks, followed by an open-label phase with individualized dose adjustments for 12 weeks. At the end of the 20-week follow-up, reductions from baseline were seen in scaling (42%), erythema (50%), and thickness of plaques (53%), with a 44% reduction in body surface area involved.[10]

TABLE 5.1
Comparison of properties of etretinate versus acitretin

Etretinate	Acitretin
Approved for psoriasis in 1986, withdrawn in 1998	Approved for psoriasis in 1997
50 times more lipophilic than acitretin	Less lipophilic
Half-life of 120 d	Half-life of 50 h
>98% eliminated 2 or more years after treatment	>98% eliminated 2 mo after treatment
Metabolized into acitretin	Small amounts may be converted into etretinate (process enhanced by ethanol)
Teratogenic	Teratogenic

Four randomized controlled trials (RCTs) evaluated the efficacy of acitretin monotherapy in comparison with etretinate monotherapy.[11–14] In one of these studies, patients treated with acitretin (n = 127) or etretinate (n = 41) were begun on an initial dose of 40 mg/d for 4 weeks with individual adjusted doses for the subsequent 8 weeks.[12] Average daily doses for acitretin and etretinate were 0.54 mg/kg/d and 0.65 mg/kg/d, respectively. After 12 weeks, 52% of acitretin and 45% of etretinate-treated subjects achieved PASI-75. A systematic literature review of these 4 RCTs of acitretin and etretinate monotherapies found similar efficacies in the treatment of psoriasis.[8,12–14]

Efficacy of acitretin in plaque psoriasis and frequency of adverse effects are dose dependent.[15] Because both therapeutic and toxic responses to acitretin vary widely among patients, a single correct dose cannot be recommended. The optimal dose range for monotherapy acitretin is usually in the range of 25 mg every other day to 50 mg daily. To avoid intolerance, acitretin may be initially dosed at 10 to 25 mg/d with gradual escalation of 10 to 25 mg every 2 to 4 weeks (maximum 75 mg/d) done according to the response of the disease and patient tolerance.[16] Another approach that can be used to achieve efficacy more quickly (for example, in patients with pustular psoriasis) is to start with 50 mg daily and reduce the dose once side effects begin to occur. At doses of 50 mg daily, however, the mucocutaneous side effects are often poorly tolerated.

Improvement while on acitretin is gradual and may take 3 to 6 months to achieve maximum disease control. Although higher doses (50–70 mg/d) may result in more rapid and complete responses, they are associated with increased adverse effects. Initial worsening of symptoms, such as burning, erythema, and plaque expansion, may occur but can improve if acitretin is continued.[17] Once the disease is adequately controlled, acitretin can be tapered to the lowest effective dose for long-term maintenance therapy.

Pustular psoriasis

Monotherapy acitretin is a first-line option in pustular psoriasis, especially palmoplantar psoriasis (PPP).[18] In a retrospective multicenter study of 385 patients with generalized pustular psoriasis (GPP), etretinate, methotrexate (MTX), cyclosporine, and PUVA were effective in 84%, 76%, 71%, and 46% of patients, respectively.[19] Acitretin can be given with an initial dose of 25 mg/d, although those with GPP may require more aggressive therapy and can be started on a higher dose (50–75 mg/d).[20] Dosing can be tapered down to the lowest effective dose as the disease is controlled. In the case of refractory PPP, combination therapy with PUVA should be considered.[21]

Erythrodermic psoriasis

Acitretin monotherapy is an efficacious treatment for erythrodermic psoriasis (EP) and should be considered when the patient has a relative or absolute contraindication to first-line agents with more rapid onset (cyclosporine or infliximab).[22] Patients can be started at an initial dose of acitretin 25 mg/d with dose escalation of 10 to 25 mg every 2 to 4 weeks.[20] EP refractory to acitretin monotherapy may require the addition of phototherapy. In the case of exfoliative EP, sequential therapy with cyclosporine may be used (Table 5.2).[23]

Combination Therapy

Acitretin is often used in combination with other therapies to increase the efficacy of treatment of plaque psoriasis. Topical therapies, conventional systemic agents, phototherapy, and biologics have been used concomitantly with acitretin to enhance efficacy and reduce the total dose requirements and adverse effects of other antipsoriatic drugs (Table 5.3).[24]

Acitretin and psoralen plus ultraviolet A

Acitretin is used in combination with PUVA (re-PUVA) to increase efficacy as well as reduce the cumulative UV-A dose, retinoid dose, and duration of therapy needed to treat plaque psoriasis.[31,32] Two randomized double-blinded studies demonstrated higher remission rates with fewer PUVA exposures and lower cumulative UV-A dose in psoriasis patients treated with re-PUVA in comparison to placebo-PUVA (Table 5.4).[31,32]

Acitretin may reduce the risk of cutaneous carcinogenicity and photoaging associated with phototherapy when used in combination with PUVA[33]. A nested cohort study analyzed 135 patients with psoriasis who were exposed to PUVA and used retinoids for at least 26 weeks in 1 year or more.[34] Each patient's tumor incidence of squamous cell carcinoma (SCC) and basal cell carcinoma (BCC) with or without retinoid use was compared. After adjusting for confounding factors, retinoid use was associated with a 30% reduction in SCC incidence (P = .002). Notably, the SCC incidence rapidly approached that of

TABLE 5.2
Sample sequential therapy with cyclosporine and acitretin*

Induction	Transitional A	Transitional B	Maintenance
Cyclosporine 5 mg/kg/d divided twice daily	Acitretin 25 mg/d (dose escalation of 10–25 mg every 2–4 wk based on patient response and side effects)	Taper cyclosporine	Acitretin continued for long term
Month 0–1	Month 2–3	Month 4–7	Month 8+

* Close monitoring of lipid profiles should be done because both drugs can cause reversible elevation of triglycerides and cholesterol.

TABLE 5.3
Studies and a review of combination therapies and recommendations

	Dose Combination	Study Design	Dose Regimen	Results	Comments & Recommendations
Topical agents	Acitretin + calcipotriol	Randomized, bilateral paired comparison[24]	40 received combination and 20 received acitretin alone for 52 wk	60% of combination arm and 40% of acitretin monotherapy arm achieved complete clearance	Ashcroft et al concluded that there is insufficient evidence to support large effects in favor of acitretin + calcipotriol in the treatment of chronic plaque psoriasis[25]
Conventional systemic agents	Acitretin + MTX	Retrospective data review[26]	18 received acitretin 25 mg (daily or alternating days) + MTX 7.5–25 mg/wk for an average 9 mo	Combination well tolerated and often effective with no new or unusual adverse effects noted, including significant hepatotoxicity	The FDA-approved acitretin prescribing information contraindicates MTX in combination with acitretin due to potential hepatotoxicity[2]
	Acitretin + cyclosporine	Review[23]	The author suggests a sequential therapy strategy for psoriasis: 1. Cyclosporine 5 mg/kg/d for month 0–1 2. Introduce and maximize acitretin dose at month 2–3 3. Taper off cyclosporine at month 4–7 4. Maintenance with acitretin after month 7	—	Skillful management of transition phases (acitretin dose escalation, cyclosporine taper) is required. If acitretin alone is inadequate, additional phototherapy or topical agents may be considered on a case-by-case basis

Biologic agents	Acitretin + etanercept	Randomized, controlled, investigator-blinded study[27]	60 patients with plaque psoriasis were studied. 22 received etanercept (25 mg twice weekly sc), 20 received acitretin (0.4 mg/kg daily), and 18 received combination etanercept (25 mg once weekly sc) plus acitretin (0.4 mg/kg daily) for 24 wk	45% of etanercept group, 30% of acitretin group, and 44% of combination group achieved PASI-75 at week 24 (P = .001 for both etanercept groups compared with acitretin alone)	Uncontrolled studies and case reports have demonstrated efficacy of treatment of plaque psoriasis with biologic plus retinoids.[28] Acitretin reduces dose requirements and increases efficacy of biologics, but cost and lack of long-term safety data are limitations
	Acitretin + infliximab	Case series[29]	4 EP patients received infliximab (5 mg/kg iv) at 0, 2, and 6 wk + acitretin (0.3–0.6 mg/kg daily)	Extremely good response of EP at 6 wk with no adverse events	This study investigates short-term infliximab therapy in EP patients. Full potential of infliximab + acitretin combination is yet to be elucidated
	Acitretin + adalimumab	Retrospective case series[30]	4 severe or recalcitrant psoriasis patients received adalimumab (40 mg weekly, or every 10 d, or every 2 wk) + acitretin (10–30 mg daily) for a mean duration of 12.9 ± 12.4 mo	3 achieved good efficacy, 1 achieved poor efficacy, 2 experienced mild side effects	—

Data from Refs.[23,24,26,27,29,30]

TABLE 5.4
Treatment outcomes of acitretin and psoralen plus UV-A combination therapy

Study	% of Patients Cleared at End Point (%)	Mean Treatment Duration (d)	Mean Number of Treatments	Cumulative UV Dose (J/cm^2)
Saurat et al,[31] 1988				
Re-PUVA	94	47.8	13.7	57.8[a]
Placebo + PUVA	80	65.4	19.9	97.2
Tanew et al,[32] 1991				
Re-PUVA	96	40.2	15.3	58.7[a]
Placebo + PUVA	80	51.0	21.4	101.5

[a] *P*<.01 versus placebo.

Data from Saurat JH, Geiger JM, Amblard P, et al. Randomized double-blind multicenter study comparing acitretin-PUVA, etretinate-PUVA and placebo-PUVA in the treatment of severe psoriasis. Dermatology 1988;177(4):218–24; and Tanew A, Guggenbichler A, Honigsmann H, et al. Photochemotherapy for severe psoriasis without or in combination with acitretin: a randomized, double-blind comparison study. J Am Acad Dermatol 1991;25(4):682–4.

preretinoid use upon discontinuation of retinoids. Systemic retinoid use in this study was not significantly associated with increased BCC incidence.

Bath or soak PUVA is a safe and effective alternative for patients who cannot tolerate the gastrointestinal and phototoxic side effects of oral PUVA.[35] Bath PUVA reduces the cumulative UV-A dose needed for disease control and the variation in psoralen plasma levels associated with gastrointestinal absorption of oral PUVA. Muchenberger and colleagues[36] treated 4 patients with erythrodermic, pustular, or plaque psoriasis with bath re-PUVA (0.5 mg/kg/d of acitretin plus bath PUVA 3–5 times/wk) and found a greater than 90% improvement after 4 weeks. Compared with 25 to 50 mg/d of acitretin required when given as monotherapy, usually 10 to 25 mg/d of acitretin is sufficient when given in combination with PUVA.[37] Patients may be begun on a daily dose of 10 to 25 mg acitretin for 1 to 2 weeks, followed by addition of PUVA treatment, which is continued until disease remission. Because retinoids thin the stratum corneum and cause an increased risk of UV radiation–induced erythema, advancement in UV-A dosimetry should be more gradual.[38] If acitretin is to be added to a patient's pre-existing PUVA regimen, UV-A dosimetry should be initially reduced by 50% to avoid burning and advanced back to baseline if no phototoxicity occurs.[39] Following the clearance of psoriasis, low-dose acitretin or PUVA alone can be considered as maintenance therapy.

Acitretin and broadband ultraviolet B phototherapy

Acitretin can be used concomitantly with broadband ultraviolet B (BBUVB) to effectively treat severe forms of plaque psoriasis. This regimen allows for increased efficacy in the treatment of plaque psoriasis with lower duration of therapy and cumulative UV dose in comparison with BBUVB alone (Table 5.5).[40–42] In the study by Ruzicka and colleagues,[40] the median cumulative BBUVB energy applied to reach PASI-75 was 41.5% lower with combination therapy in comparison to BBUVB alone. Iest and Boer[41] found that the number of BBUVB treatments to reach clearance was reduced by approximately 20% in the re-BBUVB group relative to the BBUVB group. The advantage of re-BBUVB over re-PUVA is the use of phototherapy without the need of oral psoralen and the lower risk of cutaneous carcinogenicity of BBUVB in comparison to UV-A.[21]

Physicians can start patients on 10 to 25 mg/d of acitretin for 1 week before initiating BBUVB phototherapy.[43] If acitretin is to be added to a patient's pre-existing UV-B regimen, UV-B dosimetry should be initially reduced by 50% to avoid burning and then gradually increased if no phototoxicity occurs. Following the initial clearing of psoriasis, remission can be prolonged with an additional 3 weeks of UV-B treatment.[44]

Acitretin and narrowband ultraviolet B phototherapy

Narrowband UV-B phototherapy (NBUVB) is highly effective for the treatment of plaque psoriasis and can be combined with acitretin to reduce the number of treatments for clearing. A retrospective data analysis of 40 patients on acitretin 25 mg/d plus NBUVB 3 times per week revealed that 72.5% of the patients achieved PASI-75.[45] A randomized comparison of acitretin plus NBUVB with re-PUVA revealed that both regimens

TABLE 5.5
Studies of combination acitretin with broadband ultraviolet B phototherapy

Study	Combination Treatment Regimen	Number of Patients	Mean Measure of Treatment Length	Cumulative Dose (J/cm²)	Efficacy End Points
Iest and Boer,[41] 1989	Acitretin (0.34–0.44 mg/kg) + BBUVB	9	19.3 (no. of treatments)	8.4 ± 3.7	89% obtained clearance[a]
	BBUVB	32	24.9 (no. of treatments)	11.1 ± 5.2	62.5% obtained clearance[a]
Ruzika et al,[40] 1990	Acitretin (35 mg/d × 4 wk, 25 mg/d thereafter) + BBUVB	40	48.0 (d)	8.8 ± 6.8	76% decrease in PASI 60% obtained ≥ PASI-75
	BBUVB	38	43.4 (d)	6.4 ± 5.2	35% decrease in PASI 24% obtained ≥ PASI-75

[a] Defined as 80% to 100% improvement.
Data from Ruzicka T, Sommerburg C, Braun-Falco O, et al. Efficiency of acitretin in combination with UV-B in the treatment of severe psoriasis. Arch Dermatol 1990;126(4):482–6; and Iest J, Boer J. Combined treatment of psoriasis with acitretin and UVB phototherapy compared with acitretin alone and UVB alone. Br J Dermatol 1989;120(5):665–70.

provided similar efficacy in the treatment of moderate-to-severe psoriasis.[46] Acitretin plus NBUVB dosimetry regimens can be performed similarly to that of the previously described combination phototherapy regimens.

Chemoprevention

Systemic retinoids have been widely studied for and have shown promising results on the prevention of certain cancers. The anticancer protective effects of retinoids are derived from their antiangiogenic properties and ability to induce cell proliferation, modulate growth, and induce apoptosis.[47] Retinoids reduce the risk of new primary cutaneous SCC in moderate-risk patients and immunosuppressed organ transplant patients.[48–50] Acitretin is now commonly used in practice to reduce the risk of immunosuppression-related skin cancer in transplant patients as well as to prevent and treat leukoplakia, actinic keratosis, cutaneous T-cell lymphoma, acute promyelocytic leukemia, head and neck carcinoma, nonmelanoma skin cancer, hepatocellular carcinoma, breast cancer, and neuroblastoma.[51] A nested cohort study found that oral retinoid use was associated with a 30% reduction in SCC incidence ($P = .002$) in psoriatic patients treated with PUVA.[34] Because psoriasis patients are at higher risk for malignancy, the chemopreventive properties of acitretin are added benefits to psoriatic treatment regimens.

SAFETY

Acitretin shares similar adverse effects with other systemic retinoids. Adverse effects are preventable or manageable through proper patient selection, dose adjustments, and routine monitoring. The teratogenicity of acitretin is a serious side effect that limits its use in women of reproductive potential. Most commonly reported side effects include cheilitis, xerosis, and alopecia (Table 5.6). With the exception of teratogenicity and hyperostosis, all side effects of acitretin reported in literature are dose dependent and reversible.[52] A retrospective analysis found that common adverse effects were 2 to 3 times more frequent in patients receiving 50 mg/d acitretin than 25 mg/d acitretin.[53]

Teratogenicity

Like all systemic retinoids, acitretin is labeled pregnancy category X. Major fetal abnormalities include central nervous system malformations (meningomyelocele, meningoencephalocele), craniofacial malformations (facial dysmorphia, low-set ears, high palate, anophthalmia), musculoskeletal abnormalities (multiple synostoses, syndactyly, absence of phalanges, hip malformations), and cardiovascular malformations.[2] Acitretin is contraindicated in women who are or intend on becoming pregnant during treatment or 3 years following discontinuation of treatment. Patients should not donate blood during treatment or 3 years after treatment cessation in order

TABLE 5.6
Most frequently reported adverse events during acitretin clinical trials in psoriasis patients (N = 525)

Body System	Mucous Membranes	Skin & Appendages	Musculoskeletal	Central Nervous System	Eye
>75%	Cheilitis				
50–75%		Alopecia Skin peeling			
25–50%	Rhinitis	Dry skin Nail disorder Pruritus			
10–25%	Dry mouth Epistaxis	Erythematous rash Hyperesthesia paresthesia Paronychia Skin atrophy Sticky skin (possibly due to increased mucus production)	Arthralgia Spinal hyperostosis (progression of existing lesions)	Rigors	Xerophthalmia

Acitretin dosing regimen ranged from 10 to 75 mg/d; majority received 25 to 50 mg/d. Greatest incidence of adverse events occurred in patients receiving 75 mg/d.

Data from Soriatane [package insert]. Research Triangle Park, NC; Stiefel Laboratories, Inc.; 2014. Available at: https://http://www.gsksource.com/pharma/content/dam/GlaxoSmithKline/US/en/Prescribing_Information/Soriatane/pdf/SORIATANE-PI-MG.PDF. Accessed February 21, 2016.

to reduce the risk of teratogenicity in women receiving blood donations. Available animal data cannot determine a threshold dose in human therapy below which there is no risk of teratogenicity.[54]

Ethanol is able to induce the conversion of acitretin to etretinate, which would extend the teratogenic potential for female patients because of the significantly longer elimination half-life of etretinate. Therefore, alcohol is prohibited in female patients of child-bearing potential during treatment and for 2 months after discontinuation of treatment.

Minimal studies have been done on seminal transmission of acitretin and potential risk posed on the fetus. There is currently no mandate from the FDA that prevents the exposure of women of childbearing potential to the semen of men taking acitretin. To date, available data and after-marketing surveillance have not shown any association between paternal treatment with acitretin and retinoid embryopathy.[55,56]

Mucocutaneous

Mucocutaneous adverse effects are due to decreased sebum production and impaired skin barrier function (see Table 5.6). They are also the most commonly encountered adverse effects and are dose dependent and reversible in nature. Retinoid dermatitis resembles unstable psoriasis and can develop in 25% of patients after receiving high-dose acitretin; this is a transient reaction that does not require treatment cessation.[12] Symptomatic treatment with emollients and low-strength topical corticosteroid can help relieve mucocutaneous side effects. If symptomatic measures do not help alleviate these side effects, acitretin can be tapered to a lower dose.

Nonscarring alopecia occurs more frequently in high-dose acitretin regimens (~50%–75% of patients) than low-dose regimens (~13%) and usually resolves within 6 to 8 weeks of treatment cessation.[2] Nail disorders, including onychorrhexis, onychoschizia, and periungual pyogenic granuloma, are also more common with high-dose therapy (~25%–50%) compared with low-dose therapy (0%).[20] Tapering the dose or discontinuing acitretin should be considered.

Musculoskeletal

Musculoskeletal adverse effects are uncommon but are the only significant and irreversible adverse effects that are associated with long-term systemic retinoid use. Long-term etretinate therapy has been associated with diffuse idiopathic skeletal hyperostosis syndrome (DISH), premature fusion of epiphyses, ligament calcification, osteoporosis, and periosteal thickening.[57] Retinoids are more likely to cause worsening of pre-existing skeletal overgrowth rather than de novo changes, which were seen in less than 1% of the cases studied in 3 prospective studies.[58–60]

There are conflicting reports in literature concerning the association between skeletal adverse effects and acitretin therapy. A prospective study of 51 psoriatic patients treated with acitretin (average dose 0.5 mg/kg/d) for 2 years reported 2 subjects with unusual skeletal calcifications in the forearms and hip.[61] However, a retrospective review of 49 patients on low-dose acitretin for 1 year or more revealed no radiograph-confirmed cases of DISH syndrome.[62] A prospective study measured the bone mineral density of 30 patients who took acitretin for a median of 3.6 years and found no association between daily dose of acitretin, total dose administered, and overall duration of treatment, and risk of osteopenia or osteoporosis.[63] Premature epiphyseal closure is a concern in children treated with isotretinoin, rarely with the use of etretinate, and never reported with the use of acitretin.[64]

Sustained treatment with acitretin is associated with myalgias and arthalgias, which can occur with or without the elevation of creatinine phosphokinase. Symptoms are usually mild and can be treated with oral analgesics. In severe cases, acitretin dose can be decreased by 25% until symptoms resolve.[33]

Neurologic

Pseudotumor cerebri has been associated with systemic retinoid therapy, but the association with acitretin has been unclear. Literature reveals multiple reports of pseudotumor cerebri associated with oral retinoid used concomitantly with tetracycline-class antibiotics as well as with isotretinoin monotherapy. Clinical trials (n = 525) studying the efficacy and safety of acitretin in psoriatic patients reported a rate of pseudotumor cerebri to be less than 1%.[2] One case reported new onset pseudotumor cerebri in a pediatric patient 1.5 months after the initiation of acitretin, dosed at 25 to 35 mg/d.[65] A review of 331 case reports of ocular side effects associated with retinoids (tretinoin, etretinate, acitretin) found 21 cases of intracranial hypertension, 3 of which were associated with acitretin. Based on the World Health Organization criteria, the investigators inferred a "probable" casual relationship of intracranial hypertension due to these 3 retinoids. This relationship must be inferred with caution, especially because 6 of these patients were using tetracycline or minocycline antibiotics, which are possible instigators of intracranial hypertension.[66] A review demonstrated the paucity of evidence-based data to support the casual relationship between pseudotumor cerebri secondary to acitretin.[67] The investigators concluded that further investigation is required to assess the scientific validity of this association or if its inclusion in the package insert was due to class labeling.

Patients should still be counseled for the signs and symptoms of pseudotumor cerebri (headache, diplopia, nausea, vomiting). If pseudotumor cerebri is suspected, ophthalmoscope examination can evaluate for papilledema, and the retinoid should be discontinued. Systemic retinoids should not be taken concomitantly with tetracycline class antibiotics.

Metabolic and Hepatic

During clinical trials of acitretin (dosing range 10–75 mg/d), 66% of patients experienced hypertriglyceridemia and 33% experienced hypercholesterolemia, with a lower proportion occurring in the low-dose cohort.[2,53] Initial management of hyperlipidemia consists of reduction in dietary fat intake and exercise. If lifestyle changes provide inadequate control, addition of medications can be considered (Table 5.7).[33] In the event of persistent hyperlipidemia in a patient already on a stable statin, prescription omega-3–acid ethyl esters can be added to improve lipid profile.[68]

TABLE 5.7
Management of hyperlipidemia during retinoid therapy

Hyperlipidemia	Management
Hypercholesterolemia	• Decrease dietary fat, increase exercise • Lipid-lowering agent (ie, atorvastatin 10 mg/d with individualized dose increases)
Hypertriglyceridemia	• Once medication regimen of hypertriglyceridemia optimized (gemfibrozil 600 mg twice daily) • Decrease retinoid dose by 50% if triglycerides >499 mg/dL • Discontinue retinoid if triglycerides >800 mg/dL • Reinitiate retinoid once medication regimen of hypertriglyceridemia optimized

Comment: combination therapy of a statin and fibrates (gemfibrozil) is avoided due to the increased risk of rhabdomyolysis.

Caution should be taken with patients with pre-existing liver disease before acitretin therapy. Elevations in serum transaminases occur in ~25% to 30% of patients and typically occur after 2 to 8 weeks of therapy.[33] However, these increases are often transient, reversible, and more common with high-dose regimens. A 2-year prospective study demonstrated that therapy with typical doses of acitretin (25–75 mg/d) did not induce biopsy-proven hepatotoxicity.[69] Patients should be counseled on minimizing alcohol and acetaminophen use. Retinoid dose can be decreased by 50% if liver function tests (LFTs) are 2 to 3 times normal values and discontinued if LFTs exceed 3 times normal values. Retinoid can be reinitiated at 25% of original dose once LFTs normalize.

Immunosuppression

Acitretin does not increase the risk of developing infections and internal malignancies, thus making it an ideal treatment option for psoriasis patients with HIV, cancer, or other reasons of immunosuppression. It is also safe for long-term use without time or cumulative dose limitations. An HIV patient suffering from severe psoriasis unresponsive to topical steroids and UV-B was safely and successfully treated with 21 weeks of a tapering dose of acitretin (30–10 mg/d).[70]

Ophthalmologic

Xerophthalmia and eye irritation are relatively common side effects that may require artificial tears, especially in contact lens users. Less common ophthalmologic effects are loss of night vision and color vision.

Psychiatric

Although there is a depression warning in the acitretin package insert, there is an absence of scientific evidence of acitretin-associated depression.[67] Depression may be more of a theoretic concern and class labeling. On the other hand, there have been anecdotal reports of depression, and there is no extensive scientific evidence showing that acitretin does not cause depression.[71,72]

BOX 5.1
Contraindications to acitretin therapy

Absolute contraindications:

- Pregnancy
- Women of childbearing potential who cannot guarantee adequate contraception during treatment and 3 years after treatment cessation
- Severe liver/kidney failure
- Allergy to drug components

Relative contraindications:

- Breast-feeding women
- Mild hepatic/renal impairment (adjust dose)
- Alcohol consumption
- Poorly controlled dyslipidemia
- Concomitant use of hepatotoxic drugs or drugs that interact with acitretin
- Metabolic syndrome
- Pediatric or elderly

PRECAUTIONS

Pregnancy Category X

Because of teratogenic risks, acitretin should not be used in women of childbearing potential; in rare circumstances, it could be considered in cases of recalcitrant psoriasis and presence of contraindications to other treatments (Box 5.1). These patients require 2 negative pregnancy tests before initiation of acitretin and must commit to 2 forms of contraception for at least 1 month before initiation of and during therapy and 3 years after therapy discontinuation. Because acitretin interferes with the contraceptive effect of progestin-only preparations, the "minipill" is not recommended as one of the forms of contraception. Taking St. John's wort is contraindicated in this population because reports have suggested decreased efficacy of hormonal contraceptives while taking this supplement. Breastfeeding is relatively contraindicated because trace amounts of acitretin are excreted in human milk (30–40 ng/mL).[73] Before beginning therapy, these patients should be counseled on the risks and birth defects associated with acitretin exposure.

Metabolic and Hepatic

The risk of hyperlipidemia and pancreatitis during acitretin therapy is increased in patients with a family history of hypertriglyceridemia, alcohol consumption, obesity, and diabetes; therefore, these patients may require more frequent LFT. Because hepatotoxicity is exacerbated by alcohol, diabetes, and obesity, these patients require more frequent liver function monitoring. Acitretin can alter glucose control in diabetic patients, and thus, blood sugars should be checked more frequently, especially during the initial weeks of therapy.

Drug Interactions

Acitretin has significant drug interactions that should be noted (Table 5.8). To avoid

TABLE 5.8
Notable drug interactions of acitretin

Drug	Interaction
Ethanol	Enhanced conversion of acitretin to etretinate (relevant only to women of child-bearing potential)
MTX	Increased MTX level, hepatotoxicity
Vitamin A (>4000–5000 IU/d)	Hypervitaminosis A
Microdosed progestin "minipill"	Acitretin decreases antiovulatory effect of "minipill"
Phenytoin	Acitretin reduces its protein binding, although clinical significance of this is yet unknown
Tetracylines	Increases risk of intracranial hypertension and photosensitivity
Oral corticosteroids	Hyperlipidemia, increased risk of intracranial hypertension[59]

hypervitaminosis A due to the additive effects of retinoids and vitamin A, intake of other oral retinoids and vitamin A supplements greater than the daily minimum allowance is not recommended.[2]

MONITORING

Before initiation of treatment, the physician must obtain baseline laboratory tests, perform a skin assessment, and complete a medical history with investigation of comorbidities, concomitant medications, presence of arthritis/arthralgia, and contraindications/risks (Box 5.2). Women of reproductive potential should not be treated with acitretin, but in the rare case in which no other treatment is appropriate, they are required to have 2 negative pregnancy tests before treatment initiation and monthly pregnancy testing during treatment. Follow-up laboratory tests should be obtained every month while dose adjustments are made and can be done every 3 to 6 months after dosing has stabilized and if previous laboratory work was unremarkable for hepatotoxicity or hyperlipidemia. The timing of LFT and lipid level reassessment can vary depending on patient risks and concomitant medication that can induce hepatotoxicity or dyslipidemias. One practice guideline recommends the first LFTs and lipid profile reassessment during treatment to occur between 4 to 8 weeks and then every 6 months thereafter.[74] This recommendation is based on standard clinical practice, where alterations in liver function and lipid profiles are uncommon. Unless there is evidence of bone toxicity, regular radiographic monitoring is not recommended.

BOX 5.2
Evaluation and workup for treatment with acitretin

Baseline laboratory tests before acitretin therapy

- Liver function tests
- Fasting serum triglycerides and cholesterol

Evaluation during acitretin therapy

- Mucocutaneous side effects
- Liver function tests
- Fasting serum triglycerides and cholesterol

VACCINATIONS

Acitretin is not a direct immunosuppressant and therefore does not interfere with the body's response to vaccinations, whether with toxoids, live, or attenuated vaccines. Patients may follow regular vaccination schedules while taking acitretin.

SUMMARY

Acitretin is a second-generation synthetic retinoid that is effective in treating plaque psoriasis as a monotherapy or in combination with other therapies. Monotherapy acitretin is also considered a first-line treatment for pustular psoriasis. Acitretin taken at a fixed dose of 25 mg/d obtains therapeutic response (PASI-75) in 47% of severe plaque–type patients at week 12.[75] Pregnancy is an absolute contraindication to acitretin therapy, and the authors avoid acitretin in women of child-bearing potential because there are many other therapeutic options. Although acitretin has a slow onset of action and is less effective compared with many other antipsoriatic systemic agents (MTX, cyclosporine, biologics), acitretin does achieve significant clearing, makes phototherapy more effective, and has the added benefit of being safely used in the long-term without the risk of immunosuppression.

REFERENCES

1. Lee CS, Koo J. A review of acitretin, a systemic retinoid for the treatment of psoriasis. Expert Opin Pharmacother 2005;6(10):1725–34.
2. Soriatane [package insert]. Research Triangle Park, NC; Stiefel Laboratories, Inc.; 2014. Available at: https://http://www.gsksource.com/pharma/content/dam/GlaxoSmithKline/US/en/Prescribing_Information/Soriatane/pdf/SORIATANE-PI-MG.PDF. Accessed February 21, 2016.
3. Gronhoj Larsen F, Steinkjer B, Jakobsen P, et al. Acitretin is converted to etretinate only during concomitant alcohol intake. Br J Dermatol 2000; 143(6):1164–9.
4. McNamara PJ, Jewell RC, Jensen BK, et al. Food increases the bioavailability of acitretin. J Clin Pharmacol 1988;28(11):1051–5.
5. Larsen FG, Jakobsen P, Eriksen H, et al. The pharmacokinetics of acitretin and its 13-cis-metabolite in psoriatic patients. J Clin Pharmacol 1991;31(5): 477–83.
6. Saurat JH. Retinoids and psoriasis: novel issues in retinoid pharmacology and implications for psoriasis treatment. J Am Acad Dermatol 1999;41(3 Pt 2): S2–6.
7. Tong PS, Horowitz NN, Wheeler LA. Trans retinoic acid enhances the growth response of epidermal keratinocytes to epidermal growth factor and transforming growth factor beta. J Invest Dermatol 1990; 94(1):126–31.
8. Sbidian E, Maza A, Montaudie H, et al. Efficacy and safety of oral retinoids in different psoriasis subtypes: a systematic literature review. J Eur Acad Dermatol Venereol 2011;25(Suppl 2):28–33.
9. Murray HE, Anhalt AW, Lessard R, et al. A 12-month treatment of severe psoriasis with acitretin: results of a Canadian open multicenter study. J Am Acad Dermatol 1991;24(4):598–602.
10. Olsen EA, Weed WW, Meyer CJ, et al. A double-blind, placebo-controlled trial of acitretin for the treatment of psoriasis. J Am Acad Dermatol 1989; 21(4 Pt 1):681–6.
11. Meffert H, Sonnichsen N. Acitretin in the treatment of severe psoriasis: a randomized double-blind study comparing acitretin and etretinate. Acta Derm Venereol Suppl 1989;146:176–7.
12. Kragballe K, Jansen CT, Geiger JM, et al. A double-blind comparison of acitretin and etretinate in the treatment of severe psoriasis. Results of a Nordic multicentre study. Acta Derm Venereol 1989;69(1):35–40.
13. Gollnick H, Bauer R, Brindley C, et al. Acitretin versus etretinate in psoriasis. Clinical and pharmacokinetic results of a German multicenter study. J Am Acad Dermatol 1988;19(3):458–68.
14. Ledo A, Martin M, Geiger JM, et al. Acitretin (Ro 10-1670) in the treatment of severe psoriasis. A randomized double-blind parallel study comparing acitretin and etretinate. Int J Dermatol 1988;27(9): 656–60.
15. Goldfarb MT, Ellis CN, Gupta AK, et al. Acitretin improves psoriasis in a dose-dependent fashion. J Am Acad Dermatol 1988;18(4 Pt 1):655–62.
16. Berbis P, Geiger JM, Vaisse C, et al. Benefit of progressively increasing doses during the initial treatment with acitretin in psoriasis. Dermatologica 1989;178(2):88–92.
17. Ling MR. Acitretin: optimal dosing strategies. J Am Acad Dermatol 1999;41(3 Pt 2):S13–7.
18. Geiger JM, Czarnetzki BM. Acitretin (Ro 10-1670, etretin): overall evaluation of clinical studies. Dermatologica 1988;176(4):182–90.
19. Ozawa A, Ohkido M, Haruki Y, et al. Treatments of generalized pustular psoriasis: a multicenter study in Japan. J Dermatol 1999;26(3):141–9.
20. Pang ML, Murase JE, Koo J. An updated review of acitretin–a systemic retinoid for the treatment of psoriasis. Expert Opin Drug Metab Toxicol 2008; 4(7):953–64.
21. Dogra S, Yadav S. Acitretin in psoriasis: an evolving scenario. Int J Dermatol 2014;53(5):525–38.
22. Rosenbach M, Hsu S, Korman NJ, et al. Treatment of erythrodermic psoriasis: from the medical board of the National Psoriasis Foundation. J Am Acad Dermatol 2010;62(4):655–62.
23. Koo J. Systemic sequential therapy of psoriasis: a new paradigm for improved therapeutic results. J Am Acad Dermatol 1999;41(3 Pt 2):S25–8.
24. Rim JH, Park JY, Choe YB, et al. The efficacy of calcipotriol + acitretin combination therapy for psoriasis: comparison with acitretin monotherapy. Am J Clin Dermatol 2003;4(7):507–10.
25. Ashcroft DM, Li Wan Po A, Williams HC, et al. Combination regimens of topical calcipotriene in chronic plaque psoriasis: systematic review of efficacy and tolerability. Arch Dermatol 2000;136(12):1536–43.
26. Lowenthal KE, Horn PJ, Kalb RE. Concurrent use of methotrexate and acitretin revisited. J Dermatolog Treat 2008;19(1):22–6.
27. Gisondi P, Del Giglio M, Cotena C, et al. Combining etanercept and acitretin in the therapy of chronic plaque psoriasis: a 24-week, randomized, controlled, investigator-blinded pilot trial. Br J Dermatol 2008;158(6):1345–9.
28. Cather JC, Crowley JJ. Use of biologic agents in combination with other therapies for the treatment of psoriasis. Am J Clin Dermatol 2014;15(6):467–78.
29. Takahashi MD, Castro LG, Romiti R. Infliximab, as sole or combined therapy, induces rapid clearing of erythrodermic psoriasis. Br J Dermatol 2007; 157(4):828–31.
30. Philipp S, Wilsmann-Theis D, Weyergraf A, et al. Combination of adalimumab with traditional systemic antipsoriatic drugs—a report of 39 cases. J Dtsch Dermatol Ges 2012;10(11):821–37.

31. Saurat JH, Geiger JM, Amblard P, et al. Randomized double-blind multicenter study comparing acitretin-PUVA, etretinate-PUVA and placebo-PUVA in the treatment of severe psoriasis. Dermatologica 1988;177(4):218–24.
32. Tanew A, Guggenbichler A, Honigsmann H, et al. Photochemotherapy for severe psoriasis without or in combination with acitretin: a randomized, double-blind comparison study. J Am Acad Dermatol 1991;25(4):682–4.
33. Otley CC, Stasko T, Tope WD, et al. Chemoprevention of nonmelanoma skin cancer with systemic retinoids: practical dosing and management of adverse effects. Dermatol Surg 2006;32(4):562–8.
34. Nijsten TE, Stern RS. Oral retinoid use reduces cutaneous squamous cell carcinoma risk in patients with psoriasis treated with psoralen-UVA: a nested cohort study. J Am Acad Dermatol 2003; 49(4):644–50.
35. Streit V, Wiedow O, Christophers E. Treatment of psoriasis with polyethylene sheet bath PUVA. J Am Acad Dermatol 1996;35(2 Pt 1):208–10.
36. Muchenberger S, Schopf E, Simon JC. The combination of oral acitretin and bath PUVA for the treatment of severe psoriasis. Br J Dermatol 1997;137(4): 587–9.
37. Lebwohl M. Acitretin in combination with UVB or PUVA. J Am Acad Dermatol 1999;41(3 Pt 2):S22–4.
38. Yamauchi PS, Rizk D, Kormili T, et al. Systemic retinoids. In: Weinstein GD, Gottlieb AB, editors. Therapy of moderate-to-severe psoriasis. New York: Marcel Dekker Inc; 2003. p. 137–49.
39. Busse K, Koo J. Introducing the delayed retinoid burn: a case report and discussion of this potential risk of retinoid-phototherapy combination management. J Am Acad Dermatol 2011;64(5):1011–2.
40. Ruzicka T, Sommerburg C, Braun-Falco O, et al. Efficiency of acitretin in combination with UV-B in the treatment of severe psoriasis. Arch Dermatol 1990; 126(4):482–6.
41. Iest J, Boer J. Combined treatment of psoriasis with acitretin and UVB phototherapy compared with acitretin alone and UVB alone. Br J Dermatol 1989; 120(5):665–70.
42. Lowe NJ, Prystowsky JH, Bourget T, et al. Acitretin plus UVB therapy for psoriasis. Comparisons with placebo plus UVB and acitretin alone. J Am Acad Dermatol 1991;24(4):591–4.
43. Lapolla W, Yentzer BA, Bagel J, et al. A review of phototherapy protocols for psoriasis treatment. J Am Acad Dermatol 2011;64(5):936–49.
44. Stern RS, Armstrong RB, Anderson TF, et al. Effect of continued ultraviolet B phototherapy on the duration of remission of psoriasis: a randomized study. J Am Acad Dermatol 1986;15(3):546–52.
45. Spuls PI, Rozenblit M, Lebwohl M. Retrospective study of the efficacy of narrowband UVB and acitretin. J Dermatolog Treat 2003;14(Suppl 2): 17–20.
46. Ozdemir M, Engin B, Baysal I, et al. A randomized comparison of acitretin-narrow-band TL-01 phototherapy and acitretin-psoralen plus ultraviolet A for psoriasis. Acta Derm Venereol 2008;88(6):589–93.
47. Lens M, Medenica L. Systemic retinoids in chemoprevention of non-melanoma skin cancer. Expert Opin Pharmacother 2008;9(8):1363–74.
48. George R, Weightman W, Russ GR, et al. Acitretin for chemoprevention of non-melanoma skin cancers in renal transplant recipients. Australas J Dermatol 2002;43(4):269–73.
49. Bavinck JN, Tieben LM, Van der Woude FJ, et al. Prevention of skin cancer and reduction of keratotic skin lesions during acitretin therapy in renal transplant recipients: a double-blind, placebo-controlled study. J Clin Oncol 1995;13(8):1933–8.
50. Moon TE, Levine N, Cartmel B, et al. Effect of retinol in preventing squamous cell skin cancer in moderate-risk subjects: a randomized, double-blind, controlled trial. Southwest Skin Cancer Prevention Study Group. Cancer Epidemiol Biomarkers Prev 1997;6(11):949–56.
51. Bhutani T, Koo J. A review of the chemopreventative effects of oral retinoids for internal neoplasms. J Drugs Dermatol 2011;10(11):1292–8.
52. Sarkar R, Chugh S, Garg VK. Acitretin in dermatology. Indian J Dermatol Venereol Leprol 2013; 79(6):759–71.
53. Pearce DJ, Klinger S, Ziel KK, et al. Low-dose acitretin is associated with fewer adverse events than high-dose acitretin in the treatment of psoriasis. Arch Dermatol 2006;142(8):1000–4.
54. Geiger JM, Baudin M, Saurat JH. Teratogenic risk with etretinate and acitretin treatment. Dermatology 1994;189(2):109–16.
55. Geiger JM, Walker M. Is there a reproductive safety risk in male patients treated with acitretin (neotigason/soriatane? Dermatology 2002;205(2):105–7.
56. Millsop JW, Heller MM, Eliason MJ, et al. Dermatological medication effects on male fertility. Dermatol Ther 2013;26(4):337–46.
57. Halkier-Sorensen L, Andresen J. A retrospective study of bone changes in adults treated with etretinate. J Am Acad Dermatol 1989;20(1):83–7.
58. Van Dooren-Greebe RJ, Lemmens JA, De Boo T, et al. Prolonged treatment with oral retinoids in adults: no influence on the frequency and severity of spinal abnormalities. Br J Dermatol 1996;134(1):71–6.
59. Katz HI, Waalen J, Leach EE. Acitretin in psoriasis: an overview of adverse effects. J Am Acad Dermatol 1999;41(3 Pt 2):S7–s12.
60. Orfanos CE. Retinoids: the new status. Maintenance therapy, disorders of resorption in "non-responders", interactions and interferences with drugs, treatment of children and bone toxicity,

acitetin and 13-cis-acitretin. Hautarzt 1989;40(3): 123–9 [in German].
61. Mork NJ, Kolbenstvedt A, Austad J. Efficacy and skeletal side effects of two years' acitretin treatment. Acta Derm Venereol 1992;72(6):445–8.
62. Lee E, Koo J. Single-center retrospective study of long-term use of low-dose acitretin (Soriatane) for psoriasis. J Dermatolog Treat 2004;15(1):8–13.
63. McMullen EA, McCarron P, Irvine AD, et al. Association between long-term acitretin therapy and osteoporosis: no evidence of increased risk. Clin Exp Dermatol 2003;28(3):307–9.
64. Prendiville J, Bingham EA, Burrows D. Premature epiphyseal closure–a complication of etretinate therapy in children. J Am Acad Dermatol 1986; 15(6):1259–62.
65. Sarkar S, Das K, Roychoudhury S, et al. Pseudotumor cerebri in a child treated with acitretin: a rare occurrence. Indian J Pharmacol 2013;45(1):89–90.
66. Fraunfelder FW, Fraunfelder FT. Evidence for a probable causal relationship between tretinoin, acitretin, and etretinate and intracranial hypertension. J Neuroophthalmol 2004;24(3):214–6.
67. Starling J 3rd, Koo J. Evidence based or theoretical concern? Pseudotumor cerebri and depression as acitretin side effects. J Drugs Dermatol 2005;4(6): 690–6.
68. Davidson MH, Stein EA, Bays HE, et al. Efficacy and tolerability of adding prescription omega-3 fatty acids 4 g/d to simvastatin 40 mg/d in hypertriglyceridemic patients: an 8-week, randomized, double-blind, placebo-controlled study. Clin Ther 2007;29(7):1354–67.
69. Roenigk HH Jr, Callen JP, Guzzo CA, et al. Effects of acitretin on the liver. J Am Acad Dermatol 1999; 41(4):584–8.
70. Jeong YS, Kim MS, Shin JH, et al. A case of severe HIV-associated psoriasis successfully treated with acitretin therapy. Infect Chemother 2014;46(2):115–9.
71. Elsaie ML. Suicidal tendency in a psoriasis vulgaris patient under acitretin treatment. Indian J Dermatol 2007;52:164–5.
72. Mayo KL, Gupta AK. A case of generalized erythrodermic psoriasis with suicidal ideation: a unique association. J Clin Exp Dermatol Res 2011;2:115.
73. Rollman O, Pihl-Lundin I. Acitretin excretion into human breast milk. Acta Derm Venereol 1990;70(6): 487–90.
74. Carretero G, Ribera M, Belinchon I, et al. Guidelines for the use of acitretin in psoriasis. Psoriasis Group of the Spanish Academy of Dermatology and Venereology. Actas Dermosifiliogr 2013; 104(7):598–616.
75. Dogra S, Jain A, Kanwar AJ. Efficacy and safety of acitretin in three fixed doses of 25, 35 and 50 mg in adult patients with severe plaque type psoriasis: a randomized, double blind, parallel group, dose ranging study. J Eur Acad Dermatol Venereol 2013;27(3):e305–11.

CHAPTER 6

Cyclosporine

Vidhi V. Shah, BA, Shivani P. Reddy, BS, Elaine J. Lin, MD, Jashin J. Wu, MD

KEYWORDS

• Cyclosporine • CsA • Neoral • Sandimmune • PISCES • PREWENT

KEY POINTS

- Cyclosporine (CsA) is a highly effective treatment option for patients with moderate-to-severe plaque psoriasis with a rapid onset of action.
- Its mode of action includes the formation of a CsA-cyclophilin complex, which binds to and inhibits calcineurin. Inhibition of calcineurin activity depresses T-cell differentiation and inhibits interleukin-2 activity.
- CsA is dosed at 2.5 to 5.0 mg/kg/d in 2 divided oral doses, which may be increased or decreased by 0.5 to 1.0 mg/kg/d.
- Important adverse effects of CsA therapy include the development of hypertension and nephrotoxicity; for this reason, routine monitoring of serum creatinine and blood pressure levels are indicated.

INTRODUCTION

Cyclosporine (CsA) is an effective medication used for the treatment of severe plaque psoriasis in adult patients.[1] It is commonly known for its ability to effectively prevent allograft rejection and is widely administered following kidney, liver, and heart transplantation. The capability of CsA to drastically reduce immunologic activity within short time spans has also made it a popular drug of choice for the treatment of various immune-mediated disorders, including moderate-to-severe plaque psoriasis.[2]

In 1997, the US Food and Drug Administration (FDA) officially approved CsA for the treatment of plaque psoriasis. Today, CsA is indicated for adults who are not otherwise immunosuppressed and experience severe, recalcitrant psoriasis, including patients with extensive or disabling forms of psoriasis (plaque, generalized pustular, palmoplantar, and erythrodermic) that have failed at least 1 other systemic therapy or are unable to take other systemic therapies due to contraindications or intolerable side effects. Although it has only 1 dermatologic-approved indication, CsA has been used for various off-label dermatologic disorders, including severe atopic dermatitis, chronic idiopathic uticaria refractory to treatment, and pyoderma gangrenosum.[3]

Novartis Pharmaceuticals Corporation manufactures CsA under the trade names Sandimmune (available as 25-mg or 100-mg soft gelatin capsules, 50 mL per bottle oral solution, and 5-mL sterile ampul intravenous injections) and Neoral (available as 25-mg or 100-mg soft gelatin capsules or 50 mL per bottle oral solution). Neoral and its bioequivalents include Gengraf by Abbott Laboratories Incorporated (available in 25-mg or 100-mg capsules) and the generic version "CsA USP modified." Neoral and Gengraf are newer, microemulsion formulations with better absorption and greater bioavailability than the original Sandimmune formulation.[4]

The current recommended starting dosage of CsA for patients with psoriasis is 2.5 to 3 mg/kg/d taken in 2 divided doses (1.25 mg/kg twice a day) for a short-term course of 12 to 16 weeks (Fig. 6.1). If there is no significant clinical improvement following at least 4 weeks of treatment, CsA dosages are increased in incremental dosages by 0.5 mg/kg/d until the disease is stable. The maximum dosage per day is 5.0 mg/kg. Alternatively, CsA may be started at the maximum

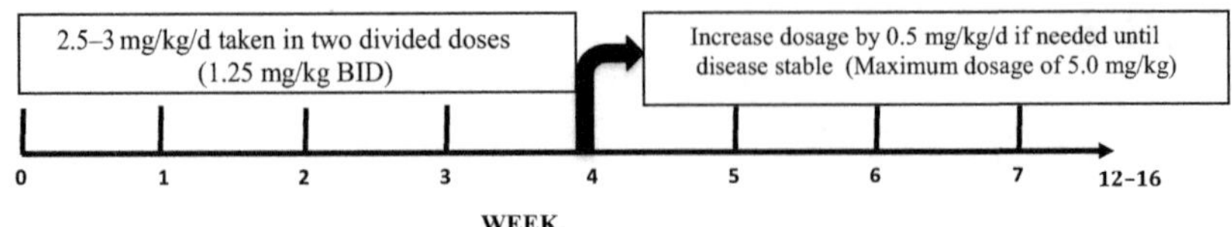

Fig. 6.1 Recommended starting regimen of CsA in incremental dosages.

dosage and be reduced in 0.5-mg/kg/d increments in severe disease. CsA is metabolized by hepatic cytochrome P450-3A, and its plasma half-life is approximately 8 hours, with a range of 5 to 18 hours.

MECHANISM OF ACTION

CsA is a lipophilic cyclic polypeptide composed of 11 amino acids.[4] It suppresses the immune system by inhibiting T-cell differentiation and activation. The drug itself binds a cytosolic protein named cyclophilin. The subsequent CsA-cyclophilin complex binds to and inhibits calcineurin. By inhibiting calcineurin, CsA blocks activation of the transcription factor, Nuclear Factor of Activated T cells (NFAT); this prevents NFAT from activating transcription of genes coding for interleukin-2 and other cytokines. The blockade of calcineurin halts signal transduction mechanisms required for the activation and differentiation of T lymphocytes (Fig. 6.2).[1] Downstream consequences of the inhibition of calcineurin include reduction of lymphocytes and macrophages in the epidermis and dermis, downregulation of cellular adhesion molecule expression in the dermal capillary endothelium, restricted activation of antigen-presenting cells, natural killer cells, and T cells, inhibition of keratinocyte proliferation, and restricted release of histamine from mast cells.[5]

EFFICACY

CsA is one of the most effective drugs for the treatment of moderate-to-severe plaque psoriasis, with rapid onset of action and powerful immunosuppressive activity. An extensive number of clinical trials have investigated the efficacy of CsA in the treatment of moderate-to-severe plaque psoriasis using various drug regimens, including monotherapy versus combination therapy; short, intermittent, and long-term therapy; and topical versus systemic therapy.

Monotherapy

Short-term therapy: for induction of remission

In an open, prospective, multicenter trial conducted by Berth-Jones and colleagues,[6] the efficacy and tolerability of intermittent CsA (Neoral) therapy were studied in 41 patients with psoriasis vulgaris. Each patient received 3 treatment periods of up to 12 weeks' duration of CsA at a divided dosage of 5 mg/kg/d. Treatment was continued until the patient achieved a 90% remission of afflicted areas or for duration of 12 weeks, whichever occurred first. Increases in blood pressure (>95 mm Hg diastolic at 2 consecutive visits), serum creatinine (>30% from baseline), or development of other adverse effects resulted in 25% dose reductions. Satisfactory clinical response to CsA was evaluated using a modified "rule of nines" criteria at the end of each treatment period. There was significant improvement in erythema, infiltration, and desquamation the end of each treatment period as compared with baseline ($P<.01$). There was a high proportion of patients achieving clinical remission following each treatment period, including 93% of patients at period 1 (mean 7.2, SD 3.0 days), 85% of patients at period 2 (mean 8.0, SD 3.2 days), and 91% of patients at period 3 (mean 7.4, SD 3.2 days). Patients experienced relapse at a median of 72 days and 53 days for periods 1 and 2, respectively. There was no significant difference between baseline and final

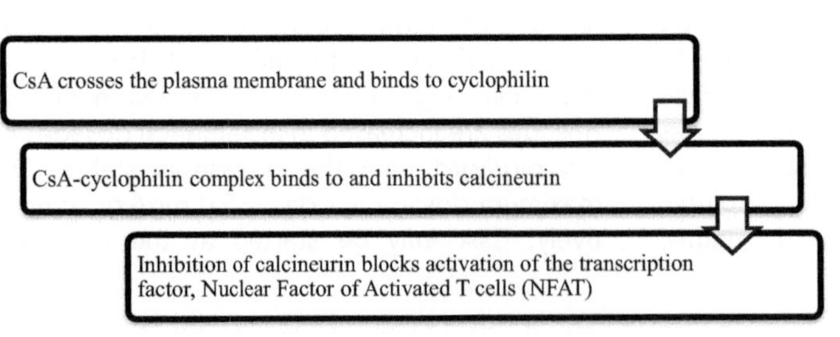

Fig. 6.2 CsA mechanism of action: CsA binds to cyclophilin, forming a CsA-cyclophilin complex that inhibits calcineurin.

follow-up for improvement or tolerability. The study concluded that intermittent courses of CsA could rapidly clear plaque psoriasis.[6]

Faerber and colleagues[7] conducted a meta-analysis of 3 major, prospective, randomized trials investigating CsA for induction of remission in 579 patients with severe plaque-type psoriasis (Table 6.1). Significant Psoriasis Area and Severity Index (PASI) reductions of 44.4%, 69.8%, and 71.5% were demonstrated in patients after 10 to 12 weeks of CsA therapy at dosages of 1.25, 2.5, and 5 mg/kg/d (mean daily dosage 0.53 mg/kg/d). Primary outcome measures included PASI and serum creatinine levels. CsA was found to be highly effective with patients reaching PASI-50 from baseline in 4.3 weeks for 5 mg/kg/d, 6.1 weeks for 2.5 mg/kg/d, and 14.1 weeks for 1.25 mg/kg/d. Moreover, CsA 1.25 mg/kg/d was found to be more efficacious than placebo, and this difference was statistically significant.[8]

Two randomized, controlled clinical trials compared the short-term effectiveness of CsA to that of methotrexate (MTX).[9] In the study by Flytstrom and colleagues,[9] 84 patients were randomized to receive either MTX or CsA for a 12-week duration. The primary endpoint was PASI-75. Patients who received CsA demonstrated greater efficacy than patients receiving MTX therapy, with 72% of CsA patients reaching significant PASI changes from baseline than 58% of MTX patients. In a similar manner, Heydendael and colleagues[10] also compared the efficacy of CsA to MTX. A total of 44 patients were treated with CsA using an initial dose of 3 mg/kg/wk for 16 weeks. In contrast to Flytstrom and colleagues, Heydendael and colleagues found no significant differences in efficacy between CsA and MTX groups.

Intermittent short-term therapy: for maintenance and prevention of relapse

In a 1-year, prospective, open, multicenter, randomized trial, the Psoriasis Intermittent Short Courses of Efficacy of Sandimmune Neoral (PISCES) studied intermittent short-term treatment of CsA in 400 patients with plaque psoriasis who were unresponsive to topical therapy. Patients were initiated at 2.5 mg/kg/d of CsA, which was increased by 0.5 to 1.0 mg/kg/d (maximum of 5 mg/kg/d) until 90% clearance of the affected areas or duration of 12 weeks, whichever occurred first. Patients who achieved satisfactory improvement (defined as PASI-75) were randomly assigned to discontinue treatment or undergo a dose reduction of 1 mg/kg/d until cessation. Patients were administered another course of CsA upon relapse and received as many treatment courses necessary for 1 year. Overall, median time to relapse was 3.6 months and 3.7 months in patients randomized to abruptly stop therapy

TABLE 6.1
Comparison of 3 major, prospective, randomized trials investigating cyclosporine for induction

	Meffert et al,[43] 1997 (*N* = 133)	**Laburte et al,[44] 1994 (*N* = 251)**	**Christophers et al,[45] 1992 (*N* = 217)**
Baseline PASI	8–25	≥18	≥15
CsA dosages (mg/kg/d)	1.25 2.5	2.5 5	1.25 2.5[a]
Duration (wk)	10	12	12–36
CsA PASI improvement from baseline (%)	27.2 51	69 89	18 56
Placebo PASI improvement from baseline (%)	5.9	NR	NR
Conclusions	CsA 1.25 mg/kg/d is superior to placebo Consider dosage reductions to 1.25 mg/kg/d once patients stable at higher doses	CsA 5 mg/kg/d is superior to 2.5 mg/kg/d in chronic plaque psoriasis	CsA 2.5 mg/kg/d is the optimal starting dosage as compared with 1.25 mg/kg/d in chronic plaque psoriasis

[a] Patients with no significant improvement had dosages doubled up to 5 mg/kg/d until response reached.
Data from Refs.[43–45]

versus those who were tapered off ($P = .04$). Mean area of skin involvement included 4%, 2.6%, 4.4%, and 4.5% at the end of treatment periods 1, 2, 3, and 4, respectively, from a baseline of 25%.[11] In an extension study, the PISCES group administered CsA to 76 patients with chronic plaque psoriasis intermittently over 2 years. Time in remission was the same whether abruptly stopping CsA or tapering over 4 weeks. Median time to relapse was 3.8 months after the first treatment, which progressively shortened after greater number of courses.[12]

The PREWENT (Psoriasis Relapse Evaluation with Week-End Neoral Treatment) study was a randomized, double-blind, multicenter, controlled study that evaluated the efficacy and tolerability of weekend CsA for the reduction of relapse rate in patients who had previously achieved remission with continuous CsA therapy. The primary endpoint was no relapse or a 75% improvement in PASI from baseline at week 24. Eighty-one patients received placebo and 162 received CsA for 2 consecutive days a week for 24 weeks. Weekend CsA reduced time to first relapse in psoriasis patients, with time to first relapse prolonged in patients receiving CsA versus placebo ($P<.05$). In addition, PASI was lower from weeks 4 to 16 in CsA recipients. In patients with moderate-severe psoriasis, the clinical success rate was increased with CsA compared with placebo (69.9% vs 46.3%; $P = .011$).[13]

Continuous long-term therapy

Smaller studies have studied the effectiveness and safety associated with CsA in continuous, long-term therapy. Chaidemenos and colleagues[14] conducted an open, randomized single-center study studying intermittent versus ongoing CsA therapy in 51 patients with chronic plaque psoriasis. Intermittent administration was less efficacious than continuous treatment (PASI-75 62% vs 92%, $P<.05$). However, patients administered continuous treatment received 139% of the mean cumulative CsA dose of intermittent therapy.

Long-term therapy should remain an option for patients who are recalcitrant to intermittent therapy. Lowe and colleagues[15] evaluated the efficacy of CsA at 12 weeks and 3 to 5 years. Forty-two patients received CsA 5 to 6 mg/kg/d for 12 weeks, and 14 of 42 patients (33.33%) received maintenance treatment for 3.5 years. At the end of 12 weeks, 36 patients (86%) were clear or almost clear of psoriatic lesions. Dosages were increased from 5 to 6 mg/kg/d in 15 patients who remained unresponsive to therapy. Sixty-seven percent of this subgroup achieved clearance within 4 weeks.

A German multicenter study assessed the results of long-term CsA therapy in 285 patients with severe psoriasis. Patients were treated with 1.25 to 5 mg/kg/d of CsA for 6 to 30 months. PASI scores were reduced by 75% to 94% from baseline; however, half of the patients experienced relapse following cessation of therapy.[16] In a 16-week unblinded study, 181 patients received 3.0 to 6.0 mg/kg/d CsA. Eighty-six percent of patients achieved a PASI-70 response. Patients entered a 24-week maintenance phase wherein they were randomly assigned to receive CsA 1.5 mg/kg/d or CsA 3 mg/kg/d or placebo. Longer time to relapse was associated with long-term maintenance therapy with CsA 3 mg/kg/d than placebo ($P<.01$). Furthermore, approximately half the patients treated with CsA 3 mg/kg/d experienced relapse as compared with placebo (42% vs 84%) at the end of the 24-week maintenance period.[17]

Additional studies have studied novel outcomes that affect the overall efficacy of CsA. Sandimmune and Neoral formulations were compared in patients with severe plaque psoriasis in a prospective, randomized, double-blind study. PASI-75 was achieved by 80% of patients in both groups by week 12. However, the Neoral group achieved a faster response and remission rates between the 2 formulations.[18] An open trial study investigated the efficacy of Neoral administered before and after meals in 37 patients with psoriasis vulgaris. CsA microemulsion of 1.5 to 3.0 mg/kg/d was administered before or after meals for 6 weeks. Giving CsA before meals improved psoriasis more than giving CsA after meals ($P<.05$).[19] Another trial evaluated the value of a fixed dose microemulsion of 100 mg/d CsA in psoriasis. Forty patients were administered either 100 mg/d CsA (group A) or 50 mg CsA twice daily (group B). PASI-50 was achieved by 82% in group A and 84% in group B. PASI-50 was significantly higher in group A than in group B at 6 weeks; however, no difference in PASI-75 and PASI-90 was seen between groups.[20]

Combination Therapy

Topical therapy

Combination treatments, including topical forms of CsA, have been studied for moderate-to-severe plaque psoriasis. Various smaller studies have evaluated topical CsA in combination with other agents, including the vitamin D analogue calcipotriol, corticosteroids, anthralin, and dithranol.[21,22] One randomized, double-blind, multicenter, placebo-controlled study evaluated the combination of topical CsA with calcipotriol ointment. Patients were randomized to receive either 2 mg/kg/d of CsA with 50 μg/g of calcipotriol ointment or 2 mg/kg/d of CsA combined with placebo ointment. More patients in the calcipotriol/CsA group (50%) achieved complete or 90% improvement in PASI scores than in the placebo/CsA group (12%).[23]

Systemic therapy

Concurrent administration of CsA with other systemic psoriasis agents, including MTX, mycophenolate mofetil (MMF), and fumaric acid esters, has been studied. The combination of 3 mg/kg/d of CsA and 7.5 to 15 mg/wk of MTX was more effective than monotherapy with either CsA or MTX alone in 19 patients with severe, recalcitrant psoriasis.[24] The addition of MFF (maximum dosage 3.0 g/d) to low-dose CsA (2.5 mg/kg/d) in 9 patients with severe, recalcitrant psoriasis resulted in moderate-to-good clinical improvement of psoriasis over 3 to 11 months.[25]

EFFICACY IN PSORIATIC ARTHRITIS

Various therapies, including corticosteroids, disease-modifying anti-rheumatic drugs (DMARDs), and biologic DMARDs, target the pain, inflammation, joint destruction, and ensuing debilities associated with psoriatic arthritis (PsA). CsA is a synthetic DMARD that has moderate efficacy for PsA spinal and joint symptoms. Most recently, the SYNERGY study conducted a large, multicenter, observational Italian study that evaluated CsA monotherapy in patients with PsA; CsA was effective in reducing all disease parameters, including PASI, the Bath Ankylosing Spondylitis Activity Index, and patient and physician global assessments.[26] Although such studies have demonstrated this drug to be effective, CsA is currently not FDA approved for the treatment of PsA, and there are currently other medications available with superior efficacy.[27,28]

SAFETY

CsA has potentially serious side effects and drug/food interactions. Patients should be well informed of the signs and symptoms of these adverse effects before beginning CsA therapy. The most important side effects are nephrotoxicity and high blood pressure, which seem to be dose and duration dependent. In general, side effects are easily reversed with cessation of therapy; however, long-term therapy may be associated with toxicity and structural abnormalities in renal microvasculature. The current guidelines recommend the administration of CsA using a short-term regimen of 2.5 to 5.0 mg/kg/d for 12 to 16 weeks. For long-term therapy, the US guidelines allow CsA use for up to 1 year, whereas the European guidelines allow its use for up to 2 years.[1]

During the clinical trials of CsA, safety problems occurred. In a study of 41 subjects, 18 patients did not complete the study, with 5 withdrawn for adverse events, including hypertension (n = 3), renal impairment (n = 1), and abdominal pain (n = 1). Less-severe side effects that were commonly encountered include paresthesia, gastrointestinal symptoms, musculoskeletal pains, influenza-like symptoms, headache, and upper respiratory tract infections. Patients during each treatment period experienced increased blood pressures and serum creatinine; however, both returned to baseline by the end of follow-up. Overall, no cumulative toxicity was appreciated.[6] Thirty-three of 400 patients were withdrawn from the study due to side effects. Adverse effects were reported in 50% of patients and included paresthesia, nausea, hypertrichosis, and headache. Most of these side effects were mild to moderate in severity; only 11 patients (3%) experienced severe side effects that included myalgia and paresthesia. No clinically significant increases in serum creatinine and/or systolic and diastolic blood pressures were appreciated during the study. Thirty-two patients (8%) experienced serum creatinine levels greater than 30% and 45 patients (12%) developed new-onset hypertension over 1 year.[11]

Nephrotoxicity

CsA exerts a constrictive effect on renal arterioles, thus contributing increased blood pressure and decreased renal function.[29] The low dosages (2.5–5 mg/kg/d) used for treatment of psoriasis run less risk of renal dysfunction than the doses used in transplant recipients. Experts recommend intermittent use of CsA over 12 weeks rather than ongoing treatment. Long-term therapy with CsA increases the chances of permanent loss of renal function. Structural and functional damage to the kidneys is a concern with continuous CsA treatment for greater than 2 years at any dosage. Patients undergoing therapy for greater than 1 year should have yearly glomerular filtration rate (GFR) monitoring and monthly creatinine levels monitored.

Patients with serum creatinine levels greater than 30% of baseline on 2 separate occasions, measured 2 weeks apart, should have CsA dosages reduced by 1 mg/kg/d and follow-up serum creatinine levels every other week for 1 month. If the serum creatinine continues to remain greater than 30% of baseline after lowering the doses after 2 similar instances, it is recommended CsA be discontinued. Patients on therapy for more than

1 year should be carefully monitored for nephrotoxicity including yearly GFR and monthly serum creatinine levels. Minimization of renal impairment may be achieved with lowering dosages and terminating therapy. Old age, obesity, pre-existing hypertension or kidney disease, and concomitant use of other nephrotoxic medications can increase the chances of CsA-induced nephrotoxicity.[1]

Hypertension

CsA has a dose- and duration-dependent effect on blood pressure that is reversible with reduction or discontinuation of therapy. CsA dosages should be reduced by 25% to 50% in patients experiencing increased blood pressure (measured at 2 separate instances). It is recommended to discontinue CsA if elevated blood pressure levels persist despite dose reductions. Various studies investigating CsA effect on blood pressure report between 5% and 26% of psoriatic patients experience increase in blood pressure after initiation of CsA therapy. Calcium-channel blockers, specifically amlodipine and isradipine, are first-line treatment choices for CsA-induced hypertension because they act to directly relax the vascular smooth muscle. Additional treatment options include angiotensin-converting enzyme inhibitors and β-blockers. Thiazide and potassium-sparing diuretics are not recommended.

Malignancies

It is difficult to determine the risk of malignancies caused by CsA in psoriasis patients because psoriasis patients have greater risk of cancer and lymphomas than the general population. B- and T-cell lymphomas are rare in CsA-treated patients. Paul and colleagues[30] prospectively followed 1252 patients for 5 years and reported no lymphoma. The connection between solid organ tumors and CsA is also unclear. Several case reports have suggested the development of organ malignancy in CsA-treated patients; however, 2 large-scale studies report the association to be unlikely. Ryan and colleagues[31] conducted a case control study and suggested that CsA in combination with another immunosuppressive therapy used together may decrease the incidence of breast and rectal cancers.

Patients should avoid simultaneous treatment of CsA and phototherapy or CsA immediately before or after psoralen and UV-A radiation (PUVA), because the risk of development of cutaneous malignancy is heightened. There is an increased risk of nonmelanoma skin cancers in patients using long-term (>2 years) CsA; patients exposed to PUVA, immunosuppressant therapy, or MTX; and patients with a history of skin cancer.

Additional Side Effects

In addition to the above-mentioned side effects, patients on CsA therapy may experience headache, tremor, paresthesia, hypertrichosis, gingival hyperplasia, worsening acne, nausea, vomiting, diarrhea, myalgia, flulike symptoms, lethargy, hypertriglyceridemia, hypomagnesemia, hyperkalemia, hyperbilirubinemia, and increased risk of infection and malignancies.[1]

PRECAUTIONS

Dermatologists should be aware of the cautions of CsA administration. Special attention should be given to patients with a history of kidney disease, pre-existing hypertension, and certain other conditions. Otherwise healthy individuals, including pregnant women, children, and elderly individuals, seeking treatment with CsA also require additional consideration (Box 6.1).

Pregnancy Category C and Lactation

There are very little data reporting CsA use in pregnant women with psoriasis. The effects of CsA in pregnancy are primarily derived from the organ transplant literature, making direct comparisons between the 2 populations difficult. In general, pregnant women who are receiving CsA treatment in the transplant population are at risk for babies with low birth weight and prematurity.[32] One retrospective study of 629 pregnant patients using 1.4 to 12 mg/kg/d CsA from week 6 through the entire pregnancy found similar rates of fetal loss and malformation to that of the general population. However, the study did find increased rates of prematurity and lower birth rates within this population.[33] Similarly, smaller studies including 1 case report[34] and retrospective analysis[35] found that low birth weight and prematurity were associated with CsA usage in pregnant patients with complicated medical history. As such, the risks and benefits of CsA should be carefully weighed before initiating therapy in pregnancy. The FDA has labeled CsA as pregnancy category C, and the general recommendation is to withhold CsA treatment in pregnant patients and only consider it in patients who have severe psoriasis recalcitrant to other medications.[32]

It is not recommended to take CsA when breast-feeding because the drug may accrue within the breast milk, although the exact levels may vary. In 1 study involving 7 breast-fed infants of mothers receiving CsA, drug levels of CsA in infants were less than 0.1 mg/kg/d, with 50 to 227 ng/mL available in daily breast milk.[36] This finding is in contrast to another study, which

BOX 6.1
Relative and absolute contraindications of cyclosporine therapy

Relative contraindications

- Patients with issues with intermittent use of medication
- Hypertension and currently on prescription medication
- Patients on nephrotoxic drugs
- Geriatric patients
- Drug-drug interactions
- Significant hepatic disease
- Gingivitis/excessive dental plaque
- Immunodeficiency
- Gout

Absolute contraindications

- Uncontrolled hypertension or diabetes
- Abnormal renal function or kidney disease
- Pregnancy and lactation
- Malignancy
- Presence of active infections
- Hypersensitivity to CsA or any of its components
- Cardiovascular issues including migraines and strokes
- Patients requiring live-attenuated vaccinations during treatment
- Noncompliant, unreliable, or unavailable patients for routine follow-up
- Concomitant PUVA or UV-B, methotrexate, or other immunosuppressive medications, coal tar, greater than 200 PUVA treatments, or radiation therapy in the past

Data from Menter A, Korman NJ, Elmets CA, et al. Guidelines of care for the management of psoriasis and psoriatic arthritis: section 4. Guidelines of care for the management and treatment of psoriasis with traditional systemic agents. J Am Acad Dermatol 2009;61:451–85; and Koo JYM, Levin EC, Leon A, et al. Moderate to severe psoriasis. 4th edition. Boca Raton (FL): CRC Press, Taylor & Francis Group; 2014. p. ix, 391.

reported substantial inconsistencies in CsA concentrations in infants receiving breast milk. Additional, long-term studies are necessary before the establishment of recommendations.[32,37] For now, pregnant women with moderate-to-severe forms of psoriasis should decide whether to terminate CsA therapy or discontinue breast-feeding.

Pediatrics

Currently, CsA is only FDA approved in adults, because the safety and efficacy of CsA in children with psoriasis has not been established yet, and there are only limited studies evaluating its use in the pediatric population. One retrospective chart review found that 17 of 22 (77%) patients were excellent responders to CsA therapy (mean dosage 3.5 $\pm$ 0.6 mg/kg/d for a mean duration of 5.7 $\pm$ 3.3 months).[38] In another case series, 15 of 38 patients (39.4%) achieved PASI-75 by week 16. Eight patients discontinued therapy secondary to abnormal laboratory values and/or adverse events, but none were serious.[39,40]

Geriatrics

Treatment of the older adults with psoriasis should involve careful assessment of baseline organ functionality, because this population generally has decreased hepatic, renal, and cardiac function. Also, the risk of drug-drug interaction effects is increased because this population is often subject to polypharmacy.

Drug and Food Interactions

CsA has significant drug interactions that should be noted and appreciated before and during therapy (Box 6.2). CsA is metabolized by cytochrome P450-3A, and several medications or dietary substances can either inhibit or enhance cytochrome P450-3A activity, which may cause an unintentional increase or decrease in serum drug concentrations. Both physicians and patients should be aware of these medications and substances that could potentially increase the risk for toxicity or reduce CsA effectiveness. Furthermore, medications or dietary substances that increase serum potassium levels, cause potential nephrotoxicity, increase or decrease immunosuppression, or directly interact with CsA itself, should be avoided. In addition, CsA can reduce the clearance of drugs such as prednisolone, statins (increased risk of rhabdomyolysis), digoxin, and colchicine.

MONITORING

Baseline Monitoring

Before initiation of treatment, the patient must have a thorough history and physical examination. The history should include past or present exposure to tuberculosis, hepatitis B or C, family history or personal history of kidney disease, diabetes, obesity, pregnancy and contraception, presence of active infection or tumors, and use of nephrotoxic drugs. Baseline blood pressure measurements as well as blood urea nitrogen

BOX 6.2
Selected medications, foods, and supplements that may interfere with cyclosporine therapy

Drugs and foods that *inhibit* cytochrome P450-3A and *increase* CsA levels

- Antifungals: ketoconazole, itraconazole, fluconazole, voriconazole
- Antibiotics: macrolides, fluoroquinolones
- Diuretics: furosemide, thiazides, carbonic anhydrase inhibitors
- Calcium channel blockers: diltiazem, nicardipine, verapamil
- Corticosteroids: methylprednisolone
- Antiemetics: metoclopramide
- Antiarrhythmic: amiodarone
- Antimalarial: hydroxychloroquine, chloroquine
- HIV protease inhibitors: ritonavir, indinavir, saquinavir, nelfinavir
- Selective serotonin re-uptake inhibitors: fluoxetine, sertraline
- Oral contraceptives
- Grapefruit and grapefruit juice

Drugs and foods that *induce* cytochrome P450-3A and *decrease* CsA levels

- Antifungals: griseofulvin
- Antibiotics: nafcillin, rifabutin, rifampin, rifapentine
- Antiepileptics: carbamazepine, phenytoin, phenobarbital, valproic acid
- Somatostatin analogues: octreotide
- Tuberculosis medication: rifampicin
- Retinoids: bexarotene
- Others: pioglitazone, rosiglitazone, phenytoin, phenobarbital, orlistat
- St. John's wort

Drugs with known nephrotoxicity

- Nonsteroidal anti-inflammatory drugs (NSAIDs): diclofenac, naproxen, sulindac, indomethacin
- Diuretics
- Antibiotics: gentamycin, aminoglycosides, amphotericin B, trimethoprim-sulfamethoxazole, vancomycin
- H-2 antagonists: cimetidine and ranitidine

Drugs, foods, and supplements that increase serum potassium

- NSAIDs: all especially indomethacin
- Angiotensin-converting inhibitors
- β-Adrenergic blockers
- Potassium-sparing diuretics
- Antiarrhythmic: digitalis

Data from Menter A, Korman NJ, Elmets CA, et al. Guidelines of care for the management of psoriasis and psoriatic arthritis: section 4. Guidelines of care for the management and treatment of psoriasis with traditional systemic agents. J Am Acad Dermatol 2009;61:451–85; and Koo JYM, Levin EC, Leon A, et al. Moderate to severe psoriasis. 4th edition. Boca Raton (FL): CRC Press, Taylor & Francis Group; 2014. p. ix, 391.

(BUN) and serum creatinine should be measured on 2 separate occasions (Table 6.2). In addition, the physician should obtain liver function tests (LFTs), complete blood count (CBC), serum magnesium, potassium, uric acid, and cholesterol lipid panel.[1]

Ongoing Monitoring

It is recommended to evaluate blood pressure and BUN/creatinine levels closely every other week in the first 3 months of CsA therapy and in monthly intervals thereafter if stable. In addition, monthly CBC, LFTs, magnesium, uric acid,

TABLE 6.2
Evaluation and workup for treatment with cyclosporine therapy

Baseline Monitoring	Ongoing Monitoring

• History and physical examination
• Blood pressure (measured on 2 separate occasions)
• Serum BUN and creatinine (measured on 2 separate occasions)
• Urinalysis[a]
• CBC
• Magnesium
• Potassium
• Uric acid
• Lipids
• Liver enzymes
• Bilirubin
• Consider purified protein derivative and pregnancy test if indicated
	• Every other week and then monthly after 3 mo if stable
	  ○ Blood pressure
	  ○ Serum BUN and creatinine
	• Monthly
	  ○ CBC
	  ○ Uric acid[a]
	  ○ Potassium
	  ○ Lipids
	  ○ Liver enzymes
	  ○ Serum bilirubin
	  ○ Magnesium

[a] Guidelines reflect official American Academy of Dermatology guidelines. Of note, the authors of this chapter do not check urinalysis, uric acid, and BUN.

Data from Menter A, Korman NJ, Elmets CA, et al. Guidelines of care for the management of psoriasis and psoriatic arthritis: section 4. Guidelines of care for the management and treatment of psoriasis with traditional systemic agents. J Am Acad Dermatol 2009;61:451–85.

potassium, and cholesterol lipid panel should be obtained. Consider calculating GFR once yearly in patients at risk for lower kidney function.[1]

VACCINATIONS

In general, it is recommended that patients on CsA should receive age-appropriate killed or inactivated vaccines. The authors of this chapter endorse annual influenza vaccinations, although previous studies in transplant patients receiving CsA report variable efficacy.[41] Concomitant administration of live-attenuated vaccinations is contraindicated with CsA therapy.[42]

SUMMARY AND RECOMMENDATIONS

There is currently a wide array of therapeutic options available for the treatment of moderate-to-severe psoriasis. Nevertheless, CsA remains a useful option owing to its reliable efficacy and rapid onset of action. This drug should be considered in patients with severe or recalcitrant psoriasis requiring intermittent, short-term therapy for either induction of remission, rescue therapy, or maintenance and prevention of relapse. Experts consider CsA especially useful as a "bridge" therapy to other medications during critical relapses. For moderate-to-severe plaque psoriasis, CsA can be started at 4 to 5 mg/kg in 2 divided doses and reduced in 0.5 mg/kg/d increments. Alternatively, CsA may be initiated at dosages of 2.5-3 mg/kg/d and be administered in 2 divided doses.[1] Patients should be continued at a stable dosage within this range for 4 weeks, after which dosages may be increased by 0.5 mg/kg/d until remission. The upper limit of CsA per day is 5.0 mg/kg and normally should not be exceeded. Physicians should expect rapid improvement within 1 to 4 weeks. Long-term treatment with CsA is not recommended, and clinicians should opt to switch to less toxic medications for continuous treatment for risk of side effects, mainly hypertension and nephrotoxicity.

REFERENCES

1. Menter A, Korman NJ, Elmets CA, et al. Guidelines of care for the management of psoriasis and psoriatic arthritis: section 4. Guidelines of care for the management and treatment of psoriasis with traditional systemic agents. J Am Acad Dermatol 2009; 61:451–85.
2. Mueller W, Herrmann B. Cyclosporin A for psoriasis. N Engl J Med 1979;301:555.
3. Wolverton SE. Comprehensive dermatologic drug therapy. 3rd edition. Edinburgh (Germany): Saunders/Elsevier; 2013. p. xxii, 826.
4. Singh AK, Narsipur SS. Cyclosporine: a commentary on brand versus generic formulation exchange. J Transpl 2011;2011:480642.
5. Wong RL, Winslow CM, Cooper KD. The mechanisms of action of cyclosporin A in the treatment of psoriasis. Immunol Today 1993;14:69–74.
6. Berth-Jones J, Henderson CA, Munro CS, et al. Treatment of psoriasis with intermittent short course cyclosporin (Neoral). A multicentre study. Br J Dermatol 1997;136:527–30.

7. Faerber L, Braeutigam M, Weidinger G, et al. Cyclosporine in severe psoriasis. Results of a meta-analysis in 579 patients. Am J Clin Dermatol 2001; 2:41–7.
8. Colombo MD, Cassano N, Bellia G, et al. Cyclosporine regimens in plaque psoriasis: an overview with special emphasis on dose, duration, and old and new treatment approaches. ScientificWorldJournal 2013;2013:805705.
9. Flytstrom I, Stenberg B, Svensson A, et al. Methotrexate vs. ciclosporin in psoriasis: effectiveness, quality of life and safety. A randomized controlled trial. Br J Dermatol 2008;158:116–21.
10. Heydendael VM, Spuls PI, Opmeer BC, et al. Methotrexate versus cyclosporine in moderate-to-severe chronic plaque psoriasis. N Engl J Med 2003;349: 658–65.
11. Ho VC, Griffiths CE, Albrecht G, et al. Intermittent short courses of cyclosporin (Neoral(R)) for psoriasis unresponsive to topical therapy: a 1-year multicentre, randomized study. The PISCES Study Group. Br J Dermatol 1999;141:283–91.
12. Ho VC, Griffiths CE, Berth-Jones J, et al. Intermittent short courses of cyclosporine microemulsion for the long-term management of psoriasis: a 2-year cohort study. J Am Acad Dermatol 2001;44: 643–51.
13. Colombo D, Cassano N, Altomare G, et al. Psoriasis relapse evaluation with week-end cyclosporine A treatment: results of a randomized, double-blind, multicenter study. Int J Immunopathol Pharmacol 2010;23:1143–52.
14. Chaidemenos GC, Mourellou O, Avgoustinaki N, et al. Intermittent vs. continuous 1-year cyclosporin use in chronic plaque psoriasis. J Eur Acad Dermatol Venereol 2007;21:1203–8.
15. Lowe NJ, Wieder JM, Rosenbach A, et al. Long-term low-dose cyclosporine therapy for severe psoriasis: effects on renal function and structure. J Am Acad Dermatol 1996;35:710–9.
16. Mrowietz U, Farber L, Henneicke-von Zepelin HH, et al. Long-term maintenance therapy with cyclosporine and posttreatment survey in severe psoriasis: results of a multicenter study. German Multicenter Study. J Am Acad Dermatol 1995;33: 470–5.
17. Shupack J, Abel E, Bauer E, et al. Cyclosporine as maintenance therapy in patients with severe psoriasis. J Am Acad Dermatol 1997;36:423–32.
18. Koo J. A randomized, double-blind study comparing the efficacy, safety and optimal dose of two formulations of cyclosporin, Neoral and Sandimmun, in patients with severe psoriasis. OLP302 Study Group. Br J Dermatol 1998;139:88–95.
19. Hashizume H, Ito T, Yagi H, et al. Efficacy and safety of preprandial versus postprandial administration of low-dose cyclosporin microemulsion (Neoral) in patients with psoriasis vulgaris. J Dermatol 2007; 34:430–4.
20. Shintani Y, Kaneko N, Furuhashi T, et al. Safety and efficacy of a fixed-dose cyclosporin microemulsion (100 mg) for the treatment of psoriasis. J Dermatol 2011;38:966–72.
21. Gottlieb SL, Heftler NS, Gilleaudeau P, et al. Short-contact anthralin treatment augments therapeutic efficacy of cyclosporine in psoriasis: a clinical and pathologic study. J Am Acad Dermatol 1995;33: 637–45.
22. Griffiths CE, Powles AV, McFadden J, et al. Long-term cyclosporin for psoriasis. Br J Dermatol 1989; 120:253–60.
23. Grossman RM, Thivolet J, Claudy A, et al. A novel therapeutic approach to psoriasis with combination calcipotriol ointment and very low-dose cyclosporine: results of a multicenter placebo-controlled study. J Am Acad Dermatol 1994;31:68–74.
24. Clark CM, Kirby B, Morris AD, et al. Combination treatment with methotrexate and cyclosporin for severe recalcitrant psoriasis. Br J Dermatol 1999;141: 279–82.
25. Ameen M, Smith HR, Barker JN. Combined mycophenolate mofetil and cyclosporin therapy for severe recalcitrant psoriasis. Clin Exp Dermatol 2001; 26:480–3.
26. Colombo D, Chimenti S, Grossi PA, et al. Efficacy of cyclosporine A as monotherapy in patients with psoriatic arthritis: a subgroup analysis of the synergy study. G Ital Dermatol Venereol 2016. [Epub ahead of print].
27. Spadaro A, Riccieri V, Sili-Scavalli A, et al. Comparison of cyclosporin A and methotrexate in the treatment of psoriatic arthritis: a one-year prospective study. Clin Exp Rheumatol 1995;13:589–93.
28. Stein CM, Pincus T. Combination treatment of rheumatoid arthritis with cyclosporine and methotrexate. Clin Exp Rheumatol 1999;17:S47–52.
29. Taler SJ, Textor SC, Canzanello VJ, et al. Cyclosporin-induced hypertension: incidence, pathogenesis and management. Drug Saf 1999;20:437–49.
30. Paul CF, Ho VC, McGeown C, et al. Risk of malignancies in psoriasis patients treated with cyclosporine: a 5 y cohort study. J Invest Dermatol 2003; 120:211–6.
31. Ryan C, Amor KT, Menter A. The use of cyclosporine in dermatology: part II. J Am Acad Dermatol 2010; 63:949–72 [quiz: 73–4].
32. Bae YS, Van Voorhees AS, Hsu S, et al. Review of treatment options for psoriasis in pregnant or lactating women: from the Medical Board of the National Psoriasis Foundation. J Am Acad Dermatol 2012;67:459–77.
33. Lamarque V, Leleu MF, Monka C, et al. Analysis of 629 pregnancy outcomes in transplant recipients treated with Sandimmun. Transplant Proc 1997;29:2480.

34. Edmonds EV, Morris SD, Short K, et al. Pustular psoriasis of pregnancy treated with ciclosporin and high-dose prednisolone. Clin Exp Dermatol 2005; 30:709–10.
35. Armenti VT, McGrory CH, Cater JR, et al. Pregnancy outcomes in female renal transplant recipients. Transplant Proc 1998;30:1732–4.
36. Nyberg G, Haljamae U, Frisenette-Fich C, et al. Breast-feeding during treatment with cyclosporine. Transplantation 1998;65:253–5.
37. Thiru Y, Bateman DN, Coulthard MG. Successful breast feeding while mother was taking cyclosporin. BMJ 1997;315:463.
38. Bulbul Baskan E, Yazici S, Tunali S, et al. Clinical experience with systemic cyclosporine A treatment in severe childhood psoriasis. J Dermatolog Treat 2016;27:328–31.
39. Di Lernia V, Stingeni L, Boccaletti V, et al. Effectiveness and safety of cyclosporine in pediatric plaque psoriasis: a multicentric retrospective analysis. J Dermatolog Treat 2015;1–4.
40. DI Lernia V, Neri I, Calzavara Pinton P, et al. Treatment patterns with systemic antipsoriatic agents in childhood psoriasis: an Italian database analysis. G Ital Dermatol Venereol 2016. [Epub ahead of print].
41. Versluis DJ, Beyer WE, Masurel N, et al. Impairment of the immune response to influenza vaccination in renal transplant recipients by cyclosporine, but not azathioprine. Transplantation 1986;42: 376–9.
42. Lebwohl M, Ellis C, Gottlieb A, et al. Cyclosporine consensus conference: with emphasis on the treatment of psoriasis. J Am Acad Dermatol 1998;39: 464–7.
43. Meffert H, Brautigam M, Farber L, et al. Low-dose (1.25 mg/kg) cyclosporin A: treatment of psoriasis and investigation of the influence on lipid profile. Acta Derm Venereol 1997;77:137–41.
44. Laburte C, Grossman R, Abi-Rached J, et al. Efficacy and safety of oral cyclosporin A (CyA; Sandimmun) for long-term treatment of chronic severe plaque psoriasis. Br J Dermatol 1994;130:366–75.
45. Christophers E, Mrowietz U, Henneicke HH, et al. Cyclosporine in psoriasis: a multicenter dose-finding study in severe plaque psoriasis. The German Multicenter Study. J Am Acad Dermatol 1992;26:86–90.

CHAPTER 7

Apremilast

Amit Om, BS, Dane Hill, MD, Steven R. Feldman, MD, PhD

KEYWORDS

• Apremilast • Plaque psoriasis • Phosphodiesterase 4 • Psoriatic arthritis

KEY POINTS

- Apremilast is the first small molecule phosphodiesterase 4 (PDE4) inhibitor approved for treatment of moderate-to-severe plaque psoriasis.
- Apremilast, in contrast to biologics, is not injectable, and its label does not require monitoring or screening for tuberculosis.
- Apremilast is the first selective PDE4 inhibitor that is US Food and Drug Administration approved for the treatment of active psoriatic arthritis.
- Apremilast has a favorable safety profile so far, and it can be used in patients with comorbidities that preclude use of other systemic medications.

INTRODUCTION

Apremilast, approved by the US Food and Drug Administration (FDA) in 2014, is the first phosphodiesterase 4 (PDE4) inhibitor approved to treat psoriatic arthritis (PsA) and moderate-to-severe psoriasis.[1–5] Biologics have revolutionized the treatment of psoriasis. They are more effective and safer than the oral options previously available. Biologics may not be the preferred systemic psoriasis treatment for every patient, however, because side effects include injection site reactions, upper respiratory tract infections, infusion reactions, and risk of reactivation of tuberculosis.[6] They may also be limited by their high cost as well as their need to be injected as the route of administration. Nevertheless, patient adherence to biologics used in psoriasis may be as low as 33%.[7] Some patients prefer an oral medication; 1 study found 93% of patients chose oral medication administration over injectable agents, assuming equal drug efficacy.[8]

Apremilast may be a good choice for patients who prefer a relatively safe oral treatment, and for patients in whom other therapies are contraindicated or become ineffective, such as those who develop antidrug antibodies against certain biologics. It is taken at home and offers the potential for better adherence for patients who may not be able to readily return to clinic for scheduled injections. It is an acceptable therapy for patients with certain medical comorbidities, especially renal, hepatic, or hematologic, where some biologics or traditional systemic psoriasis therapies may be contraindicated. It is also an acceptable therapy for patients with compromised immunity, such as those with human immunodeficiency virus (HIV). In addition, apremilast can be safely combined with several systemic psoriasis treatments for greater efficacy.[1]

Apremilast is being tested for treatment of other diseases. Currently, there are clinical trials testing apremilast in patients affected by cutaneous lupus, lichen planus, cutaneous sarcoidosis, atopic dermatitis, ankylosing spondylitis, prostatitis, vulvodynia, osteoarthritis, rheumatoid arthritis, Behcet disease, and rosacea, because these diseases are thought to be affected to some degree by the same pathways apremilast acts on.[9]

MECHANISM OF ACTION

Apremilast is a selective inhibitor of PDE4. Phosphodiesterases facilitate the breakdown of cyclic adenosine 3′,5′-monophosphate (cAMP).[2] Thus, by blocking PDE4, intracellular cAMP levels increase, reducing proinflammatory mediators, such as interferon-γ, tumor necrosis factor-α (TNF-α), interleukin-12 (IL-12), IL-17, and IL-23. Increasing cAMP levels also increase anti-inflammatory cytokines such as IL-10 (Fig. 7.1).[10] Specifically, the increased intracellular accumulation of cAMP activates protein kinase A (PKA)

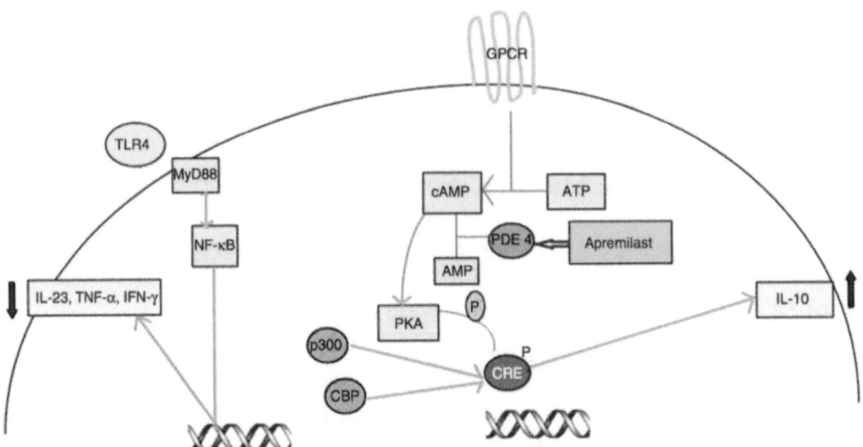

Fig. 7.1 Mechanism of action of apremilast. Apremilast blocks PDE4, thus increasing the intracellular cAMP, which ultimately activates PKA and leads to an anti-inflammatory effect.

and phosphorylates the cAMP-response element binding protein, which suppresses the transcription of numerous proinflammatory cytokines, exerting an overall anti-inflammatory effect.[11] The increased cAMP downregulates myeloid dendritic cells as well as T helper 1 and T helper 2 immune responses. This downregulation decreases immune cell infiltration in the epidermis and dermis of psoriatic lesions and causes a reduction in gene expression of numerous cytokines (IL-12/IL-23p40, IL-22, IL-8, β-defensin 4, myxovirus resistance protein 1, IL-17A, and IL-23p19).[12] The systemic effects of PDE4 inhibition may lead to some of the side effects seen with apremilast, such as weight loss.[13] In contrast to TNF-α inhibitors, such as infliximab or adalimumab, which bind directly to TNF-α, PDE4 inhibitors inhibit TNF-α production at the level of gene expression and do not completely suppress TNF-α levels; this leads to a decrease of proinflammatory mediators, but not complete inhibition.[14]

EFFICACY

The efficacy of apremilast on plaque psoriasis has been tested in 2 separate phase 3 trials. ESTEEM 1 and ESTEEM 2 included 1257 patients 18 years of age or older with moderate-to-severe plaque psoriasis. Moderate-to-severe plaque disease was defined by body surface area involvement of 10% or greater; static Physicians' Global Assessment (sPGA) score of 3 or greater (moderate or severe disease); Psoriasis Area and Severity Index (PASI) score 12 or greater; and candidates for phototherapy or systemic therapy.[2] Both studies assessed the proportion of patients who achieved PASI-75 at week 16 and those who achieved an sPGA score of either 0 (cleared disease) or 1 (minimal disease) at week 16. In the ESTEEM 1 trial, a total of 844 patients were studied over 52 weeks, divided into 3 periods. Period A looked at apremilast 30 mg twice daily versus placebo from 0 to 16 weeks; patients were randomized 2:1, apremilast:placebo. Period B ranged from week 16 to 32 and replaced the initial placebo with apremilast. Period C rerandomized patients who started with apremilast initially and showed a PASI-75 or greater at week 32 to placebo or apremilast (Fig. 7.2). At 16 weeks, more patients who received apremilast achieved a PASI-75 compared with placebo (33.1% vs 5.3%, respectively; $P<.001$). Furthermore, more patients who received apremilast (21.7%) achieved an sPGA score of 0 or 1 compared with placebo (3.9%). Achieved response rates were maintained well at week 32.[12] Long-term efficacy was reported as the percentage of patients who were still on drug. Of the 844 original patients randomized, 314 patients that had received at least 1 dose of apremilast discontinued the study by week 52, with 124 patients citing "lack of efficacy" as the reason for discontinuing. When determining long-term efficacy rates, those with PASI-75 out of the only the remaining patients in the study were used in calculating reported PASI-75 rates, which yielded a higher efficacy rate than would have been reported if all patients who started on drug were included in the denominator. In ESTEEM 1, of all the patients exposed to apremilast at any period of the study, including those who discontinued the study, 18.7% were at PASI-75 at week 52.

In the ESTEEM 2 trial, a total of 411 patients were studied. Patients were initially randomized

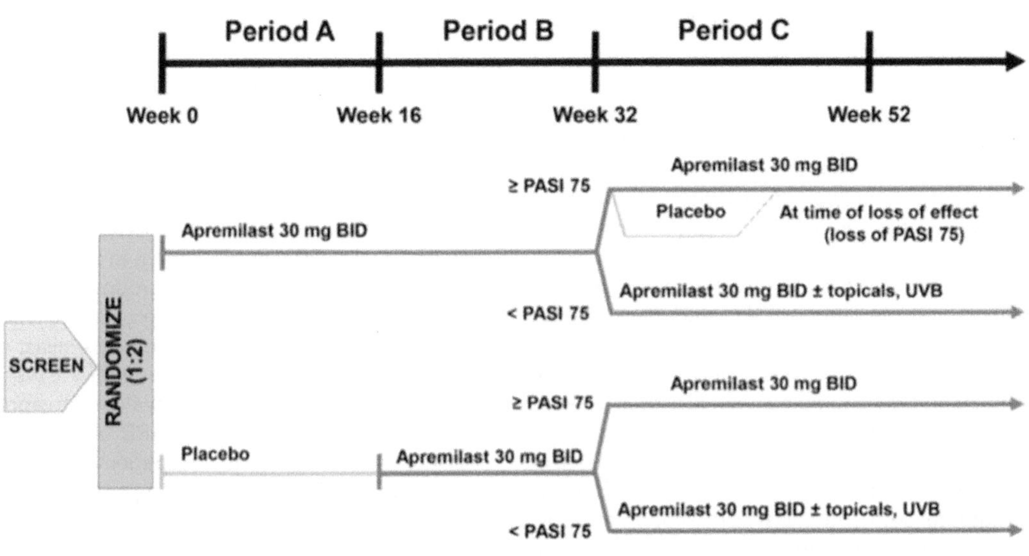

Fig. 7.2 Study design of ESTEEM-1. Period A: Patients were randomized to either apremilast 30 mg twice daily or placebo for the first 16 weeks. Period B: At 16 weeks, all patients were given apremilast 30 mg twice daily until week 32. Period C: At this point, in the initial group randomized to apremilast 30 mg twice daily, patients were further randomized to either apremilast 30 mg twice daily or placebo if more than a PASI-75 response was achieved. If loss of effect occurred in the placebo group, they were reinstated on apremilast 30 mg twice daily.

2:1, apremilast:placebo, and at week 16, all patients were switched to apremilast. At week 32, patients were evaluated for PASI-50 or greater, and patients who met these criteria were randomized 1:1 to receive apremilast or placebo (Fig. 7.3). At week 16, more patients who received apremilast achieved a PASI-75 compared with placebo (28.8% vs 5.8%). In addition, more patients who

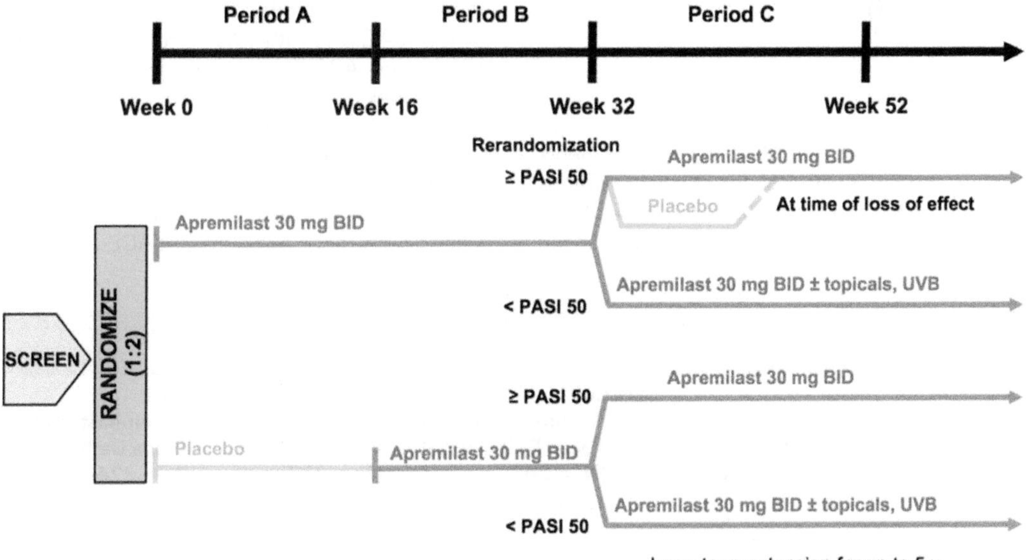

Fig. 7.3 Study design of ESTEEM-2. Period A: Patients were randomized to either apremilast 30 mg twice daily or placebo for the first 16 weeks. Period B: At 16 weeks, all patients were given apremilast 30 mg twice daily until week 32. Period C: At this point, in the initial group randomized to apremilast 30 mg twice daily, patients were further randomized to either apremilast 30 mg twice daily or placebo if more than a PASI-50 response was achieved. If loss of effect occurred in the placebo group, they were reinstated on apremilast 30 mg twice daily.

received apremilast achieved an sPGA of clear or almost clear compared with placebo (20.4% vs 4.4%, respectively; *P*<.001). The response was sustained over 52 weeks without significant adverse effects[15] (Table 7.1). As with ESTEEM 1, the long-term results from the ESTEEM 2 study were reported based only on the subjects remaining in the study. Of the original 411 randomized patients, 115 that had received at least 1 dose of the drug discontinued the study before 1 year. Of the 115 patients that discontinued, 47 cited "lack of efficacy" as the reason.

Apremilast has been retrospectively studied in combination with multiple systemic psoriasis treatments, including narrowband (NB)-UV-B, methotrexate, acitretin, cyclosporine, etanercept, adalimumab, infliximab, or ustekinumab. Efficacy was greater with apremilast combination therapy than with either treatment modality alone.[1] It was slightly less effective than etanercept 50 mg in clearing psoriasis, as measured by PASI-75 response at 16 weeks. In an ongoing phase III trial comparing apremilast to etanercept and placebo, 48% of etanercept patients and 40% of apremilast patients achieved PASI-75 at week 16.[16] The higher efficacy rate in this study (40%) than in the ESTEEM trials may be due to a less severe population because these patients were biologically naïve (whereas in ESTEEM, many of the subjects had previously failed biological treatment). A single case report combining apremilast and adalimumab resulted in an almost clearing of severe, biologic-resistant plaque psoriasis.[17]

EFFICACY IN PSORIATIC ARTHRITIS

The efficacy in PsA has been studied in 3 trials, known as the PALACE-1, -2, and -3 trials. Patients 18 years and older with PsA for at least 6 months were included. Subjects had to have been inadequately treated with disease-modifying antirheumatic drugs (DMARDs) and have a swollen joint count (SJC) greater than or equal to 3 and tender joint count (TJC) greater than or equal to 3.[18] The design of the study was similar to the ESTEEM trials: patients were initially randomized (1:1:1) to placebo, apremilast 20 mg twice daily, or apremilast 30 mg twice daily. After 16 weeks, if patients did not experience a greater than or equal to 20% improvement in SJC or TJC and were initially in the placebo group, they were rerandomized to apremilast 20 mg or 30 mg twice daily. If the patient was already on apremilast at 16 weeks, the course was continued. At week 24, all patients on placebo were switched to apremilast. Concurrent biologic DMARD use was not allowed. PALACE-3 required patients to have one greater than or equal to 2 cm psoriatic lesion as well as the SJC and TJC criteria.[18]

The primary endpoint in the studies was ACR20, which means a 20% improvement in modified American College of Rheumatology (ACR) response criteria at week 16.[19] A 50% and 70% improvement in response criteria (ACR50 and ACR70, respectively) were additional endpoints. In PALACE-1, 38.1% patients on apremilast 30 mg twice daily achieved ACR20 versus 19.0% placebo at week 16. In addition, 16.1% achieved ACR50 and 4.2% achieved ACR70 at 16 weeks. At week 24, 45.3% of patients achieved ACR20. By week 52, 54.6%, 24.6%, and 13.8% of patients achieved ARC20, ARC50, and ARC70, respectively.[20] In PALACE-2, at week 16, 32.1% of patients on apremilast versus 18.9% on placebo achieved ACR20, with 10.5% and 1.2% achieving ARC50 and ARC70, respectively. In PALACE-3, at 16 weeks 40.7% of patients on apremilast achieved ACR20, whereas 18.3% on placebo did so, with 15% and 3.6% achieving ARC50 and ARC70, respectively[14] (Table 7.2). The ARC20 response was sustained through 52 weeks as well: 52.6% and 63% in PALACE-2 and -3,

TABLE 7.1
Clinical response at 16 weeks of apremilast versus placebo in ESTEEM-1 and ESTEEM-2 trials

Clinical Response	ESTEEM-1 Placebo, N (%) (N = 282)	ESTEEM-1 Apremilast 30 mg Twice Daily, N (%) (N = 562)	ESTEEM-2 Placebo, N (%) (N = 137)	ESTEEM-2 Apremilast 30 mg Twice Daily, N (%) (N = 274)
PASI-75	15 (5.3)	186 (33.1)	8 (5.8)	79 (28.8)
sPGA of clear or almost clear	11 (3.9)	122 (21.7)	6 (4.4)	56 (20.4)

Data from Papp K, Reich K, Leonardi C, et al. Apremilast, an oral phosphodiesterase 4 (PDE4) inhibitor, in patients with moderate to severe plaque psoriasis: results of a phase III, randomized, controlled trial (Efficacy and Safety Trial Evaluating the Effects of Apremilast in Psoriasis [ESTEEM] 1). J Am Acad Dermatol 2015;73(1):37–49; and Paul C, Cather J, Gooderham M, et al. Efficacy and safety of apremilast, an oral phosphodiesterase 4 inhibitor, in patients with moderate-to-severe plaque psoriasis over 52 weeks: a phase III, randomized controlled trial (ESTEEM 2). Br J Dermatol 2015;173(6):1387–99.

TABLE 7.2
Clinical response at 16 weeks of apremilast versus placebo in PALACE-1, -2, and -3 trials

Patients Achieving ACR Response at Week 16	PALACE-1 Study		PALACE-2 Study		PALACE-3 Study	
	Placebo ± DMARDs (N = 168)	Apremilast[a] ± DMARDs (N = 168)	Placebo ± DMARDs (N = 159)	Apremilast[a] ± DMARDs (N = 162)	Placebo ± DMARDs (N = 169)	Apremilast[a] ± DMARDs (N = 167)
ACR20, %	19	38[b]	19	32[b]	18	41[b]
ACR50, %	6	16	5	11	8	15
ACR70, %	1	4	1	1	2	4

[a] Apremilast 30 mg twice daily.
[b] Significantly different from placebo (*P*<.05).
Data from Refs.[14,18,19]

respectively.[14] At week 52, ARC50 and ARC70 responses were well maintained at 18.6% and 6.8%, respectively, in PALACE-2, and 30.2% and 10.4%, respectively, in PALACE-3.

In 2 additional randomized trials, apremilast was statistically superior to placebo in achieving and maintaining ARC20.[21–27] Despite long-term efficacy of achieving ARC20 and improving PsA symptoms in several studies, apremilast may not reduce radiographic evidence of joint disease progression. Among patients with active PsA not well-controlled with methotrexate, apremilast was not more effective than placebo after 1 year at reducing joint disease, as measured with MRI.[28] Apremilast was effective against joint disease in 1 study of patients with ankylosing spondylitis, suggesting further radiographic studies are needed to assess the effect of apremilast on long-term joint disease.[29]

SAFETY

The therapeutic dosing of apremilast is 30 mg twice daily. To reduce gastrointestinal (GI) upset, apremilast is given a starter pack to up-titrate using the following schedule: day 1: 10 mg (AM); day 2: 10 mg (AM) and 10 mg (PM); day 3: 10 mg (AM) and 20 mg (PM); day 4: 20 mg (AM) and 20 mg (PM); day 5: 20 mg (AM) and 30 mg (PM); and day 6: 30 mg (AM) and 30 mg (PM).[2] The medication can be taken with food without any decrease in absorption.[30]

Some of the metabolic pathways used in the breakdown of apremilast involve the cytochrome P450 (CYP450) system. As such, the concentration of apremilast will be reduced by inducers of CYP450, such as phenytoin, rifampicin, and St John's wort. Therefore, when using with other CYP450 enzyme inducers, patients and providers should be cognizant of the reduced effect. On the other hand, inhibitors of CYP450, such as ketoconazole, do not significantly increase the concentration.[31] The elimination half-life is about 9 hours.[18] Apremilast metabolites are excreted in the urine. For patients with renal impairment (defined as creatinine clearance <30 mL per minute), the recommended dose is 30 mg daily, as opposed to twice daily. Initially, when starting the medicine, titrate using the AM schedule only as above.[9] Because of the renal clearance, there is no need to adjust the dose for hepatic impairment.[13]

The major side effects seen in trials have been diarrhea, nausea, and weight loss. No significant serious infections and no reactivation of tuberculosis have been reported.[10]

Apremilast has a favorable safety profile to this point, even in combination with other drugs for psoriasis.[1] Many psoriasis patients on biologics become refractory to treatment. Up to 20% to 30% of patients on biologic agents can experience "biologic fatigue"; therefore, combining therapies may be a beneficial approach.[32] In 1 study combining apremilast with another therapy (either NB-UV-B, methotrexate, acitretin, cyclosporine, etanercept, adalimumab, infliximab, or ustekinumab), 14 patients of 81 (17%) discontinued treatment before completion of 12 weeks of apremilast therapy. Of the subjects who completed the 12-week trial, 25% experienced nausea and diarrhea, while 15% had weight loss.[1]

PRECAUTIONS

The most common side effects associated with apremilast are diarrhea in 14% of patients, nausea in 12%, headache in 10%, and upper respiratory tract infections in 10%[14] (Box 7.1). The GI side effects were usually mild and self-limited. The median onset of diarrhea was 9 days and lasted an average of 29.5 days. The median onset of nausea was 10 days and lasted an average of 17 days.[15] The most serious side effects were GI clostridial

BOX 7.1
Side effects of apremilast

Common side effects (>3%)
Diarrhea
Nausea
Upper respiratory tract infections
Headaches
Weight loss
Abdominal pain
Vomiting
Fatigue
Dyspepsia
Decreased appetite

Rare side effects (<2%)
Insomnia
Back pain
Migraine
Bronchitis
Tooth abscess
Folliculitis
Severe diarrhea
Severe nausea
GI clostridial infection
Pneumonia

Do not use apremilast in pregnancy due to teratogenicity. It is OK during breast-feeding.

infection in 1 patient and pneumonia in another.[19] Discontinuation due to side effects was rare and occurred in 7% of patients taking apremilast.[30] Patients stopped in 1.6% of cases due to nausea, 1.0% due to diarrhea, and 0.8% due to headache, and 4.1% of placebo patients discontinued.[2]

Weight loss of 5% to 10% was observed in 12% of patients treated with 30 mg twice daily versus 5% treated with placebo. Weight loss greater than 10% was seen in 2% of patients on apremilast versus 1% of patients on placebo.[20] This weight loss was noted in patients at any time during the controlled period of the trial. The weight loss is unrelated to diarrhea,[33–35] but may be viewed as a beneficial side effect by some patients.[14] Apremilast is associated with a slightly increased risk of depression. In the 3 PALACE trials, 1.0% of patients treated with apremilast reported depression or depressed mood compared with 0.8% treated with placebo, although 4 patients (0.3%) in the apremilast group discontinued treatment because of depression or depressed mood compared with none among placebo-treated patients.[2,20]

In the PALACE trials for PsA, the most common adverse effects were similar to those in the plaque psoriasis studies: GI symptoms such as diarrhea and nausea.[20] Diarrhea was reported in 14.3% of patients, and 12.6% reported nausea.[14] Although 57.1% experienced some weight loss, 75.8% of patients remained within 5% of baseline weight.[14] Discontinuation was infrequent and due to diarrhea (1.8%), nausea (1.8%), and headache (1.2%) in PALACE-1 trial.[2]

MONITORING

Before initiating therapy, a thorough history should be taken, and education provided to patients about potential side effects. There is no requirement to screen for tuberculosis. In patients with a history of moderate-severe renal impairment, a creatinine clearance should be obtained at baseline.

Apremilast is contraindicated in patients with a known hypersensitivity to apremilast or to any of the ingredients in the formulation.[2] Pregnancy is a contraindication; however, apremilast is acceptable to use while breast-feeding.[2] With a half-life of up to about 9 hours, becoming pregnant would result in little to no apremilast exposure after 3 days of stopping treatment.

VACCINATIONS

There is currently no indication to avoid inactivated or live vaccines while on apremilast. Although no trials have studied this, specifically, patients in large clinical trials incidentally given live vaccines while on apremilast did not experience more side effects than those not given apremilast.[13]

SUMMARY AND RECOMMENDATIONS

- Approved in 2014, apremilast is the first and only PDE4 inhibitor for both PsA and moderate-to-severe plaque psoriasis.
- Apremilast is an appropriate first-line systemic treatment for moderate-to-severe psoriasis. It is an especially good choice for patients who would prefer a relatively safe oral treatment and who are not concerned about the lower efficacy rate compared with biologics.
- Apremilast is an efficacious option compared with placebo, offering statistically significant PASI-75 scores in 2 psoriasis trials used for approval.

- Because apremilast is an oral medication, it is beneficial for those averse to injections, and it has a potential role in the pediatric population in the future.
- It is acceptable for use in patients with other comorbidities (renal, hepatic, or hematologic diseases), or in patients with compromised immunity, such as those with HIV.
- The side-effect profile is advantageous in that the major effects only include diarrhea, nausea, and slight weight loss. It is also safe to use in combination with other psoriasis therapies.
- Apremilast is an effective and safe therapy for treatment of psoriatic arthritis, especially for those patients who have failed DMARDs and biologics.
- Currently, studies are being done to expand its use to other diseases, such as ankylosing spondylitis, lichen planus, cutaneous lupus, and cutaneous sarcoidosis.

REFERENCES

1. AbuHilal M, Walsh S, Shear N. Use of apremilast in combination with other therapies for treatment of chronic plaque psoriasis: a retrospective study. J Cutan Med Surg 2016;20(4):313–6.
2. Fala L. Otezla (apremilast), an oral PDE-4 inhibitor, receives FDA approval for the treatment of patients with active psoriatic arthritis and plaque psoriasis. Am Health Drug Benefits 2015;8(Special Feature): 105–10.
3. Menter A, Korman N, Elmets C, et al. Guidelines of care for the management of psoriasis and psoriatic arthritis. J Am Acad Dermatol 2011;65(1): 137–74.
4. Menter A, Korman N, Elmets C, et al. Guidelines of care for the management of psoriasis and psoriatic arthritis. J Am Acad Dermatol 2009;60(4):643–59.
5. Lebwohl M. A clinician's paradigm in the treatment of psoriasis. J Am Acad Dermatol 2005; 53(1):S59–69.
6. Scherer K, Spoerl D, Bircher AJ. Adverse drug reactions to biologics. J Dtsch Dermatol Ges 2010;8(6): 411–26.
7. Thorneloe R, Bundy C, Griffiths C, et al. Adherence to medication in patients with psoriasis: a systematic literature review. Br J Dermatol 2012;168(1): 20–31.
8. Utz K, Hoog J, Wentrup A, et al. Patient preferences for disease-modifying drugs in multiple sclerosis therapy: a choice-based conjoint analysis. Ther Adv Neurol Disord 2014;7(6):263–75.
9. Otezla® [package insert]. Summit, NJ: Celgene Corporation; 2014.
10. Papp K, Kaufmann R, Thaçi D, et al. Efficacy and safety of apremilast in subjects with moderate to severe plaque psoriasis: results from a phase II, multicenter, randomized, double-blind, placebo-controlled, parallel-group, dose-comparison study. J Eur Acad Dermatol Venereol 2012;27(3): e376–83.
11. Perez-Aso M, Montesinos M, Mediero A, et al. Apremilast, a novel phosphodiesterase 4 (PDE4) inhibitor, regulates inflammation through multiple cAMP downstream effectors. Arthritis Res Ther 2015;17(1):249.
12. Papp K, Reich K, Leonardi C, et al. Apremilast, an oral phosphodiesterase 4 (PDE4) inhibitor, in patients with moderate to severe plaque psoriasis: results of a phase III, randomized, controlled trial (Efficacy and Safety Trial Evaluating the Effects of Apremilast in Psoriasis [ESTEEM] 1). J Am Acad Dermatol 2015;73(1):37–49.
13. Summary of the risk management plan (RMP) for Otezla (apremilast) [Internet]. 1st edition. European Medicines Agency; Celgene Europe Limited; 2016. Available at: http://www.ema.europa.eu/docs/en_GB/document_library/EPAR_-_Risk-management-plan_summary/human/003746/WC500177381.pdf.
14. Busa S, Kavanaugh A. Drug safety evaluation of apremilast for treating psoriatic arthritis. Expert Opin Drug Saf 2015;14(6):979–85.
15. Paul C, Cather J, Gooderham M, et al. Efficacy and safety of apremilast, an oral phosphodiesterase 4 inhibitor, in patients with moderate-to-severe plaque psoriasis over 52 weeks: a phase III, randomized controlled trial (ESTEEM 2). Br J Dermatol 2015; 173(6):1387–99.
16. Positive Results from Phase III Study Evaluating Oral OTEZLA® (Apremilast) or Injectable Etanercept versus Placebo in Patients with Moderate to Severe Plaque Psoriasis Presented at AAD. Available at: http://ir.celgene.com/releasedetail.cfm?releaseid=902701. Accessed April 6, 2016.
17. Danesh MJ, Beroukhim K, Nguyen C, et al. Apremilast and adalimumab: a novel combination therapy for recalcitrant psoriasis. Dermatol Online J 2015; 21(6).
18. Deeks E. Apremilast: a review in psoriasis and psoriatic arthritis. Drugs 2015;75(12):1393–403.
19. Kavanaugh A, Mease PJ, Gomez-Reino JJ, et al. Treatment of psoriatic arthritis in a phase 3 randomised, placebo-controlled trial with apremilast, an oral phosphodiesterase 4 inhibitor. Ann Rheum Dis 2014;73:1020–6.
20. Danesh M, Beroukhim K, Nguyen C, et al. Apremilast and adalimumab: a novel combination therapy for recalcitrant psoriasis. Dermatol Online J 2015; 21(6).
21. Menter A, Gottlieb A, Feldman S, et al. Guidelines of care for the management of psoriasis and

psoriatic arthritis. J Am Acad Dermatol 2008;58(5): 826–50.

22. Menter A, Korman N, Elmets C, et al. Guidelines of care for the management of psoriasis and psoriatic arthritis. J Am Acad Dermatol 2009;61(3):451–85.
23. Roenigk H, Auerbach R, Maibach H, et al. Methotrexate in psoriasis: revised guidelines. J Am Acad Dermatol 1988;19(1):145–56.
24. Maza A, Montaudié H, Sbidian E, et al. Oral cyclosporin in psoriasis: a systematic review on treatment modalities, risk of kidney toxicity and evidence for use in non-plaque psoriasis. J Eur Acad Dermatol Venereol 2011;25:19–27.
25. Sandoval L, Pierce A, Feldman S. Systemic therapies for psoriasis: an evidence-based update. Am J Clin Dermatol 2014;15(3):165–80.
26. FDA approves new psoriasis drug Cosentyx [Internet]. Fda.gov. 2015. Available at: http://www.fda.gov/NewsEvents/Newsroom/PressAnnouncements/ucm430969.htm. Accessed March 31, 2016.
27. Gooderham M, Papp K. Apremilast in the treatment of psoriasis and psoriatic arthritis. Skintherapyletter.com. 2016. Available at: http://www.skintherapyletter.com/2015/20.5/1.html. Accessed March 31, 2016.
28. Schett G, Wollenhaupt J, Papp K, et al. Oral apremilast in the treatment of active psoriatic arthritis: results of a multicenter, randomized, double-blind, placebo-controlled study. Arthritis Rheum 2012;64(10):3156–67.
29. Genovese MC, Jarosova K, Cieślak D, et al. Apremilast in patients with active rheumatoid arthritis: a phase II, multicenter, randomized, double-blind, placebo-controlled, parallel-group study. Arthritis Rheumatol 2015;67:1703–10.
30. Pathan E, Abraham S, Van Rossen E, et al. Efficacy and safety of apremilast, an oral phosphodiesterase 4 inhibitor, in ankylosing spondylitis. Ann Rheum Dis 2013;72:1475–80.
31. Zerilli T, Ocheretyaner E. Apremilast (Otezla): a new oral treatment for adults with psoriasis and psoriatic arthritis. P T 2015;40(8):495–500.
32. New drugs: apremilast. Aust Prescr 2015;38(4): 177–82.
33. Levin E, Gupta R, Brown G, et al. Biologic fatigue in psoriasis. J Dermatolog Treat 2014;25(1):78–82.
34. Reich K, Langley R, Lebwohl M, et al. Cardiovascular safety of ustekinumab in patients with moderate to severe psoriasis: results of integrated analyses of data from phase II and III clinical studies. Br J Dermatol 2011;164(4):862–72.
35. Abdulrahim H, Thistleton S, Adebajo A, et al. Apremilast: a PDE4 inhibitor for the treatment of psoriatic arthritis. Expert Opin Pharmacother 2015; 16(7):1099–108.

CHAPTER 8

Etanercept

Shivani P. Reddy, BS, Vidhi V. Shah, BA, Elaine J. Lin, MD, Jashin J. Wu, MD

KEYWORDS

• Etanercept • Enbrel • TNF-α • OBSERVE-5 • Biologic

KEY POINTS

- Etanercept is a soluble human dimeric fusion protein that competitively binds and inhibits tumor necrosis factor.
- Etanercept improved psoriatic skin lesions in phase 2 and phase 3 clinical trials.
- Etanercept can be used in pediatric and geriatric populations and is pregnancy category B.
- The most common side effects of etanercept are injection-site reactions and infection.

INTRODUCTION

Etanercept, a tumor necrosis factor (TNF) inhibitor, was a significant advancement in treatment of moderate-to-severe psoriasis. A quantum leap forward, etanercept provided a combination of efficacy and short- and long-term safety that was unmatched by the other available options at that time, better than systemic therapies, such as methotrexate (MTX), cyclosporine, and psoralen and UV-A radiation (PUVA).[1] Etanercept was the first TNF inhibitor approved by the US Food and Drug Administration (FDA) for plaque psoriasis (May 2004) and is also approved for the treatment of rheumatoid arthritis (RA), polyarticular juvenile idiopathic arthritis, psoriatic arthritis, and ankylosing spondylitis.[2] It is effective for erythrodermic and pustular psoriasis as well.[3]

The current recommended dosing of etanercept is 50 mg twice weekly (BIW) for the first 12 weeks, followed by a 50-mg weekly maintenance dose (Fig. 8.1).[2] If the patient prefers, doses of 25 mg weekly or 50 mg weekly are efficacious as well.[2] Etanercept is effective in the pediatric psoriasis population, at a dose of 0.8 mg/kg (up to a maximum of 50 mg) once weekly.[4] Etanercept is available as a single-use prefilled syringe and a single-use prefilled SureClick autoinjector, which patients may subcutaneously self-inject after appropriate training if deemed capable by the dermatologist.[2]

Recommended injection sites for etanercept include the abdomen (excluding a 2-inch circumference surrounding the navel), the front of the middle thighs, and the outer upper arms. Injection sites should be rotated each time, and areas of bruised or tender skin, or psoriatic lesions, should be avoided.[2]

The half-life of etanercept is 4.3 days, the shortest of all the TNF inhibitors approved for psoriasis,[5] which is a potential advantage in the setting of adverse events (AEs).[1] Concentrations peak in the system at 48 to 60 hours with a bioavailability of 58%.[5] Metabolism of etanercept is not decreased in the setting of renal or hepatic impairment,[6] and no dose adjustment is needed when administered alongside MTX, warfarin, or digoxin.[7–9]

Mechanism of Action

Etanercept, a fully soluble, human dimeric fusion protein, functions as a TNF inhibitor by competitively binding to TNF and preventing its activation of the inflammatory cascade. Etanercept is composed of 2 extracellular ligand-binding domains of the TNF p75 receptor linked to the Fc portion of human immunoglobulin G1 (IgG1) by 3 disulfide bonds.[2] Etanercept is a soluble form of the p75 receptor that inhibits TNF-α, and to some extent TNF-β, by blocking its interaction with cell-surface TNF receptors.[2] Etanercept is different from adalimumab and infliximab, which are monoclonal antibodies to TNF.[1] The dimeric structure of etanercept allows it to bind TNF at an affinity that is 50 to 1000 times greater than naturally occurring TNF receptors (Fig. 8.2).[10]

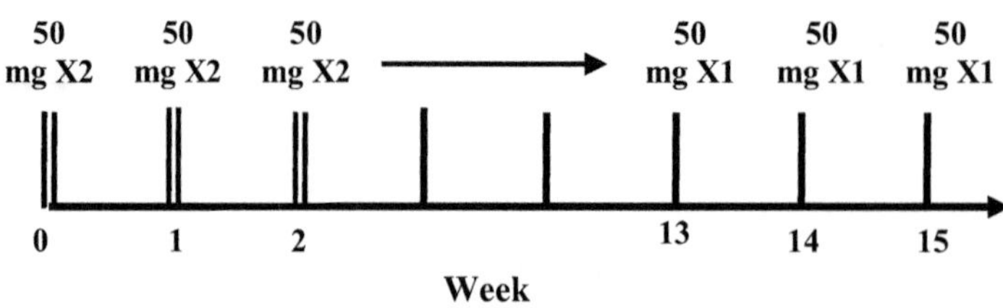

Fig. 8.1 Dosing of etanercept therapy for moderate-to-severe psoriasis. Recommended dosing of etanercept for the treatment of plaque psoriasis is 50 mg BIW for the first 12 weeks, followed by a 50-mg weekly maintenance dose.

Etanercept is a very large, complex glycoprotein. A batch of etanercept contains multiple variants with subtle differences; those variants can vary from batch to batch.[11] Etanercept is a mixture, and the mixture changes over time. Understanding that there is variation in the brand name etanercept product may be important in considering how etanercept biosimilars should be perceived.

By binding and sequestering TNF, etanercept modulates biologic responses involved in the pathogenesis of psoriasis, such as the expression of adhesion molecules that function in leukocyte migration (E-selectin and intercellular adhesion molecule-1), serum cytokine levels, and serum matrix metalloproteinase-3 levels.[2]

EFFICACY

Etanercept therapy improves psoriatic skin lesions considerably. Patients may show some loss of response after 12 weeks of therapy with the recommended step-down from 50 mg BIW to 50 mg weekly dosing.[12] Clearance is better maintained with uninterrupted therapy, although rebound does not typically occur with discontinuation of therapy.[13–15] There is a potential for loss of efficacy of etanercept therapy over long periods of time, possibly because of antibody development or poor adherence.[12]

Pivotal Trials

US psoriasis pivotal trial

A 24-week, phase 3, double-blinded study across 47 sites in the United States assessed the clinical response of etanercept monotherapy in patients with psoriasis (Fig. 8.3).[16] The primary measure of efficacy was the percentage of patients in each of the treatment groups who achieved a Psoriasis Area Severity Index (PASI) 75 score by week 12. The study population consisted of 652 patients with a mean psoriasis duration of 18.7 years,

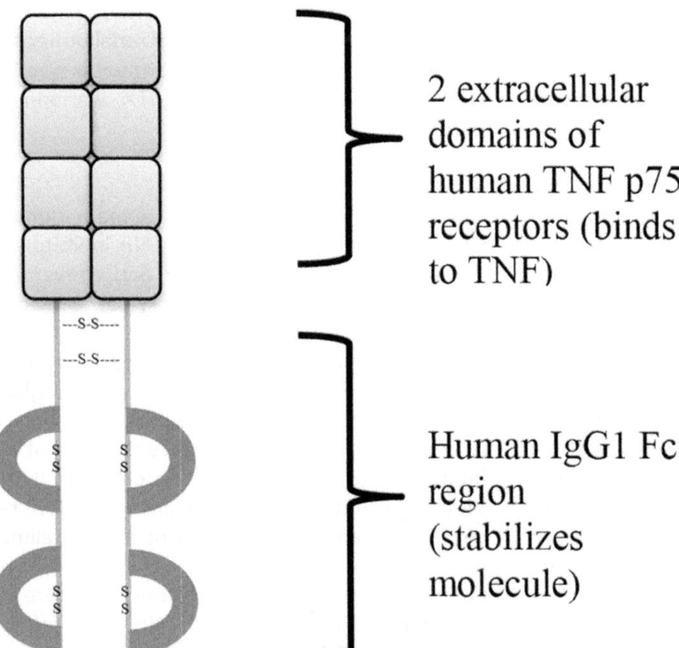

Fig. 8.2 Structure of etanercept.

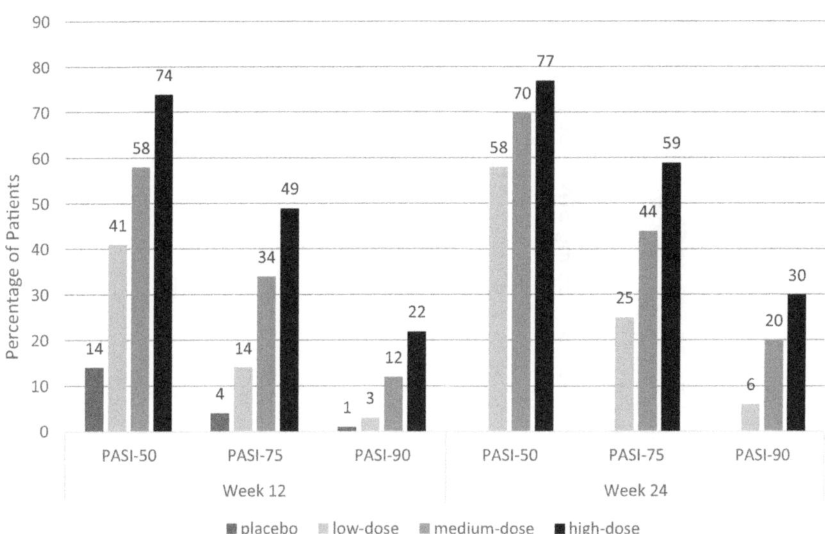

Fig. 8.3 Clinical responses to etanercept therapy from the US pivotal trial. Efficacy outcomes after 12 and 24 weeks of treatment with either placebo or low-dose (25 mg weekly), medium-dose (25 mg BIW), or high-dose etanercept therapy (50 mg BIW), defined as percentage of patients with psoriasis who met specified PASI response criteria for improvement (PASI-50, -75, -90).

a mean affected body surface area (BSA) of 28.7%, and a mean baseline PASI of 18.4.

During the first 12 weeks of this study, patients were randomized to receive either placebo, low-dose etanercept (25 mg weekly), medium-dose etanercept (25 mg BIW), or high-dose etanercept (50 mg BIW), in order to assess dose-dependent responses to therapy. At week 12, the placebo group then began to receive medium-dose etanercept as well.

By week 12, PASI-75 was achieved by 4% of patients in the placebo group, 14% of patients in the low-dose group, 34% of patients in the medium-dose group, and 49% of patients in the high-dose group ($P<.001$ for all compared with placebo). Statistically significant differences were noted from the placebo group as early as week 4 in the high-dose group, and week 8 in the medium-dose group. Mean levels of improvement as assessed by PASI score in the 4 groups by week 12 were 14.0% in the placebo group, 40.9% in the low-dose group, 52.6% in the medium-dose group, and 64.2% in the high-dose group.

At week 24, PASI-75 was achieved by 25% of the low-dose group, 44% of the medium-dose group, and 59% of the high-dose group (there was no placebo control in the second half of this study). From the original placebo group, 33% of patients had achieved PASI-75 after crossover to etanercept therapy starting week 12, consistent with the medium-dose group at week 12 (34%).

This pivotal trial demonstrated significant dose-dependent increases in etanercept efficacy after 12 weeks of therapy, and continued improvement in psoriatic skin lesions with continued therapy. An extension of this study aimed to determine whether etanercept could be used in an intermittent treatment paradigm by assessing how long psoriasis stayed under control after withdrawal of therapy, and once relapsed, whether control of psoriasis could be re-established with reinitiation of therapy.[17] Patients from the initial study who achieved at least PASI-50 by week 24 discontinued etanercept therapy until they experienced relapse of disease (loss of $\geq$50% of week 24 PASI improvement). They were then reinitiated on etanercept at their originally randomized dose (25 mg BIW or 50 mg BIW or 25 mg weekly). Patients relapsed on average 3 months after withdrawal from etanercept therapy. After 12 weeks of re-treatment, efficacy data were similar to that of the initial 12 weeks (Table 8.1). Re-treatment of psoriasis with etanercept appeared effective and well-tolerated.

Global psoriasis pivotal trial

Etanercept was tested in a 24-week, global phase 3 randomized controlled trial across 50 sites in the United States, Canada, and Western Europe to further investigate the efficacy after dose reduction (Fig. 8.4).[13] The primary endpoint in this study was achievement of PASI-75 after 12 weeks of study. Secondary efficacy endpoints at week 12

TABLE 8.1
Pivotal trial safety data (percentage of patients)

	US Pivotal Trial							Global Pivotal Trial					
		Week 12			Week 24			Week 12			Week 24		
	Placebo	LD	MD	HD	LD	MD	HD	Placebo	25 mg BIW	50 mg BIW	Placebo	25 mg BIW	50 mg BIW
Injection-site reaction	7	11	17	13	14	20	16	6	13	18	10	5	4
Headache	7	3	12	7	5	12	9	8	12	11	3	5	6
Upper respiratory infection (URI)	11	10	9	5	14	14	12	13	13	13	16	16	13
Accidental injury	4	4	3	4	7	7	7	6	4	7	6	4	5
Flulike syndrome	—	—	—	—	—	—	—	2	5	4	2	6	3
Sinusitis	1	0	0	0	6	6	5	—	—	—	—	—	—
Myalgia	2	2	4	2	5	7	4	—	—	—	—	—	—
Nausea	1	3	2	2	5	3	3	—	—	—	—	—	—
Rash	2	3	2	3	2	4	6	—	—	—	—	—	—
Asthenia	3	4	4	2	6	7	3	—	—	—	—	—	—

Abbreviations: HD, high-dose group; LD, low-dose group; MD, medium-dose group.

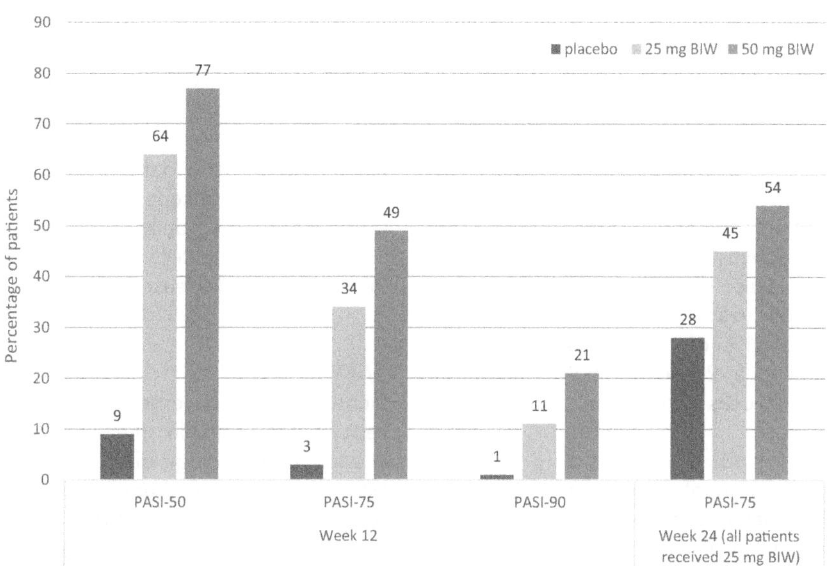

Fig. 8.4 Clinical responses to etanercept therapy from the global psoriasis pivotal trial. Efficacy outcomes after 12 and 24 weeks of treatment with either placebo or etanercept. During the first 12 weeks, patients received doses of either 25 mg BIWor 50 mg BIW etanercept. From weeks 12 to 24, all patients received etanercept 25 mg BIW. Efficacy was defined as percentage of patients with psoriasis who met specified PASI response criteria for improvement (PASI-50, -75, -90).

were achievement of PASI-50 and PASI-90, and percentage improvement from baseline PASI. The study population consisted of 583 patients with a median duration of psoriasis of 19 years, median BSA affected of 23%, and median baseline PASI of 16.4. During the first 12 weeks of this study, patients were randomly assigned to receive placebo, etanercept 25 mg BIW, or etanercept 50 mg BIW. During the second 12 weeks, all study patients received etanercept 25 mg BIW.

By week 12, 49% of patients in the etanercept 50-mg BIW group and 34% of patients in the 25-mg BIW group achieved PASI-75, in comparison to 3% of patients in the placebo group (*P*<.0001). Subgroup analyses based on baseline covariates, such as PASI, age, sex, race, prior systemic or phototherapy, and BSA, revealed no significant impact of these factors on treatment efficacy. Statistically significant differences in PASI-75 responses were seen as soon as week 4 between the etanercept 50-mg BIW group (10%) and placebo group (2%), and as soon as week 8 between the etanercept 25-mg BIW group (20%) and placebo group (3%). By week 12, the mean percentage improvement from baseline PASI was 68% in the etanercept 50-mg BIW group, 57% in the 25-mg BIW group, and 0.2% in the placebo group.

By week 24, PASI-75 was achieved by 54% of patients in the group following a dose reduction from 50 mg BIW to 25 mg BIW, 45% of patients continuing on 25 mg BIW, and 38% of patients that received 25 mg BIW after the initial 12 weeks of placebo treatment. Remarkably, of the 88 patients that had not achieved PASI-75 by week 12, 28 (32%) of them did achieve this by week 24.

This pivotal trial demonstrated statistically and clinically significant dose-dependent improvements in psoriasis with etanercept therapy. This study was also the first to systematically examine the maintenance of etanercept efficacy following a dose reduction and to have found that most patients were able to maintain PASI-75. The results of this study are similar to the findings of Leonardi and colleagues,[16] whose study was conducted with the same doses.

Efficacy in Pediatric and Geriatric Populations

Etanercept is effective in children with moderate-to-severe psoriasis. During a 48-week study in which pediatric patients were given 0.8 mg/kg weekly of etanercept, 57% of patients achieved PASI-75 by week 12 as opposed to 11% of patients receiving placebo.[4] From weeks 12 to 36, all patients received open-label etanercept, and PASI-75 response rates after 36 weeks were 68% and 65% for patients initially randomized to etanercept and placebo, respectively. During weeks 36 to 48, withdrawal effects were studied when patients were randomly reassigned to receive etanercept or placebo. Forty-two percent of patients in the placebo group lost adequate response after withdrawing etanercept therapy, but reached similar response rates as the initial etanercept group with 4 to 8 weeks of retreatment. A continuation of this study as a 5-year open-label extension study demonstrated that PASI-75 and PASI-90 scores were achieved and maintained in approximately 60% to 70%, and 30% to 40% of the pediatric patients through the 5 years, respectively.[18]

Etanercept is also effective for psoriasis in patients aged 65 years or older, with PASI-75 achieved by 54.1% of patients at 12 weeks, 78.7% of patients at 24 weeks, and 83.6% of patients after 156 weeks of treatment.[19]

Efficacy with Combination Therapy

Combination therapy of systemic and/or topical agents with etanercept has the potential to maximize efficacy, particularly in patients who have failed monotherapy etanercept or who lost adequate response after dose reduction.

Corticosteroids can increase the speed of therapeutic response in patients using etanercept, and the European Dermatology Expert Group recommends concomitant use, especially at the start of therapy.[20]

The UNITE (Utilization of narrowband ultraviolet light B therapy and etanercept for the treatment of psoriasis) study showed that narrowband-UV-B light therapy 3 times weekly combined with etanercept 50 mg BIW in moderate-to-severe patients with psoriasis yielded a PASI-75 response in 84.4% of patients after 12 weeks.[21] The combination therapy in this study was well tolerated, without an increase in photosensitivity, although caution should still be taken in patients with a known or suspected history of skin cancer.

Studies focusing on the combined use of etanercept and MTX have mostly been conducted in RA and psoriatic arthritis patients. The TEMPO (Trial of Etanercept and Methotrexate with Radiographic Patient Outcomes) and COMET (Combination of methotrexate and etanercept in active, early, moderate to severe rheumatoid arthritis) trials both found combination therapy to be generally safe and well tolerated.[22,23] Zachariae and colleagues[24] studied the combined use of these 2 agents in plaque patients with psoriasis who previously failed MTX monotherapy. They found higher proportions of patients to achieve PASI-50/75/90 and Physician Global Assessment scores of clear or almost clear in the combination therapy group as opposed to the etanercept/MTX taper groups, with little differences in AEs.

Data on the combined use of acitretin and etanercept are limited to case series showing no adverse effects[25]; thus, further long-term studies are needed to gain conclusive evidence. A pilot trial showed that PASI-75 responses after 24 weeks was achieved in 45% of patients treated with etanercept 25 mg BIW, 30% of patients treated with 0.4 mg/kg acitretin daily, and 44% of patients treated with etanercept 25 mg once weekly plus acitretin 0.4 mg/kg daily.[26] The combined use of acitretin and etanercept may be useful in patients looking to take decreased doses of etanercept.

SAFETY

General safety concerns with the use of etanercept therapy include infection (bacterial, viral, and fungal), neurologic disease (multiple sclerosis, MS), heart disease, drug-induced lupuslike syndromes, lymphoma (although the risk of lymphoma may be more closely related to having an immune disease and not a direct effect of the drug), melanoma and nonmelanoma skin cancer (NMSC), hematologic disease, and more. Etanercept is pregnancy category B and is considered safe in pregnant women if used with caution. The most common side effect of etanercept is injection site reaction, occurring in up to 37% of patients.[12] These reactions include erythema, itching, hemorrhage, pain, and/or swelling, which are generally mild to moderate and do not require discontinuation of the drug. Precaution should be taken in latex-sensitive patients, because the needle cover of the prefilled etanercept syringe contains latex.[12]

Clinical Trial Safety Data

In the US pivotal trial safety analysis, etanercept was generally well tolerated, with similar AE and infection rates across all treatment dose groups and no reported cases of tuberculosis (TB) or opportunistic infection (see Table 8.1).[16] Twenty-seven patients withdrew because of AEs, and 16 patients withdrew because of inefficacy. The global pivotal trial safety analysis also found similar rates of AEs and infections in the treatment groups over 24 weeks.[13] Two patients withdrew from the study because of infection and 9 patients discontinued because of AEs, 5 of which were thought to be drug related.

In the pediatric population, Paller and colleagues[4] reported 3 serious AEs, including an ovarian cyst that required surgical removal, gastroenteritis complicated by dehydration, and serious pneumonia in an asthmatic patient that required discontinuation of etanercept therapy. In the 5-year open-label extension study, no new safety concerns were reported in 181 patients that participated.[18] Through 264 weeks, 89% of patients experienced an AE, most commonly upper respiratory infections (37.6%), nasopharyngitis (26%), and headache (21.5%). There were 8 serious adverse events (SAEs) in 7 patients, only 1 of which (cellulitis) was considered treatment related.

Esposito and colleagues[19] reported a favorable risk:benefit profile of etanercept therapy in the geriatric population. Of the 15 out of 61 patients who withdrew from the study, 2 cases were due to AEs: 1 case was due to repeated episodes of tachycardia after etanercept administration, and 1 case was due to gastric cancer.

OBSERVE-5 Observational Registry Data

The OBSERVE-5 (Observational postmarketing safety surveillance registry of etanercept for the treatment of psoriasis) FDA-mandated phase 4 surveillance registry assessed long-term safety and effectiveness of etanercept therapy in 2510 patients across 375 sites for 5 years.[27] Patients with moderate-to-severe psoriasis were assessed at 6-month intervals for up to 5 years for SAEs, serious infectious events (SIEs) including any infection requiring hospitalization, and events of medical interest (EMIs).

SAEs were those that were fatal, life-threatening, required hospitalization, resulted in disability/incapacity, or were a congenital anomaly/birth defect or a significant medical hazard. EMIs included malignancies (including basal cell and squamous cell carcinomas), TB, opportunistic infections, central nervous system (CNS) demyelinating disorders, lupus disease, coronary artery disease, and worsening psoriasis.

Of the 2510 patients, 418 reported an SAE during the study (Table 8.2). The most common noninfectious SAEs were myocardial infarction (MI; 0.7%), coronary artery disease (0.6%), and osteoarthritis (0.6%). There were 120 patients that reported an SIE, the most being pneumonia (1.2%) and cellulitis (0.9%). There were 604 patients that had 1 or more EMI, 159 of which were considered to be etanercept related.

Patients in the OBSERVE-5 registry were compared with patients in the Truven Health MarketScan Commercial Claims and Encounters and MarketScan Medicare Supplemental

TABLE 8.2
Pediatric safety data (number of events)

	48-wk Study (n = 315)		
	Etanercept (n = 210)	**Placebo (n = 105)**	**5-y Study (n = 181)**
Total number AEs	914	144	161
URI	90	13	144
Headache	54	18	55
Nasopharyngitis	52	10	93
Influenza	23	3	28
Streptococcal pharyngitis	22	1	36
Cough	20	2	26
Vomiting	20	2	—
Skin papilloma	16	0	17
Injection-site reaction	62	5	16
Severe AE (excluding infection)	3	3	8 (serious, including infection) Cellulitis (1) Infectious mononucleosis (1) Osteonecrosis (2) Thyroid cyst (1) Postoperative intestinal obstruction (1) Anxiety (1) Abortion-induced (1)
Infection	378	58	2
Severe	4	0	
Serious	3	0	

databases, which provided age- and sex-standardized expected incidence rates or AEs as compared with patients on nonbiologic oral medications (MTX, cyclosporine). Based on this database, observed rates of malignancies, lymphomas, NMSC, and infections requiring hospitalization in OBSERVE-5 patients were not higher than expected.

Overall, this long-term safety assessment found low incidences of SAEs, SIEs, and EMIs, with decreasing incremental yearly incidences—thus, greater exposure to etanercept was not associated with an increased incidence rate of these events (Table 8.3).

PRECAUTIONS

Special attention should be given to patient populations with a history of TB, malignancy, demyelinating disorders, and congestive heart failure (CHF), given the role of TNF in such disease pathogenesis. Etanercept is contraindicated in patients with sepsis.[2]

Serious Infections

Patients using etanercept are at increased risk for serious infection (bacterial, viral, fungal, and parasitic). Risk may be increased with concomitant use of MTX, corticosteroids, and other immunosuppressants, in patients greater than 65 years, or in patients with underlying predisposing medical conditions. The use of etanercept with concomitant abatacept and anakinra is not recommended, because RA patients had an increased risk of serious infection with such therapy.[2,28]

Etanercept should be withheld in patients requiring antibiotics, discontinued in those with serious or opportunistic infections, and should not be initiated in patients with active infection (systemic or localized). Risks and benefits should be discussed before initiating therapy in patients with recurrent/chronic infection.[2,12,28]

Tuberculosis

Reports of reactivation of TB or new-onset TB infection have been seen with patients receiving etanercept therapy, although the risk of reactivation of latent TB is lower with etanercept in comparison to the monoclonal antibody TNF inhibitors (adalimumab, infliximab) due to its soluble TNF receptor fusion protein quality.[29] Patients should be evaluated based on risk factors for TB and screened for latent TB before initiation and during therapy. In patients on etanercept, a purified protein derivative (PPD) screen with 5-mm or greater induration is considered positive, even in those with a history of BCG vaccination.[12]

TB treatment should be given to any patient with a history of active or latent TB, in whom completion of a treatment course cannot be confirmed. Etanercept therapy can be initiated after 1 to 2 months of latent TB treatment, although reactivation of TB remains a possibility despite prophylactic treatment. A TB expert should be consulted in the case of any questions or hesitations.

Opportunistic infections

Opportunistic infections, such as aspergillosis, blastomycosis, candidiasis, histoplasmosis, legionellosis, listeriosis, coccidioidomycosis, cryptococcosis, and pneumocystis, may present in patients receiving etanercept therapy as disseminated rather than localized infection. If the symptomatic patient resides or travels to regions of endemic mycoses, it is important to consider empiric antifungal therapy while waiting on a diagnostic workup. Antigen and antibody testing may be negative in patients with active histoplasmosis.[2,12]

TABLE 8.3
OBSERVE-5 safety data

SAEs (n = 418)	SIEs (n = 120)	EMIs (n = 604)
Treatment emergent	Treatment emergent	Malignancy (122)
Pneumonia (30)	Pneumonia (30)	NMSC (66)
Cellulitis (22)	Cellulitis (22)	Coronary artery disease (49)
MI (17)	Diverticulitis (11)	Worsening of psoriasis (13)
Coronary artery disease (14)	Staphylococci infection (7)	CNS demyelinating disorder (3)
Osteoarthritis (14)	Sepsis (5)	Lymphoma (2)
Diverticulitis (11)	Appendicitis (4)	TB (2)
Treatment related	Bronchitis (4)	Lupus disease (1)
Pneumonia (8)	Herpes zoster (4)	Opportunistic infection (1)
Cellulitis (8)		Coccidioidomycosis (0)
		Histoplasmosis (0)

Malignancies

Although the FDA label for etanercept describes precaution for lymphoproliferative malignancy, melanoma, and NMSC in patients using TNF inhibitor therapy, the OBSERVE-5 trial did not show an increased rate of malignancy in patients using etanercept as compared with the general population.[27] In addition, there is an inherent increased risk of Hodgkin lymphoma and cutaneous T-cell lymphoma in patients with psoriasis that should be acknowledged.[30,31] Dermatologists should take precaution in watching for signs and symptoms of these particular malignancies in patients.

Lymphoproliferative malignancy

The observed rates of lymphoproliferative malignancies in patients with psoriasis using etanercept were similar to those of the Marketscan database (patients receiving nonbiologic oral agents) and were as expected based on the Surveillance, Epidemiology, and End Results database (did not increase with increasing etanercept dosage or exposure).[27,32] There have, however, been resolved cases of lymphoma reported in patients stopping TNF inhibitors such as etanercept and infliximab.[33]

Nonmelanoma skin cancer

An increased incidence of NMSC was reported from studies in patients with psoriasis receiving etanercept therapy.[32] This rate may be associated with the use of high-dose PUVA, cyclosporine, MTX, and immunosuppressants concurrently or before etanercept therapy.[34] In addition, there have been significant associations reported with melanoma and TNF inhibitor therapy.[35] Regular skin examinations should be performed for all patients, and precaution should be taken in patients with a history of skin cancer.

Heart Failure

Although the role of TNF in CHF is much debated, 2 randomized controlled trials, RENAISSANCE/RECOVER (Randomised Etanercept North AmerIcan Strategy to Study Antagonism of CytokinEs/Research into Etanercept Cyt-Okine Antagonism in VentriculaR dysfunction trial) and ATTACH (Anti-TNF alpha Therapy Against Chronic Heart Failure),[36,37] suggest dose-dependent worsening of CHF prognosis with TNF inhibitors. Etanercept should be withdrawn with new-onset or worsening symptoms in patients with pre-existing CHF. There have been rare reports of new-onset CHF in patients without pre-existing cardiovascular disease. Patients diagnosed with class 3 or 4 CHF or ejection fraction less than 50% should avoid etanercept use, and those diagnosed with class 1 or 2 CHF should undergo echo testing.[12,38,39]

Hepatitis B Virus Reactivation

TNF is thought to promote viral clearance in hepatitis B. If a patient receiving etanercept therapy develops hepatitis B virus (HBV) reactivation, therapy should be stopped immediately and antiviral therapy should ensue.[2]

Patients should be monitored for signs and symptoms of HBV infection during and for 6 months after stopping therapy.[40] This monitoring includes liver function tests (LFTs), hepatitis B surface antigen, hepatitis B envelope antigen, and HBV DNA counts in patients at risk for reactivation.[40] No definitive information is available regarding treating HBV carriers using antiviral therapy along with etanercept, or regarding resuming etanercept therapy after the control of reactivated HBV infection.

Neurologic Events

TNF inhibitors have been associated with new-onset or exacerbation of CNS demyelinating disorders (ie, MS, optic neuritis) and peripheral demyelinating diseases such as Guillain-Barré syndrome.[12,41,42] Etanercept should not be initiated in patients with a personal history of or first-degree relative with MS,[43,44] or other demyelinating disorders. Adverse neurologic events have been reported to resolve with termination of therapy.[41]

Hematologic Events

Isolated cases of aplastic anemia, pancytopenia, isolated leukopenia, and thrombocytopenia have been reported with TNF inhibitor use.[45,46] Patients who experience pallor, easy bruising, bleeding, or persistent fever should seek immediate attention. Etanercept therapy should be discontinued if significant hematologic abnormalities occur[2,12] and should not be initiated in patients with concurrent anakinra because there have been reports of such patients developing neutropenia.[47]

Allergic Reactions

There is a small risk (<0.2%) for the development of an anaphylactic reaction or other serious allergic reaction with etanercept use.[2] If this occurs, etanercept should be discontinued and appropriate therapy should ensue.

Autoimmunity

A recent study found that 26.7% of etanercept-treated patients formed autoantibodies.[48] There is a risk for formation of autoantibodies with etanercept therapy that may rarely (<0.1%) result in the development of a lupuslike syndrome or autoimmune hepatitis.[2] If these conditions develop, etanercept should be discontinued and the patient should be further evaluated. The development of autoantibodies with initiation of TNF inhibitor therapy may be a marker for forthcoming treatment failure.[49]

Granulomatosis with Polyangiitis

The use of etanercept is not recommended in patients with granulomatosis with polyangiitis,[2] as 1 study showed that the addition of etanercept to standard therapy for granulomatosis with polyangiitis was associated with an increased incidence of noncutaneous solid malignancies.[50] This risk could not be attributed to etanercept, however, as placebo patients had a similar risk of solid malignancy as etanercept-treated patients when compared with the general population.[50] Clinical outcomes of these patients were not improved with the addition of etanercept in comparison to standard therapy alone.

Severe Alcoholic Hepatitis

Precaution should be taken when administering etanercept to patients with moderate-to-severe alcoholic hepatitis.[2] A study involving 48 hospitalized patients treated with etanercept or placebo for moderate-to-severe alcoholic hepatitis demonstrated significantly higher mortalities in patients treated with etanercept after 6 months of use.[51]

MONITORING

The information presented is primarily based on psoriasis guidelines from the American Academy of Dermatology (AAD).[12]

A thorough history and physical examination should be taken before initiation of etanercept therapy, including TB exposure, chronic/recurrent infections, malignancy, neurologic and cardiac history, and a thorough review of systems. Routine follow-up examinations should adequately monitor patients for side effects and AEs.[52]

Aside from baseline TB test, annual monitoring for TB, and a baseline hepatitis profile, routine laboratory testing beyond that for concomitant therapies or comorbidities is generally not supported.[53] The highest grade US Preventive Services Task Force evidence for screening studies is grade B for TB testing (interferon-γ release assay is preferred over tuberculin skin testing), and HBV/hepatitis C virus screening is supported only by grade C evidence.[54] The AAD recommends baseline PPD, LFTs, and complete blood count (CBC). For ongoing monitoring, the AAD recommends yearly PPD and periodic LFTs, CBC, history, and physical examinations (Table 8.4).[12]

The Centers for Disease Control and Prevention recommends TB testing before the therapy initiation as well.[55] Positive skin test findings should be followed with a chest radiograph—if negative, patients should be treated for latent TB (6–9 months of 300 mg isoniazid daily and/or 4 months of 600 mg daily rifampicin),[56] and if positive, patients should receive therapy for active TB. Biologic therapy may be started after 1 to 2 months of prophylactic treatment if the patient is adherent to and tolerating the prophylactic regimen.[57] If a patient has a positive PPD because of prior BCG vaccination, blood tests can be obtained measuring interferon production on stimulation with TB antigens that are not present in BCG. Most guidelines perform annual TB skin testing in patients receiving etanercept to screen for the TB reactivation, especially in those at risk (ie, health care workers, travelers to endemic areas).

The authors of this section recommend initial baseline monitoring that includes a QuantiFERON-TB Gold (QFT), LFTs, CBC, and hepatitis B and hepatitis C profile. QFT should be repeated annually.

VACCINATIONS

Because of the possibility that biologic agents may impair the body's immunologic response to vaccinations, administration of vaccinations should be carefully considered in patients receiving biologic therapy (Table 8.5). Live vaccines (measles, mumps, and rubella [MMR], varicella, zoster, intranasal influenza, and so forth) are contraindicated within 1 month of treatment.[58] However, scientifically based/standardized recommendations for administering

TABLE 8.4
Monitoring recommendations from the American Academy of Dermatology

	Monitoring
History and physical	Baseline and routine
CBC	Baseline and periodically
LFTs	Baseline and periodically
TB skin test	Baseline and annually after
Hepatitis profile	Not specified

Data from Menter A, Gottlieb A, Feldman SR, et al. Guidelines of care for the management of psoriasis and psoriatic arthritis: section 1. Overview of psoriasis and guidelines of care for the treatment of psoriasis with biologics. J Am Acad Dermatol 2008;58(5):826–50.

TABLE 8.5
Vaccination recommendations from the National Psoriasis Foundation

Vaccination	Before Therapy	During Therapy
Live vaccines (MMR, varicella, herpes zoster, intranasal influenza, oral typhoid, yellow fever, oral polio, smallpox, BCG, rotavirus)	Contraindicated within 1 mo	Contraindicated
Influenza	Vaccinate with inactivated or live	Yearly immunization with inactivated vaccine
Chicken pox	If negative serology, vaccinate	Contraindicated
Zoster	Before therapy: 1 dose for adults $\geq$50 y	Contraindicated
Human papillomavirus	Unvaccinated males/female patients up to age 26	Same
Hepatitis A	Vaccinate if high risk (diabetes, liver disease, intravenous drug users, homosexual men, and so forth)	Same; consider obtaining postvaccination serology
Hepatitis B	Serology, risk factor assessment. Offer vaccination if necessary	High-dose vaccine Consider obtaining serology postvaccination
Pneumococcal	Pneumococcal polysaccharide vaccine (PPSV23) vaccine recommended	Pneumococcal conjugate vaccine followed by PPSV23 if not given before
Haemophilus influenzae type b	Vaccinate if unvaccinated	Same
MMR	Vaccinate if negative, or seronegative to any component	Contraindicated
Tetanus diphtheria booster/ tetanus diphtheria pertussis vaccine	Booster every 10 y and high-risk wounds Offer before therapy, substitute 1 dose with TDAP	Same
Meningococcal	Assess risk factors, vaccinate if high risk (asplenia, complement deficient, group living)	Same
Poliomyelitis	Assess risk factors, vaccinate if high risk (health care worker, laboratory worker)	Same

biologically inactive or recombinant vaccines to patients on biologic agents are lacking. Non-live vaccinations may have the potential to achieve adequate immune response, although antibody titers may not achieve optimal levels and may decrease more rapidly if given during biologic therapy.

It is preferable to complete all age-appropriate immunizations according to current immunization guidelines before initiating biologic therapy. The production of antibodies from the vaccine generally occurs in the 2-week period from primary immunization, but could take more than 6 weeks to peak. A period of 4 times the half-life of etanercept (17 days) has been suggested to allow for the return of the immune system to its baseline before vaccination with live vaccines.

TUMOR NECROSIS FACTOR INHIBITOR THERAPY AND CARDIOVASCULAR RISK REDUCTION

Recent evidence suggests that TNF inhibitor therapy has the potential to reduce cardiovascular risk by lowering systemic inflammation. A retrospective study at Kaiser Permanente Southern

California concluded that TNF inhibitor use was associated with a significant reduction in MI risk (50%) and incidence (55%) compared with topical treatments for psoriasis,[59] and a 5-year Danish follow-up study found that patients treated with TNF inhibitors had a significant reduction in cardiovascular risk compared with other therapies (interleukin-12/23, cyclosporine, retinoids).[60] However, there have been studies reporting that there is not a reduced MI risk in patients with psoriasis receiving systemic psoriasis therapy (including TNF inhibitor therapy); thus, further investigation is warranted to determine the potential for risk reduction.[61]

SUMMARY

Etanercept is effective for the treatment of moderate-to-severe plaque psoriasis. This drug should be considered in patients who are candidates for systemic therapy or phototherapy, although among the TNF inhibitors, adalimumab and infliximab therapy are more effective than etanercept therapy when compared with placebo.[62,63] The authors consider etanercept to be second-line biologic therapy because of lowest efficacy of all approved and marketed biologics. Etanercept has a lower risk for serious infections such as TB in comparison to other TNF inhibitors and may be a more practical choice in those at increased risk for immunosuppression. The response to etanercept therapy is varied, and typically continuous therapy is necessary for optimal clearance of psoriatic skin lesions. With the exception of TB screening, there is a lack of evidence-based guidelines for consistent monitoring of patients using etanercept.[54] Based on clinical experience, the authors of this section recommend baseline screening for TB and hepatitis B and annual screening solely for TB.

REFERENCES

1. Nguyen TU, Koo J. Etanercept in the treatment of plaque psoriasis. Clin Cosmet Investig Dermatol 2009;2:77–84.
2. Research Center for Drug Evaluation and "Therapeutic Biologic Applications (BLA)—Etanercept Product Approval Information—Licensing Action 12/2/98." WebContent. Available at: http://www.fda.gov/Drugs/DevelopmentApprovalProcess/HowDrugsareDevelopedandApproved/ApprovalApplications/TherapeuticBiologicApplications/ucm080536.htm. Accessed January 30, 2016.
3. Levin EC, Debbaneh M, Koo J, et al. Biologic therapy in erythrodermic and pustular psoriasis. J Drugs Dermatol 2014;13(3):342–54.
4. Paller AS, Siegfried EC, Langley RG, et al. Etanercept treatment for children and adolescents with plaque psoriasis. N Engl J Med 2008;358(3):241–51.
5. Zhou H. Clinical pharmacokinetics of etanercept: a fully humanized soluble recombinant tumor necrosis factor receptor fusion protein. J Clin Pharmacol 2005;45(5):490–7.
6. Don BR, Spin G, Nestorov I, et al. The pharmacokinetics of etanercept in patients with end-stage renal disease on haemodialysis. J Pharm Pharmacol 2005; 57(11):1407–13.
7. Zhou H, Mayer PR, Wajdula J, et al. Unaltered etanercept pharmacokinetics with concurrent methotrexate in patients with rheumatoid arthritis. J Clin Pharmacol 2004;44(11):1235–43.
8. Zhou H, Parks V, Patat A, et al. Absence of a clinically relevant interaction between etanercept and digoxin. J Clin Pharmacol 2004;44(11): 1244–51.
9. Zhou H, Patat A, Parks V, et al. Absence of a pharmacokinetic interaction between etanercept and warfarin. J Clin Pharmacol 2004;44(5):543–50.
10. Mohler KM, Torrance DS, Smith CA, et al. Soluble tumor necrosis factor (TNF) receptors are effective therapeutic agents in lethal endotoxemia and function simultaneously as both TNF carriers and TNF antagonists. J Immunol 1993;151(3):1548–61.
11. Schiestl M, Stangler T, Torella C, et al. Acceptable changes in quality attributes of glycosylated biopharmaceuticals. Nat Biotechnol 2011;29(4):310–2.
12. Menter A, Gottlieb A, Feldman SR, et al. Guidelines of care for the management of psoriasis and psoriatic arthritis: section 1. Overview of psoriasis and guidelines of care for the treatment of psoriasis with biologics. J Am Acad Dermatol 2008;58(5): 826–50.
13. Papp KA, Tyring S, Lahfa M, et al. A global phase III randomized controlled trial of etanercept in psoriasis: safety, efficacy, and effect of dose reduction. Br J Dermatol 2005;152(6):1304–12.
14. Gordon K, Korman N, Frankel E, et al. Efficacy of etanercept in an integrated multistudy database of patients with psoriasis. J Am Acad Dermatol 2006;54(3 Suppl 2):S101–11.
15. Moore A, Gordon KB, Kang S, et al. A randomized, open-label trial of continuous versus interrupted etanercept therapy in the treatment of psoriasis. J Am Acad Dermatol 2007;56(4):598–603.
16. Leonardi CL, Powers JL, Matheson RT, et al. Etanercept as monotherapy in patients with psoriasis. N Engl J Med 2003;349(21):2014–22.
17. Gordon KB, Gottlieb AB, Leonardi CL, et al. Clinical response in psoriasis patients discontinued from and then reinitiated on etanercept therapy. J Dermatolog Treat 2006;17(1):9–17.
18. Paller AS, Siegfried EC, Pariser DM, et al. Long-term safety and efficacy of etanercept in children and

adolescents with plaque psoriasis. J Am Acad Dermatol 2016;74(2):280–7.e3.

19. Esposito M, Giunta A, Mazzotta A, et al. Efficacy and safety of subcutaneous anti-tumor necrosis factor-alpha agents, etanercept and adalimumab, in elderly patients affected by psoriasis and psoriatic arthritis: an observational long-term study. Dermatology 2012;225(4):312–9.
20. Boehncke W-H, Brasie RA, Barker J, et al. Recommendations for the use of etanercept in psoriasis: a European dermatology expert group consensus. J Eur Acad Dermatol Venereol 2006;20(8):988–98.
21. Kircik L, Bagel J, Korman N, et al. Utilization of narrow-band ultraviolet light B therapy and etanercept for the treatment of psoriasis (UNITE): efficacy, safety, and patient-reported outcomes. J Drugs Dermatol 2008;7(3):245–53.
22. Klareskog L, van der Heijde D, de Jager JP, et al. Therapeutic effect of the combination of etanercept and methotrexate compared with each treatment alone in patients with rheumatoid arthritis: double-blind randomised controlled trial. Lancet 2004;363(9410):675–81.
23. Emery P, Breedveld FC, Hall S, et al. Comparison of methotrexate monotherapy with a combination of methotrexate and etanercept in active, early, moderate to severe rheumatoid arthritis (COMET): a randomised, double-blind, parallel treatment trial. Lancet 2008;372(9636):375–82.
24. Zachariae C, Mørk N-J, Reunala T, et al. The combination of etanercept and methotrexate increases the effectiveness of treatment in active psoriasis despite inadequate effect of methotrexate therapy. Acta Derm Venereol 2008;88(5):495–501.
25. Conley J, Nanton J, Dhawan S, et al. Novel combination regimens: biologics and acitretin for the treatment of psoriasis– a case series. J Dermatolog Treat 2006;17(2):86–9.
26. Gisondi P, Del Giglio M, Cotena C, et al. Combining etanercept and acitretin in the therapy of chronic plaque psoriasis: a 24-week, randomized, controlled, investigator-blinded pilot trial. Br J Dermatol 2008;158(6):1345–9.
27. Kimball AB, Rothman KJ, Kricorian G, et al. OBSERVE-5: observational postmarketing safety surveillance registry of etanercept for the treatment of psoriasis final 5-year results. J Am Acad Dermatol 2015;72(1):115–22.
28. Bresnihan B, Cunnane G. Infection complications associated with the use of biologic agents. Rheum Dis Clin North Am 2003;29(1):185–202.
29. Fallahi-Sichani M, Flynn JL, Linderman JJ, et al. Differential risk of tuberculosis reactivation among anti-TNF therapies is due to drug binding kinetics and permeability. J Immunol 2012;188(7):3169–78.
30. Gelfand JM, Berlin J, Van Voorhees A, et al. Lymphoma rates are low but increased in patients with psoriasis: results from a population-based cohort study in the United Kingdom. Arch Dermatol 2003;139(11):1425–9.
31. Gelfand JM, Shin DB, Neimann AL, et al. The risk of lymphoma in patients with psoriasis. J Invest Dermatol 2006;126(10):2194–201.
32. Pariser DM, Leonardi CL, Gordon K, et al. Integrated safety analysis: Short- and long-term safety profiles of etanercept in patients with psoriasis. J Am Acad Dermatol 2012;67(2):245–56.
33. Brown SL, Greene MH, Gershon SK, et al. Tumor necrosis factor antagonist therapy and lymphoma development: twenty-six cases reported to the Food and Drug Administration. Arthritis Rheum 2002;46(12):3151–8.
34. Paul CF, Ho VC, McGeown C, et al. Risk of malignancies in psoriasis patients treated with cyclosporine: a 5 y cohort study. J Invest Dermatol 2003;120(2):211–6.
35. Nardone B, Hammel JA, Raisch DW, et al. Melanoma associated with tumour necrosis factor-α inhibitors: a Research on Adverse Drug events And Reports (RADAR) project. Br J Dermatol 2014;170(5):1170–2.
36. Coletta AP, Clark AL, Banarjee P, et al. Clinical trials update: RENEWAL (RENAISSANCE and RECOVER) and ATTACH. Eur J Heart Fail 2002;4(4):559–61.
37. Chung ES, Packer M, Lo KH, et al. Randomized, double-blind, placebo-controlled, pilot trial of infliximab, a chimeric monoclonal antibody to tumor necrosis factor-alpha, in patients with moderate-to-severe heart failure: results of the anti-TNF Therapy Against Congestive Heart Failure (ATTACH) trial. Circulation 2003;107(25):3133–40.
38. Desai SB, Furst DE. Problems encountered during anti-tumour necrosis factor therapy. Best Pract Res Clin Rheumatol 2006;20(4):757–90.
39. Khanna D, McMahon M, Furst DE. Safety of tumour necrosis factor-alpha antagonists. Drug Saf 2004;27(5):307–24.
40. Motaparthi K, Stanisic V, Van Voorhees AS, et al. From the Medical Board of the National Psoriasis Foundation: recommendations for screening for hepatitis B infection prior to initiating anti-tumor necrosis factor-alfa inhibitors or other immunosuppressive agents in patients with psoriasis. J Am Acad Dermatol 2014;70(1):178–86.
41. Mohan N, Edwards ET, Cupps TR, et al. Demyelination occurring during anti-tumor necrosis factor alpha therapy for inflammatory arthritides. Arthritis Rheum 2001;44(12):2862–9.
42. TNF neutralization in MS: results of a randomized, placebo-controlled multicenter study. The Lenercept Multiple Sclerosis Study Group and the

University of British Columbia MS/MRI Analysis Group. Neurology 1999;53(3):457–65.
43. Barcellos LF, Kamdar BB, Ramsay PP, et al. Clustering of autoimmune diseases in families with a high-risk for multiple sclerosis: a descriptive study. Lancet Neurol 2006;5(11):924–31.
44. Dyment DA, Sadovnick AD, Willer CJ, et al. An extended genome scan in 442 Canadian multiple sclerosis-affected sibships: a report from the Canadian Collaborative Study Group. Hum Mol Genet 2004;13(10):1005–15.
45. Kuruvilla J, Leitch HA, Vickars LM, et al. Aplastic anemia following administration of a tumor necrosis factor-alpha inhibitor. Eur J Haematol 2003;71(5): 396–8.
46. Vidal F, Fontova R, Richart C. Severe neutropenia and thrombocytopenia associated with infliximab. Ann Intern Med 2003;139(3):W-W63.
47. Genovese MC, Cohen S, Moreland L, et al. Combination therapy with etanercept and anakinra in the treatment of patients with rheumatoid arthritis who have been treated unsuccessfully with methotrexate. Arthritis Rheum 2004;50(5):1412–9.
48. Bardazzi F, Odorici G, Virdi A, et al. Autoantibodies in psoriatic patients treated with anti-TNF-α therapy. J Dtsch Dermatol Ges 2014;12(5):401–6.
49. Pink AE, Fonia A, Allen MH, et al. Antinuclear antibodies associate with loss of response to antitumour necrosis factor-alpha therapy in psoriasis: a retrospective, observational study. Br J Dermatol 2010;162(4):780–5.
50. Silva F, Seo P, Schroeder DR, et al. Solid malignancies among etanercept-treated patients with granulomatosis with polyangiitis (Wegener's): long-term followup of a multicenter longitudinal cohort. Arthritis Rheum 2011;63(8):2495–503.
51. Boetticher NC, Peine CJ, Kwo P, et al. A randomized, double-blinded, placebo-controlled multicenter trial of etanercept in the treatment of alcoholic hepatitis. Gastroenterology 2008;135(6): 1953–60.
52. Lebwohl M, Bagel J, Gelfand JM, et al. From the Medical Board of the National Psoriasis Foundation: monitoring and vaccinations in patients treated with biologics for psoriasis. J Am Acad Dermatol 2008;58(1):94–105.
53. van Lümig PPM, Driessen RJB, Roelofs-Thijssen MA, et al. Relevance of laboratory investigations in monitoring patients with psoriasis on etanercept or adalimumab. Br J Dermatol 2011;165(2):375–82.
54. Ahn CS, Dothard EH, Garner ML, et al. To test or not to test? An updated evidence-based assessment of the value of screening and monitoring tests when using systemic biologic agents to treat psoriasis and psoriatic arthritis. J Am Acad Dermatol 2015; 73(3):420–8.e1.
55. CDC—Tuberculosis (TB) [Internet]. Available at: http://www.cdc.gov/tb/?404;http://www.cdc.gov:80/tb/pubs/LTBI/pdf/TargetedLTBI05.pdf. Accessed February 1, 2016.
56. Targeted tuberculin testing and treatment of latent tuberculosis infection. American Thoracic Society. MMWR Recomm Rep 2000;49(RR-6):1–51.
57. Doherty SD, Van Voorhees A, Lebwohl MG, et al. National Psoriasis Foundation consensus statement on screening for latent tuberculosis infection in patients with psoriasis treated with systemic and biologic agents. J Am Acad Dermatol 2008;59(2): 209–17.
58. Wine-Lee L, Keller SC, Wilck MB, et al. From the Medical Board of the National Psoriasis Foundation: vaccination in adult patients on systemic therapy for psoriasis. J Am Acad Dermatol 2013;69(6): 1003–13.
59. Wu JJ, Poon K-YT, Channual JC, et al. Association between tumor necrosis factor inhibitor therapy and myocardial infarction risk in patients with psoriasis. Arch Dermatol 2012;148(11):1244–50.
60. Ahlehoff O, Skov L, Gislason G, et al. Cardiovascular outcomes and systemic anti-inflammatory drugs in patients with severe psoriasis: 5-year follow-up of a Danish nationwide cohort. J Eur Acad Dermatol Venereol 2015;29(6):1128–34.
61. Abuabara K, Lee H, Kimball AB. The effect of systemic psoriasis therapies on the incidence of myocardial infarction: a cohort study. Br J Dermatol 2011;165(5):1066–73.
62. Bissonnette R, Bolduc C, Poulin Y, et al. Efficacy and safety of adalimumab in patients with plaque psoriasis who have shown an unsatisfactory response to etanercept. J Am Acad Dermatol 2010;63(2):228–34.
63. Reich K, Nestle FO, Papp K, et al. Infliximab induction and maintenance therapy for moderate-to-severe psoriasis: a phase III, multicentre, double-blind trial. Lancet 2005;366(9494):1367–74.

CHAPTER 9

Infliximab

Catherine Ni, MD, Shivani P. Reddy, BS, Jashin J. Wu, MD

KEYWORDS

• Infliximab • TNF-α • Psoriasis • SPIRIT • EXPRESS • EXPRESS II • IMPACT

KEY POINTS

- Infliximab is a safe and effective therapy for the treatment of moderate-to-severe psoriasis.
- The mechanism of action of infliximab is inhibition of tumor necrosis factor-α, thereby inhibiting the inflammatory cascade leading to psoriatic skin lesions.
- Pivotal trials on infliximab therapy for the treatment of psoriasis and psoriatic arthritis include SPIRIT, EXPRESS, EXPRESS II, and IMPACT.
- Infliximab is generally safe and well-tolerated. Annual tuberculosis screening is recommended with infliximab use.

INTRODUCTION

Standard therapies for the treatment of severe psoriasis have traditionally been limited to methotrexate (MTX), cyclosporine, acitretin, psoralen and UV-A radiation (PUVA), and UV-B phototherapy. Tumor necrosis factor (TNF) inhibitors have been approved for use in severe psoriasis and represent a convenient, targeted systemic agent that can achieve rapid clinical improvement with less potential for drug-related toxicities in both the short and the long term.[1] Infliximab is a chimeric immunoglobulin 1 (IgG1) monoclonal antibody that targets TNF-α. Multiple randomized, controlled trials have evaluated the efficacy and safety of infliximab in psoriasis and psoriatic arthritis (PsA). In 2006, the US Food and Drug Administration approved infliximab for the treatment of chronic, severe plaque psoriasis and PsA.[2] Infliximab is also approved for use in rheumatoid arthritis, Crohn disease, ulcerative colitis, and ankylosing spondylitis and is used off-label in the treatment of neutrophilic and bullous dermatoses, connective tissue diseases such as dermatomyositis and scleroderma, and hidradenitis suppurativa.[3]

The current recommended dosing of infliximab for chronic, severe psoriasis and PsA is 5 mg/kg given as an intravenous (IV) induction regimen at weeks 0, 2, 6, followed by maintenance dosing of 5 mg/kg at 8-week intervals afterward (Fig. 9.1).[4] Patients who develop neutralizing antibodies to infliximab are less likely to maintain a response than those who are antibody negative, but the formation of antibodies does not necessarily determine clinical responsiveness.[5,6] When the clinical response to infliximab is waning, the frequency of infusions may need to be increased or low-dose MTX may be prescribed concurrently to decrease the formation of antibodies against infliximab and therefore maintain clinical efficacy (Table 9.1).[2]

MECHANISM OF ACTION

Infliximab is a chimeric monoclonal antibody composed of a constant human IgG1 region and a variable murine region. It has high binding affinity and specificity for TNF-α, forming complexes with both soluble and transmembrane forms of TNF-α, thus preventing its downstream effects.[7] The binding to transmembrane TNF-α mediates complement and antibody-dependent cytotoxicity of cell lines that express TNF-α, namely macrophages and monocytes.[8]

TNF-α is found in high levels in the skin lesions and plasma of psoriasis patients and plays a key role in pathogenesis of psoriasis. TNF-α upregulates vascular endothelial growth factor, induces keratinocyte proliferation, stimulates lymphocyte migration, and increases the expression of proinflammatory cytokines.[2] By inhibiting TNF-α, infliximab inhibits key steps in the pathogenesis of psoriasis and normalizes keratinocyte differentiation.

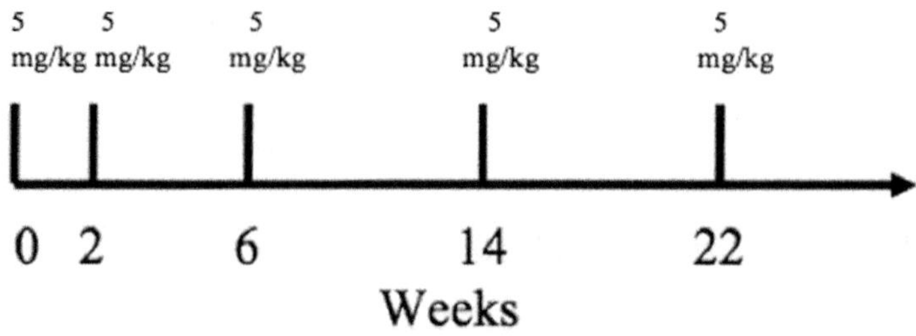

Fig. 9.1 Infliximab dosing regimen for psoriasis.

EFFICACY

The efficacy of infliximab in the treatment of psoriasis has been evaluated in multiple randomized, controlled trials. The Study of Psoriasis with Infliximab Induction Therapy (SPIRIT), European Infliximab for Psoriasis Efficacy and Safety Study (EXPRESS), and European Infliximab for Psoriasis Efficacy and Safety Study II (EXPRESS II) trials found that infliximab induces rapid, efficacious, and sustainable clinical response for the treatment of moderate-to-severe plaque psoriasis.

TABLE 9.1
Summary of clinical trials

Study	Study Population	Dose and Timing	Results
SPIRIT (phase 2, Gottlieb 2004)	• n = 249 • Severe plaque psoriasis, ≥6 mo • PASI ≥12, BSA ≥10%	• 3 mg/kg infliximab (n = 99) • 5 mg/kg infliximab (n = 99) • Placebo (n = 51) • Weeks 0, 2, 6 • Additional infusion at week 26 if static PGA of moderate/severe	PASI-75 week 10: 3 mg/kg 72%, 5 mg/kg 88%, placebo 6% (*P*<.001) DLQI % improvement week 10: 3 mg/kg 84%, 5 mg/kg 91%, placebo 0% (*P*<.001)
EXPRESS (phase 3, Reich 2005)	• n = 387 • Moderate-to-severe plaque psoriasis ≥6 mo • PASI ≥12, BSA ≥10%	• 5 mg/kg infliximab (n = 301) • Placebo (n = 77) • Weeks 0, 2, 6, every 8 wk through week 46 • At week 24, placebo patients crossed over to infliximab	PASI-75 week 10: infliximab 80%, placebo 3% (*P*<.0001) PASI-75 week 24: infliximab 82%, placebo 4% (*P*<.0001) PASI-75 week 50: infliximab 61%
EXPRESS II (phase 3, Menter 2007)	• n = 835 • Moderate-to-severe plaque psoriasis • PASI ≥12, BSA ≥10%	• 3 mg/kg infliximab (n = 313) • 5 mg/kg infliximab (n = 314) • Placebo (n = 208) • Infliximab groups randomized at weeks 14 to q 8 wk continuous OR intermittent, as-needed therapy • Placebo group crossed over at week 16 to infliximab 5 mg/kg at weeks 16, 18, 22, then q8 wk	PASI-75 week 10: 3 mg/kg 70%, 5 mg/kg 76%, placebo 2% (*P*<.001) PASI-75 week 50: • 3 mg/kg continuous: 44% • 3 mg/kg intermittent: 25% • 5 mg/kg continuous: 55% • 5 mg/kg intermittent: 38%
IMPACT (Antoni 2008)	• n = 104 • PsA ≥6 mo • Failed prior treatment with 1 or more DMARD	• Infliximab 5 mg/kg (n = 52) • Placebo (n = 52) • Weeks 0, 2, 6, 14 • Placebo crossed over to infliximab at week 50 • Long-term extension to week 98 (n = 69)	Week 50 infliximab: • ACR20: 73% • ACR50: 50% • ACR70: 31% Week 98 infliximab: • ACR20: 62% • ACR50: 45% • ACR70: 35%

Data from Refs.[1,5,6,15]

Study of Psoriasis with Infliximab Induction Therapy

The SPIRIT trial was a multicenter double-blinded, placebo-controlled phase 2 trial that randomized 249 patients to receive IV infusions of infliximab or placebo.[1] Selected patients had plaque psoriasis for at least 6 months, Psoriasis Area Severity Index (PASI) ≥12 or more, and 10% or greater body surface area (BSA) affected. The primary endpoint was the proportion of patients who achieved PASI-75 at week 10. Patients were randomly assigned in a 1:2:2 ratio to infusions of infliximab 3 mg/kg, 5 mg/kg, or placebo and were treated at weeks 0, 2, and 6, and followed to week 30.

Responses were seen after the first infusion of infliximab. By week 2, 34% and 40% of patients in the infliximab 3 and 5 mg/kg groups had achieved PASI-50, compared with 4% in the placebo group. At week 10, 72% of the 3-mg/kg group and 88% of the 5-mg/kg group achieved PASI-75 compared with 6% of placebo. These results correlated with Physician's Global Assessment (PGA) findings, with 72% and 90% of the infliximab 3- and 5-mg/kg groups, respectively, achieving PGAs of minimal (PGA = 1) or cleared (PGA = 0) psoriasis by week 10. Improvements in quality of life were also noted–the median change in Dermatology Life Quality Index (DLQI) from baseline to week 10 was −8 and −10 for the 3- and 5-mg/kg groups, respectively, compared with 10 in the placebo group.

To assess the safety of re-treatment, patients with PGA ≥ 3 were eligible for a single IV infusion of their assigned treatment at week 26. A month after re-treatment, 38%, 64%, and 18% of patients in the 3-mg/kg, 5-mg/kg, and placebo group had a PsA less than 3 (considered mild, minimal, or clear psoriasis).

Patients were followed up to 20 weeks to assess the duration of response. The maximum response was achieved at week 10 for both the 3- and the 5-mg/kg groups. The response began to decline at week 10 in the 3-mg/kg group and week 14 in the 5-mg/kg group.

In summary, SPIRIT demonstrated that infliximab induction therapy resulted in significant improvement in psoriasis for most patients in the study. After 3 doses of infliximab, the response rates in this study were similar to those seen with cyclosporine,[9,10] and greater than those achieved by other biologics.[11–13] The response seen at week 4, with about one-third and one-half of patients in the 3- and 5-mg/kg infliximab groups, was only seen after 12 or more weeks of therapy with other biologics.[11–13] The improvement in quality of life, as measured by DLQI, was also greater than other biologics or hospital-based treatment (Fig. 9.2).[1]

European Infliximab for Psoriasis Efficacy and Safety Study I

The EXPRESS I trial was a multicenter, double-blinded, phase 3 trial that evaluated the efficacy of infliximab induction and maintenance therapy for moderate-to-severe psoriasis.[5] The primary endpoint was the percentage of patients achieving PASI-75 at week 10. The secondary endpoints were PASI-50 and -90 at week 10. Selected patients had moderate-to-severe plaque psoriasis, PASI ≥12, BSA ≥10%, and were candidates for phototherapy and systemic therapy.

In the EXPRESS I trial, 378 patients were randomized to infusions of infliximab 5 mg/kg or placebo. Infusions were given at weeks 0, 2, 6, and then every 8 weeks up to week 46. Patients in the placebo group received placebo infusions at weeks 0, 2, 6, 14, 22 and then crossed over in a double-blinded fashion to receive infliximab 5 mg/kg at weeks 24, 26, 30, and every 8 weeks through week 46.

At week 10, 80% of patients achieved PASI-75 and 57% achieved PASI-90 in the infliximab

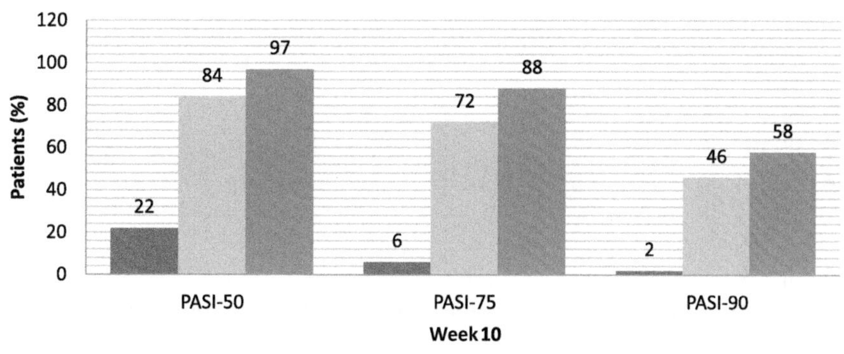

Fig. 9.2 Efficacy data of SPIRIT trial.

group. Only 3% and 1% of the placebo group achieved PASI-75 and PASI-90, respectively. This response was maintained at week 24. By week 50, PASI-75 and PASI-90 had dropped to 61% and 45%, respectively. Similarly, 83% of patients attained a PGA of clear or minimal psoriasis by week 10, which dropped to 53% at week 50. This decline in clinical response was associated with low infliximab serum concentrations due to the development of anti-infliximab antibodies. Within the group of patients who achieved PASI-75 at week 10, only 39% who were antibody positive maintained this response through week 50 versus 81% and 96% of the antibody-negative and inconclusive patients, respectively. Being antibody positive did not preclude those patients from having a clinical response, although fewer antibody-positive patients achieved PASI-75 or a maintained clinical response.

Maintenance of clinical response was related to the ability to achieve stable serum concentrations of infliximab. Of the patients who maintained their PASI response through week 50, median preinfusion serum infliximab concentrations were 1.0 μg/mL or greater at weeks 30 and later. The patients who lost response by week 50 had median preinfusion serum infliximab concentrations 1.0 μg/mL or less. Among the patients who achieved PASI-75 at week 10, 89% of patients maintained this response at 6 months and 65% maintained this response at 1 year. No dose escalation or additional therapy was needed, apart from low-potency topical corticosteroids on the face or groin.

In summary, the EXPRESS trial demonstrated the efficacy, rapid onset, and maintenance of therapeutic benefit of infliximab as monotherapy in moderate-to-severe psoriasis. By week 6, about two-thirds of patients achieved PASI-75 and one-third achieved PASI-90, with proportions of these patients continuing to increase during the course of the study. By week 10, one-fourth of patients reported complete clearing. This study also demonstrated that maintenance treatment with infliximab 5 mg/kg every 8 weeks was effective in maintaining clinical response and well tolerated in most patients (Fig. 9.3).

European Infliximab for Psoriasis Efficacy and Safety Study II

The EXPRESS II trial was a phase 3, randomized, double-blinded placebo-controlled trial that investigated the benefit of regular versus on-demand maintenance regimens of infliximab.[6] The EXPRESS II trial was the first biologic study to directly compare maintenance regimens of continuous, every-8-week therapy versus intermittent, as-needed therapy.

The primary endpoint was the percentage of patients achieving PASI-75 at week 10. Other endpoints were improvement in the PGA and DLQI by week 10, and the average percentage improvement from baseline PASI between weeks 16 and 30 and weeks 16 and 50.

All patients had moderate-to-severe psoriasis, with a PASI ≥12 and 10% or greater BSA involvement. This study consisted of 835 patients who were assigned to infliximab 3 mg/kg, 5 mg/kg, or placebo at weeks 0, 2, and 6. At week 14, patients were randomized again to either continuous maintenance therapy or as-needed intermittent therapy at the same dose as the induction phase. In the maintenance group, patients received their assigned infliximab doses at 8-week intervals (weeks 14, 22, 30, 38). In the as-needed group, infliximab was given when the PASI improvement from baseline dropped to less than 75% at the weekly study visits. If PASI improvement was at least 75%, placebo was given. The placebo group was crossed over at

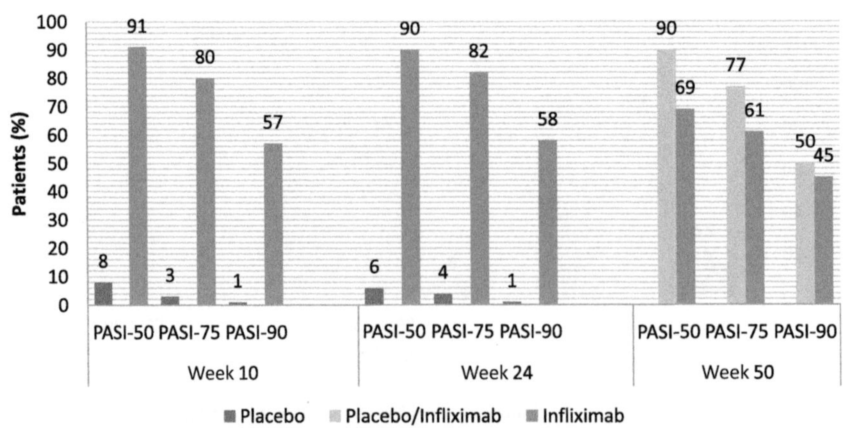

Fig. 9.3 Efficacy data of EXPRESS I trial.

week 16 to receive infliximab 5 mg/kg at weeks 16, 18, 22, and every 8 weeks until week 46.

At week 10, 70% and 75% of the 3-mg/kg and 5-mg/kg group had achieved PASI-75 versus 1.9% in the placebo group. PASI-90 was achieved by 37% and 45% of the 3-mg/kg and 5-mg/kg group versus 0.5% in the placebo group.

Efficacy for the maintenance phase was evaluated from week 14 through week 50. Among the week 10 PASI-75 responders, response was better maintained in the every-8-week continuous maintenance group as compared with the as-needed intermittent group. In the patients receiving 3 mg/kg, the median of the average percentage improvement in PASI was 80.6% for the every-8-week group versus 72.4% for the as-needed group. In the patients receiving 5 mg/kg, the median of the average percentage improvement in PASI was 89.6% versus 76.4% for the every-8-week group versus as-needed group. Among the week 10 PASI-75 nonresponders, 59.0% eventually achieved responder status at some point during the maintenance phase across all groups.

This study concluded that the patients in the 5-mg/kg every-8-week continuous therapy group maintained PASI responses better than the 5-mg/kg intermittent treatment group and 3-mg/kg groups. Of the patients assigned to 3 mg/kg, those who received infliximab every 8 weeks maintained PASI responses better than the intermittent treatment group as well. Although infliximab has been shown to provide excellent initial control, a maintenance regimen is important in sustaining adequate response. At the same time, long-term drug exposure should be limited by choosing the lowest effective dose or least frequent interval of drug administration (Fig. 9.4).

EFFICACY IN PSORIATIC ARTHRITIS

Treatment options for PsA are wide ranging, with nonsteroidal anti-inflammatory drugs (NSAIDs) being used for mild cases and disease-modifying antirheumatic drugs (DMARDs) for more severe cases. However, many patients do not respond significantly, and thus, the anti-TNF agents are becoming increasingly popular.

The Infliximab Multinational PsA Controlled Trial (IMPACT) study was a phase 3, double-blinded, randomized, controlled trial that assessed the efficacy of infliximab for PsA in patients who had failed prior treatment with DMARDs or NSAIDs.[14,15] The primary endpoint was American College of Rheumatology (ACR)-20 response at week 98. This study recruited 104 patients with active peripheral polyarticular joint involvement and was conducted in 3 stages. During stage 1, patients were assigned to placebo or infliximab 5 mg/kg at weeks 0, 2, 6, and 14. Stage 2 began at week 16, when the placebo group was crossed over to infliximab 5 mg/kg every 8 weeks through week 46. The original infliximab group continued to receive infliximab 5 mg/kg every 8 weeks until week 46. Stage 3 was an open-label extension from week 54 to week 98, during which patients received infliximab 5 mg/kg every 8 weeks.

At week 14, 58% of patients in the infliximab group and 11% in the placebo group achieved ACR20 response. By week 50, 74% of patients had achieved 20% or greater improvement in their ACR criteria. At week 98, 62% maintained this ACR20 response, with 45% and 35% achieving ACR50 and ACR70. At week 98, 82% or more of patients showed articular improvement, as evidenced by a moderate or good disease activity score (DAS) 28 response. DAS28 improved 48% and 43% from baseline at weeks

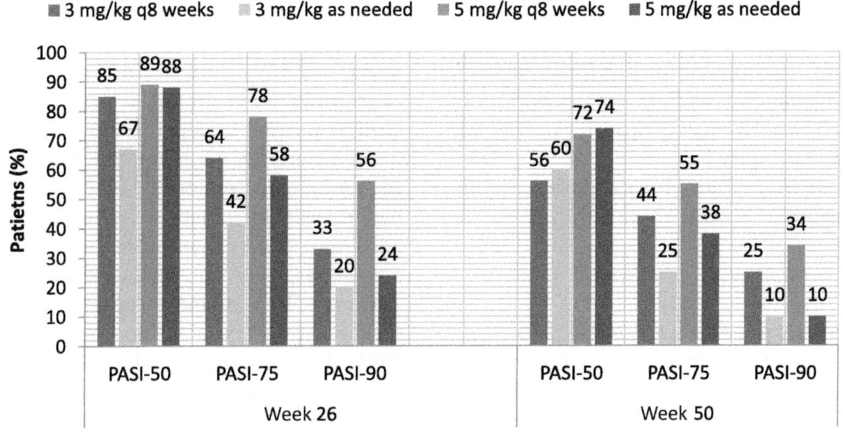

Fig. 9.4 Efficacy data of EXPRESS II trial.

50 and 98, respectively. Physical function also improved, with Health Assessment Questionnaire scores approaching normal levels of functioning by week 50 (49% improvement from mean baseline of 1.1). Average annual radiographic progression was also significantly reduced in the infliximab group as compared with placebo. The modified van der Heijde-Sharp (vdH-S score) was used to score bone erosion, joint space narrowing, and total radiographic scores in 40 joints in both hands and 12 joints in both feet. At baseline, the mean estimated annual progression was 5.74 modified vdH-S points. At year 2 of infliximab treatment, the mean estimated progression was significantly reduced to 0.65 modified vdH-S points. One drawback of the modified vdH-S scoring system is that changes in just 1 joint of a patient may result in a higher score and overemphasize the disease course. This data together indicate that infliximab 5 mg/kg was able to maintain a significant, sustained clinical improvement in treatment-refractory PsA.

SAFETY

Infliximab is very well tolerated by most patients. Because of TNF's role in mounting an immune response, the most common risk with TNF inhibitors is that of infection and malignancy. Sepsis, invasive fungal infections, opportunistic infections, and reactivation of latent tuberculosis (TB) are more serious infections that have been reported. Lymphoma and nonmelanoma skin cancer (NMSC) are also concerns with the administration of TNF antagonists.

The most common side effects in randomized clinical trials were upper respiratory infections, headaches, and infusion reactions.[1,5,6] Those with antibodies to infliximab were seen to be especially prone to infusion reactions.[16] Other adverse events (AEs) include hepatitis B, multiple sclerosis (MS) and demyelinating disorders, congestive heart failure (CHF), drug-induced lupus, blood dyscrasias, and hypersensitivity reactions. Worsening of CHF was reported in one study in the 10-mg/kg group.[17] Infliximab is pregnancy category B.[4]

Safety data from clinical trials are presented in later discussion.

Study of Psoriasis with Infliximab Induction Therapy

Patients were assessed through week 30 for AEs.[1] The rate of AEs was slightly higher in the 3-mg/kg and 5-mg/kg groups as compared with placebo (78%, 79%, and 63%, respectively). However, the fact that patients in the infliximab group received a larger number of infusions and were followed for longer was not adjusted for. Of the 12 patients who reported serious AEs, 4 were considered by Gottlieb and colleagues[1] to be related to infliximab. One patient reported squamous cell carcinoma, and 1 patient reported cholecystitis and cholelithiasis in the 3 mg/kg group. In the 5-mg/kg group, 1 patient reported diverticulitis, sepsis, and pyelonephritis.

The rate of infusion reactions was 18%, 22%, and 2% in the 3-mg/kg, 5-mg/kg, and placebo groups, respectively. Symptoms included headache, flushing, chills, nausea, dyspnea, site infiltrations, and taste perversion. Most were mild or moderate in severity.

The re-treatment infusions were well tolerated, with no delayed-type hypersensitivity reactions reported. At week 26, the incidence of infusion reactions was 2 to 3 times higher for patients with antibodies to infliximab versus antibody-negative patients. Despite this, the presence of antibodies was poorly predictive of infusion reactions during the study, because most antibody-positive patients did not have infusion reactions.

Laboratory values were for the most part unchanged, with the exception of elevated alanine aminotransferase (placebo 16%, infliximab 34%) and aspartate aminotransferase (placebo 14%, infliximab 24%).

Antinuclear antibodies (ANA) were also measured in this study, because of previous studies that detected newly positive ANAs in patients receiving infliximab. The incidence of newly positive ANA was 22% to 25% in the SPIRIT trial, which is lower than previous trials of infliximab in rheumatoid arthritis and Crohn disease. No patients developed drug-induced lupus or lupuslike syndrome.

European Infliximab for Psoriasis Efficacy and Safety Study I

The proportion of patients who reported AEs was slightly higher in the infliximab versus placebo group (82% vs 71%).[5] Three serious infections were reported in the infliximab group; 1 patient died as a result of sepsis and necrotizing fasciitis from a burn on his hand, for which he did not seek medical attention for 1 week. Three delayed hypersensitivity reactions were reported in the infliximab group. Symptoms included myalgias, arthralgias, fever, and rash, which improved within 2 weeks. Two patients reported lupuslike syndrome with arthralgias and anti-double-stranded DNA. Four serious infusion reactions were reported in infliximab patients. There were no cases of TB, demyelinating events, heart failure, or malignancies other than skin cancer.

European Infliximab for Psoriasis Efficacy and Safety Study II

The safety profile of infliximab in this study was similar to that of previous trials.[6] Across the 4 different treatment regimens, the safety profile was similar. There were no additional safety concerns for the 5-mg/kg group over the 3-mg/kg group. Two cases of TB were reported in patients who originally had negative purified protein derivative (PPD) tests, emphasizing the importance of thorough screening at baseline for TB risk factors and consideration of chest radiographs.[18] Twelve malignancies were reported in the infliximab group. One patient developed squamous cell carcinoma and 9 developed basal cell carcinomas. All 10 of these patients had previous exposure to narrowband UV-B and/or PUVA. Two patients in the infliximab group reported lupuslike syndrome. One patient developed prolonged muscle weakness and peripheral neuropathy, which subsequently resolved. One patient with no prior cardiac history died of a fatal myocardial infarction 9 months after discontinuing infliximab. Five patients reported serious infusion reactions in the combined infliximab treatment groups. Nine reported delayed hypersensitivity reactions, with myalgias and/or arthralgias, and fever and/or rash.

Psoriasis Longitudinal Assessment and Registry

Psoriasis Longitudinal Assessment and Registry (PSOLAR) is the largest intercontinental registry for patients with psoriasis on biologic therapy.[19] Conducted from 2007 to 2013, PSOLAR enrolled 12,095 patients who received either infliximab, ustekinumab, other biologic agents, or nonbiologic agents. Rates of all-cause mortality, major adverse cardiovascular events (MACE), malignancies (excluding MNSC), and serious infections were reported.

Although incidence rates for all-cause mortality, MACE, and malignancy were comparable across the biologic groups, rates of death and MACE were higher in the nonbiologic group. Although oral immunomodulator use (defined as either MTX or cyclosporine) increased risk of MACE, infliximab and other biologics did not predict MACE. Higher rates of serious infections were reported in the infliximab group and other biologics group, as compared with the ustekinumab and nonbiologic groups. PSOLAR concluded that no additional safety precautions were identified for infliximab, other biologic agents, or immunomodulators. The association between TNF inhibitors and risk of serious infection is consistent with previous studies and already detailed in prescribing information. Safety data from PSOLAR will continue to be reported to regulatory agencies annually (Table 9.2).

PRECAUTIONS

It is important that dermatologists are wary of precautions in infliximab administration. Special

TABLE 9.2
Safety data from Psoriasis Longitudinal Assessment and Registry

	Infliximab	Ustekinumab	Other Biologics	Nonbiologics	Total
All-cause mortality	0.35 (21)	0.43 (30)	0.42 (55)	0.70 (39)	0.46 (145)
Cardiovascular	0.08 (5)	0.13 (9)	0.10 (13)	0.22 (12)	0.12 (39)
Other	0.17 (10)	0.23 (16)	0.23 (30)	0.32 (18)	0.23 (74)
Unexplained death	0.10 (6)	0.07 (5)	0.09 (12)	0.16 (9)	0.10 (32)
MACE	0.38 (23)	0.33 (23)	0.33 (43)	0.45 (25)	0.36 (114)
Cardiovascular death	0.08 (5)	0.13 (9)	0.10 (13)	0.22 (12)	0.12 (39)
Nonfatal cerebrovascular accident	0.12 (7)	0.10 (7)	0.11 (14)	0.11 (6)	0.11 (34)
Nonfatal myocardial infarction	0.18 (11)	0.10 (7)	0.14 (19)	0.14 (8)	0.14 (45)
Malignancy excluding NMSC	0.58 (35)	0.53 (37)	0.74 (98)	0.81 (45)	0.68 (215)
Serious infections and infestations	2.73 (67)	1.0 (56)	1.80 (186)	1.26 (169)	1.5 (478)

Data from Gottlieb AB, Kalb RE, Langley RG, et al. Safety observations in 12095 patients with psoriasis enrolled in an international registry (PSOLAR): experience with infliximab and other systemic and biologic therapies. J Drugs Dermatol 2014;13(12):1441–8.

attention should be given to patient populations with a history of TB, malignancy, demyelinating disorders, CHF, and certain other conditions, given the role of TNF in such disease pathogenesis.

Infection

Patients using infliximab are at increased risk for serious infection (bacterial, viral, fungal, and parasitic). Risk is increased with concomitant use of MTX, corticosteroids, and other immunosuppressants, or in patients with underlying predisposing medical conditions. The use of infliximab with concomitant abatacept and anakinra is not recommended, because patients with rheumatoid arthritis had an increased risk of serious infection with such therapy.[4,20]

Infliximab should be withheld in patients requiring antibiotics, discontinued in those with serious or opportunistic infections, and should not be initiated in patients with active infection (systemic or localized). Risks and benefits should be discussed before initiating therapy in patients with recurrent/chronic infection, and careful monitoring should take place.[4,21,22]

Tuberculosis

Patients receiving infliximab therapy are at increased risk for the development of TB or reactivation of latent TB (pulmonary and extrapulmonary TB). Patients should be evaluated based on risk factors for TB and screened for latent TB before initiation and during therapy. A PPD screen with 5-mm or greater induration is considered positive, even in those with a history of BCG vaccination.[22]

TB treatment should be given to any patient with a history of active or latent TB, in whom completion of a treatment course cannot be confirmed as well as in patients with risk factors for TB infection but a negative screen. Infliximab therapy can be initiated after 1 to 2 months of latent TB treatment, although reactivation of TB remains a possibility despite prophylactic treatment. A TB expert should be consulted in the case of any questions or hesitations.[4]

Opportunistic Infections

Opportunistic infections, such as aspergillosis, blastomycosis, candidiasis, histoplasmosis, legionellosis, listeriosis, coccidioidomycosis, cryptococccosis, and pneumocystis, are more likely to present in this population and may present with disseminated rather than localized infection. If the symptomatic patient resides or travels to regions of endemic mycoses, it is important to consider empiric antifungal therapy while waiting on a diagnostic workup. Consider that antigen and antibody testing may be negative in patients with active histoplasmosis.[4,22]

Malignancy

An increased incidence rate for melanoma and NMSC has been shown in psoriasis patients using infliximab.[4] This rate is associated with the use of high-dose psoralen and PUVA, cyclosporine, MTX, and immunosuppressants for NMSC.[23] Patients with a personal history of malignancy should take special precaution.

Increased rates of lymphoma have been reported in patients receiving either etanercept or infliximab for psoriasis.[24] There is also, however, a general increased risk of Hodgkin lymphoma and cutaneous T-cell lymphoma in psoriasis patients that should be acknowledged.[25,26]

Hepatitis B

TNF is thought to promote viral clearance in hepatitis B.[22] If a patient receiving infliximab therapy develops hepatitis B virus (HBV) reactivation, therapy should be stopped immediately and antiviral therapy should ensue.[4]

Patients should be monitored for signs and symptoms of HBV infection during and for 6 months after stopping therapy. This monitoring includes liver function tests (LFTs), hepatitis B surface antigen, hepatitis B envelope antigen, and HBV DNA counts in patients at risk for reactivation.[27] No definitive information is available regarding treating HBV carriers with antiviral therapy along with infliximab or regarding resuming infliximab therapy after the control of reactivated HBV infection.

Multiple Sclerosis and Demyelinating Disorders

TNF inhibitors have been associated with new-onset or exacerbation of central nervous system demyelinating disorders (MS, optic neuritis) and peripheral demyelinating diseases such as Guillain-Barré syndrome.[22,28] It should not be initiated in patients with a history of MS (including in a first-degree relative, given the increased risk)[29,30] or other demyelinating disorders. Associated neurologic symptoms have been reported to resolve with termination of therapy.[28]

Congestive Heart Failure

Although the role of TNF in CHF is much debated, 2 randomized, controlled trials, RENAISSANCE/RECOVER (Randomized Etanercept North American Strategy to Study Antagonism of Cytokines/Research into Etanercept: Cytokine Antagonism in Ventricular Dysfunction) and ATTACH (Anti-TNF Therapy

Against Congestive Heart Failure), have shown trends toward a worse CHF prognosis that was dose-dependent with TNF inhibitors. Infliximab should be withdrawn with new-onset or worsening symptoms in patients with pre-existing CHF.[17,31] Patients diagnosed with class 3 or 4 CHF or ejection fraction less than 50% should avoid infliximab use, and class 1 or 2 CHF should undergo echocardiographic testing.[22,32,33]

Drug-induced Lupus

Infliximab therapy can lead to autoantibody formation, although few of these patients develop clinical symptoms. It has been suggested that the development of autoantibodies with initiation of anti-TNF therapy is a marker for forthcoming treatment failure.[34]

A recent study found that 48% of infliximab-treated patients formed autoantibodies.[35] If a patient experiences signs and symptoms of a lupuslike syndrome, the dermatologist should assess circulating ANA and discontinue therapy.[22]

Blood Dyscrasias

Isolated cases of aplastic anemia, pancytopenia, isolated leukopenia, and thrombocytopenia have been reported with TNF-inhibitor use.[36,37] Patients experiencing pallor, easy bruising, bleeding, or persistent fever should seek immediate attention. Infliximab therapy should be discontinued with significant hematologic abnormalities.[4,22]

Hypersensitivity Reactions

There have been rare reported cases of anaphylaxis, angioneurotic edema, allergic rash, fixed drug reactions, urticaria, serum sickness, and non-specified drug reactions. Immediately discontinue infliximab therapy if this occurs and start appropriate therapy.[4]

MONITORING

The information presented is primarily based on psoriasis guidelines from the American Academy of Dermatology (AAD).[38]

A thorough history and physical examination should be taken before initiation of infliximab therapy, including TB exposure, chronic/recurrent infections, malignancy, neurologic and cardiac history, and a thorough review of systems. Routine follow-up examinations should adequately monitor patients for side effects and AEs.[39]

Aside from baseline TB test, annual monitoring for TB, and a baseline hepatitis B test, routine laboratory testing beyond that for concomitant therapies or comorbidities is generally not supported.[40] The highest grade US Preventative Services Task Force evidence of screening studies is grade B for TB testing (interferon-γ release assay is preferred over tuberculin skin testing). There have been reports of treatment with infliximab $\pm$ MTX leading to reactivation of chronic hepatitis B infection. It is unclear how TNF-α affects hepatitis C, and data from small scale studies are insufficient to refute or support the need to monitor for hepatitis B virus (HCV). Based on evidence from these small studies, HBV/HCV screening is only supported by grade C evidence.[41] The AAD recommends baseline PPD, LFTs, complete blood count (CBC), hepatitis profile, history, and physical examinations for patients on infliximab.

The Centers for Disease Control and Prevention recommends TB testing before the therapy initiation.[18] Positive skin test findings should be followed with a chest radiograph—if negative, patients should be treated for latent TB (6–9 months of 300 mg isoniazid daily and/or 4 months of 600 mg daily rifampicin),[42] and if positive, patients should receive therapy for active TB. Biologic therapy may be started after 1 to 2 months of prophylactic treatment if the patient is adherent to and tolerating the prophylactic regimen.[43] If a patient has a positive PPD due to prior BCG vaccination, blood tests can be obtained measuring interferon production on stimulation with TB antigens that are not present in BCG. Most guidelines perform annual TB skin testing in patients receiving infliximab to screen for the TB reactivation, especially in those at risk (ie, health care workers, travelers to endemic areas).

The authors of this section recommend initial baseline monitoring that includes a QuantiFERON-TB Gold (QFT), LFTs, CBC, and hepatitis B and hepatitis C profile. QFT should be repeated annually (Table 9.3).

TABLE 9.3
Monitoring recommendations from the American Academy of Dermatology

	Monitoring
History and physical	Baseline and routine
CBC	Baseline and periodically
LFTs	Baseline and periodically
TB skin test	Baseline and annually after
Hepatitis B serology	Before initiation of therapy

Data from Menter A, Gottlieb A, Feldman SR, et al. Guidelines of care for the management of psoriasis and psoriatic arthritis: section 1. Overview of psoriasis and guidelines of care for the treatment of psoriasis with biologics. J Am Acad Dermatol 2008;58(5):841.

VACCINATIONS

Because of the possibility that biologic agents may impair the body's immunologic response to vaccinations, administration of vaccinations should be carefully considered in patients receiving biologic therapy (Table 9.4). Live vaccines (measles, mumps, and rubella [MMR], varicella, zoster, intranasal influenza, and so forth) are contraindicated within 1 month of treatment.[44] However, scientifically based/standardized recommendations for administering biologically inactive or recombinant vaccines to patients on biologic agents are lacking. Non-live vaccinations may have the potential to achieve adequate immune response, although antibody titers may not achieve optimal levels and may decrease more rapidly if given during biologic therapy.

It is preferable to complete all age-appropriate immunizations according to current immunization guidelines before initiating biologic therapy. The production of antibodies from the vaccine generally occurs in the 2-week period from primary

TABLE 9.4
Vaccination recommendations from the National Psoriasis Foundation

Vaccination	Before Therapy	During Therapy
Live vaccines (MMR, varicella, herpes zoster, intranasal influenza, oral typhoid, yellow fever, oral polio, smallpox, BCG, rotavirus)	Contraindicated within 1 mo	**Contraindicated
Influenza	Vaccinate with inactivated or live	Yearly immunization with inactivated vaccine
Chicken pox	If negative serology, vaccinate	**Contraindicated
Zoster	Before therapy: 1 dose for adults ≥50 y	**Contraindicated
Human papillomavirus	Unvaccinated male/female patients up to age 26	Same
Hepatitis A	Vaccinate if high risk (diabetes, liver disease, IV drug users, homosexual men, and so forth)	Same; consider obtaining postvaccination serology
Hepatitis B	Serology, risk factor assessment. Offer vaccination if necessary	High-dose vaccine Consider obtaining serology postvaccination
Pneumococcal	Pneumococcal polysaccharide vaccine (PPSV23) vaccine recommended	Pneumococcal conjugate vaccine followed by PPSV23 if not given before
Haemophilus influenzas type b	Vaccinate if unvaccinated	Same
MMR	Vaccinate if negative, or seronegative to any component	**Contraindicated
Tetanus-diphtheria/ diphtheria-tetanus-acellular pertussis (TDAP)	Booster every 10 y and high-risk wounds Offer before therapy, substitute 1 dose with TDAP	Same
Meningococcal	Assess risk factors, vaccinate if high risk (asplenia, complement deficient, group living)	Same
Poliomyelitis	Assess risk factors, vaccinate if high risk (health care worker, laboratory worker)	Same

** Vaccination can be considered on case-by-case basis in consultation with experts.

Adapted from Lebwohl M. Psoriasis. Lancet 2003;361(9364):1197–204; and Wine-Lee L, Keller SC, Wilck MB, et al. *From* the Medical Board of the National Psoriasis Foundation: vaccination in adult patients on systemic therapy for psoriasis. J Am Acad Dermatol 2013;69(6):1007.

immunization, but could take more than 6 weeks to peak. A period of 4 times the half-life of infliximab (56 days) has been suggested to allow for the return of the immune system to its baseline before vaccination with live vaccines (see Table 9.4).

SUMMARY AND RECOMMENDATIONS

The efficacy of infliximab in the treatment of moderate-to-severe plaque psoriasis has been documented in multiple randomized, controlled trials. Infliximab is notable for its ability to achieve rapid clinical response, with an onset of action that is faster than other biologics.[45] Multiple meta-analyses evaluating etanercept, infliximab, adalimumab, and ustekinumab found that infliximab is most efficacious, with a higher proportion of patients achieving PASI-75.[46–49] Continuous maintenance therapy with infliximab was also found to be more effective than as-needed, intermittent therapy.[22] The authors consider infliximab to be third- or fourth-line biologic therapy for patients with chronic, severe plaque psoriasis who are candidates for systemic therapies.[4,50] Infliximab's main advantage is that it is the only biologic that is dosed based on exact weight. Thus, very obese patients are more likely to clear on infliximab compared with other biologics. Further studies comparing the efficacy of infliximab directly to systemic therapies and other biologics as well as infliximab as combination therapy (in particular with MTX) for psoriasis are warranted.

REFERENCES

1. Gottlieb AB, Evans R, Li S, et al. Infliximab induction therapy for patients with severe plaque-type psoriasis: a randomized, double-blind, placebo-controlled trial. J Am Acad Dermatol 2004;51(4):534–42.
2. Gall JS, Kalb RE. Infliximab for the treatment of plaque psoriasis. Biologics 2008;2(1):115–24.
3. Fathi R, Armstrong AW. The role of biologic therapies in dermatology. Med Clin North Am 2015;99(6):1183–94.
4. FDA. Highlights of prescribing information. 2013. Available at: http://www.accessdata.fda.gov/drugsatfda_docs/label/2013/103772s5359lbl.pdf. Accessed January 30, 2016.
5. Reich K, Nestle FO, Papp K, et al. Infliximab induction and maintenance therapy for moderate-to-severe psoriasis: a phase III, multicentre, double-blind trial. Lancet 2005;366(9494):1367–74.
6. Menter A, Feldman SR, Weinstein GD, et al. A randomized comparison of continuous vs. intermittent infliximab maintenance regimens over 1 year in the treatment of moderate-to-severe plaque psoriasis. J Am Acad Dermatol 2007;56(1):31.e1-15.
7. Knight DM, Trinh H, Le J, et al. Construction and initial characterization of a mouse-human chimeric anti-TNF antibody. Mol Immunol 1993;30(16):1443–53.
8. Scallon BJ, Moore MA, Trinh H, et al. Chimeric anti-TNF-α monoclonal antibody cA2 binds recombinant transmembrane TNF-α and activates immune effector functions. Cytokine 1995;7(3):251–9.
9. Ellis CN, Fradin MS, Messana JM, et al. Cyclosporine for plaque-type psoriasis. Results of a multidose, double-blind trial. N Engl J Med 1991;324(5):277–84.
10. Koo J. A randomized, double-blind study comparing the efficacy, safety and optimal dose of two formulations of cyclosporin, Neoral and Sandimmun, in patients with severe psoriasis. OLP302 Study Group. Br J Dermatol 1998;139(1):88–95.
11. Mease PJ, Goffe BS, Metz J, et al. Etanercept in the treatment of psoriatic arthritis and psoriasis: a randomised trial. Lancet 2000;356(9227):385–90.
12. Lebwohl M. Psoriasis. Lancet 2003;361(9364):1197–204.
13. Ellis CN, Krueger GG, Alefacept Clinical Study Group. Treatment of chronic plaque psoriasis by selective targeting of memory effector T lymphocytes. N Engl J Med 2001;345(4):248–55.
14. Antoni C, Krueger G, de Vlam K, et al. Infliximab improves signs and symptoms of psoriatic arthritis: results of the IMPACT 2 trial. Ann Rheum Dis 2005;64(8):1150–7.
15. Antoni CE, Kavanaugh A, van der Heijde D, et al. Two-year efficacy and safety of infliximab treatment in patients with active psoriatic arthritis: findings of the Infliximab Multinational Psoriatic Arthritis Controlled Trial (IMPACT). J Rheumatol 2008;35(5):869–76.
16. Lecluse LLA, Piskin G, Mekkes JR, et al. Review and expert opinion on prevention and treatment of infliximab-related infusion reactions. Br J Dermatol 2008;159(3):527–36.
17. Chung ES, Packer M, Lo KH, et al, Anti-TNF Therapy Against Congestive Heart Failure Investigators. Randomized, double-blind, placebo-controlled, pilot trial of infliximab, a chimeric monoclonal antibody to tumor necrosis factor-alpha, in patients with moderate-to-severe heart failure: results of the anti-TNF Therapy Against Congestive Heart Failure (ATTACH) trial. Circulation 2003;107(25):3133–40.
18. CDC - Tuberculosis (TB). Available at: http://www.cdc.gov/tb/?404;http://www.cdc.gov:80/tb/pubs/LTBI/pdf/TargetedLTBI05.pdf. Accessed February 6, 2016.
19. Gottlieb AB, Kalb RE, Langley RG, et al. Safety observations in 12095 patients with psoriasis enrolled in an international registry (PSOLAR): experience

with infliximab and other systemic and biologic therapies. J Drugs Dermatol 2014;13(12):1441–8.
20. Kimball AB, Rothman KJ, Kricorian G, et al. OBSERVE-5: observational postmarketing safety surveillance registry of etanercept for the treatment of psoriasis final 5-year results. J Am Acad Dermatol 2015;72(1):115–22.
21. Bresnihan B, Cunnane G. Infection complications associated with the use of biologic agents. Rheum Dis Clin North Am 2003;29(1):185–202.
22. Menter A, Korman NJ, Elmets CA, et al. Guidelines of care for the management of psoriasis and psoriatic arthritis: section 4. Guidelines of care for the management and treatment of psoriasis with traditional systemic agents. J Am Acad Dermatol 2009; 61(3):451–85.
23. Paul CF, Ho VC, McGeown C, et al. Risk of malignancies in psoriasis patients treated with cyclosporine: a 5 y cohort study. J Invest Dermatol 2003;120(2):211–6.
24. Brown SL, Greene MH, Gershon SK, et al. Tumor necrosis factor antagonist therapy and lymphoma development: twenty-six cases reported to the Food and Drug Administration. Arthritis Rheum 2002;46(12):3151–8.
25. Gelfand JM, Berlin J, Van Voorhees A, et al. Lymphoma rates are low but increased in patients with psoriasis: results from a population-based cohort study in the United Kingdom. Arch Dermatol 2003;139(11):1425–9.
26. Gelfand JM, Shin DB, Neimann AL, et al. The risk of lymphoma in patients with psoriasis. J Invest Dermatol 2006;126(10):2194–201.
27. Motaparthi K, Stanisic V, Voorhees ASV, et al. From the Medical Board of the National Psoriasis Foundation: recommendations for screening for hepatitis B infection prior to initiating anti-tumor necrosis factor-alfa inhibitors or other immunosuppressive agents in patients with psoriasis. J Am Acad Dermatol 2014;70(1):178–86.
28. Mohan N, Edwards ET, Cupps TR, et al. Demyelination occurring during anti-tumor necrosis factor alpha therapy for inflammatory arthritides. Arthritis Rheum 2001;44(12):2862–9.
29. Barcellos LF, Kamdar BB, Ramsay PP, et al. Clustering of autoimmune diseases in families with a high-risk for multiple sclerosis: a descriptive study. Lancet Neurol 2006;5(11):924–31.
30. Dyment DA, Sadovnick AD, Willer CJ, et al. An extended genome scan in 442 Canadian multiple sclerosis-affected sibships: a report from the Canadian Collaborative Study Group. Hum Mol Genet 2004;13(10):1005–15.
31. Coletta AP, Clark AL, Banarjee P, et al. Clinical trials update: RENEWAL (RENAISSANCE and RECOVER) and ATTACH. Eur J Heart Fail 2002; 4(4):559–61.
32. Desai SB, Furst DE. Problems encountered during anti-tumour necrosis factor therapy. Best Pract Res Clin Rheumatol 2006;20(4):757–90.
33. Khanna D, McMahon M, Furst DE. Safety of tumour necrosis factor-alpha antagonists. Drug Saf 2004; 27(5):307–24.
34. Pink AE, Fonia A, Allen MH, et al. Antinuclear antibodies associate with loss of response to antitumour necrosis factor-alpha therapy in psoriasis: a retrospective, observational study. Br J Dermatol 2010;162(4):780–5.
35. Bardazzi F, Odorici G, Virdi A, et al. Autoantibodies in psoriatic patients treated with anti-TNF-α therapy. J Dtsch Dermatol Ges 2014;12(5):401–6.
36. Kuruvilla J, Leitch HA, Vickars LM, et al. Aplastic anemia following administration of a tumor necrosis factor-alpha inhibitor. Eur J Haematol 2003;71(5): 396–8.
37. Vidal F, Fontova R, Richart C. Severe neutropenia and thrombocytopenia associated with infliximab. Ann Intern Med 2003;139(3):W-W63.
38. Menter A, Gottlieb A, Feldman SR, et al. Guidelines of care for the management of psoriasis and psoriatic arthritis: section 1. Overview of psoriasis and guidelines of care for the treatment of psoriasis with biologics. J Am Acad Dermatol 2008;58(5):826–50.
39. Lebwohl M, Bagel J, Gelfand JM, et al. From the Medical Board of the National Psoriasis Foundation: monitoring and vaccinations in patients treated with biologics for psoriasis. J Am Acad Dermatol 2008;58(1):94–105.
40. Van Lümig PPM, Driessen RJB, Roelofs-Thijssen MA, et al. Relevance of laboratory investigations in monitoring patients with psoriasis on etanercept or adalimumab. Br J Dermatol 2011;165(2):375–82.
41. Ahn CS, Dothard EH, Garner ML, et al. To test or not to test? An updated evidence-based assessment of the value of screening and monitoring tests when using systemic biologic agents to treat psoriasis and psoriatic arthritis. J Am Acad Dermatol 2015; 73(3):420–8.e1.
42. Targeted tuberculin testing and treatment of latent tuberculosis infection. American Thoracic Society. MMWR Recomm Rep 2000;49(RR-6):1–51.
43. Doherty SD, Voorhees AV, Lebwohl MG, et al. National Psoriasis Foundation consensus statement on screening for latent tuberculosis infection in patients with psoriasis treated with systemic and biologic agents. J Am Acad Dermatol 2008;59(2): 209–17.
44. Wine-Lee L, Keller SC, Wilck MB, et al. From the Medical Board of the National Psoriasis Foundation: vaccination in adult patients on systemic therapy for psoriasis. J Am Acad Dermatol 2013; 69(6):1003–13.
45. Nast A, Jacobs A, Rosumeck S, et al. Efficacy and safety of systemic long-term treatments for

moderate-to-severe psoriasis: a systematic review and meta-analysis. J Invest Dermatol 2015;135(11): 2641–8.

46. Schmitt J, Rosumeck S, Thomaschewski G, et al. Efficacy and safety of systemic treatments for moderate-to-severe psoriasis: meta-analysis of randomized controlled trials. Br J Dermatol 2014; 170(2):274–303.
47. Signorovitch JE, Betts KA, Yan YS, et al. Comparative efficacy of biological treatments for moderate-to-severe psoriasis: a network meta-analysis adjusting for cross-trial differences in reference arm response. Br J Dermatol 2015;172(2):504–12.
48. Reich K, Burden AD, Eaton JN, et al. Efficacy of biologics in the treatment of moderate to severe psoriasis: a network meta-analysis of randomized controlled trials. Br J Dermatol 2012; 166(1):179–88.
49. Lin VW, Ringold S, Devine EB. Comparison of ustekinumab with other biological agents for the treatment of moderate to severe plaque psoriasis: a Bayesian Network Meta-analysis. Arch Dermatol 2012;148(12):1403–10.
50. Yawalkar N. Management of psoriasis. Bern, Switzerland: Karger Medical and Scientific Publishers; 2009.

CHAPTER 10

Adalimumab

Shivani P. Reddy, BS, Elaine J. Lin, MD, Vidhi V. Shah, BA,
Jashin J. Wu, MD

KEYWORDS

• Adalimumab • TNF-α • Psoriasis • CHAMPION • REVEAL • ADEPT • ESPRIT

KEY POINTS

- Adalimumab is a safe and effective therapy for the treatment of moderate-to-severe psoriasis.
- The mechanism of action of adalimumab is inhibition of tumor necrosis factor-α (TNF-α), thereby inhibiting the inflammatory cascade leading to psoriatic skin lesions.
- Pivotal trials on adalimumab therapy for the treatment of psoriasis and psoriatic arthritis include CHAMPION, REVEAL, and ADEPT.
- Adalimumab is generally safe and well-tolerated. Annual tuberculosis screening is recommended with adalimumab use.

INTRODUCTION

The advent of adalimumab therapy has greatly advanced the effectiveness of skin clearance in moderate-to-severe plaque psoriasis. Originally developed for the treatment of rheumatoid arthritis (RA)[1] and psoriatic arthritis (PsA), adalimumab improves skin lesions in patients with psoriasis. Adalimumab was approved by the US Food and Drug Administration (FDA) for the treatment of moderate-to-severe chronic plaque psoriasis in 2008 and has since become a widely used therapy in the United States and abroad. It is also effective in erythrodermic and generalized pustular psoriasis[2] and is additionally FDA approved for the treatment of RA, juvenile idiopathic arthritis, PsA, ankylosing spondylitis, adult Crohn disease, pediatric Crohn disease, ulcerative colitis, and hidradenitis suppurativa.[3]

The current recommended dosing of adalimumab for psoriasis is subcutaneous (SC) injection of an 80-mg loading dose at baseline, 40 mg the following week, and maintenance on 40 mg every other week (EOW) thereafter (Fig. 10.1).[3] No definitive conclusions have been made regarding off-label omission of the loading dose.[4] After a single dose, adalimumab levels peak in the bloodstream at approximately 5.5 days, with a half-life of approximately 2 weeks.[1]

Available methods of SC injections include a pen and syringe, each containing 0.8 mL of 40 mg adalimumab. Self-injection is permitted so long as the dermatologist has carefully explained and evaluated the patient's ability to do so. Injection sites should be alternated and should not be chosen in regions of bruised or tender skin. Patients tend to prefer the pen over the syringe, as it less painful, more convenient, faster, and safer.[5]

MECHANISM OF ACTION

Adalimumab is the first fully human recombinant immunoglobulin G1 monoclonal antibody that binds and neutralizes soluble and membrane-bound tumor necrosis factor (TNF), so that it cannot interact with p55 and p75 cell-surface TNF receptors. It also induces apoptosis in mononuclear cells with TNF receptors.[6]

In regards to the pathogenesis of psoriasis and PsA, adalimumab inhibits specific events such as the release of serum cytokines (interleukin-6), acute phase reactants of inflammation, matrix metalloproteases, other markers of cartilage and synovium turnover, and the expression of adhesion molecules responsible for leukocyte migration.[6] The inhibition of these events is thought to prevent epidermal cell hyperproliferation leading to psoriatic skin lesions.

EFFICACY

Clinical trials on adalimumab therapy for psoriasis demonstrated remarkable results that led to its

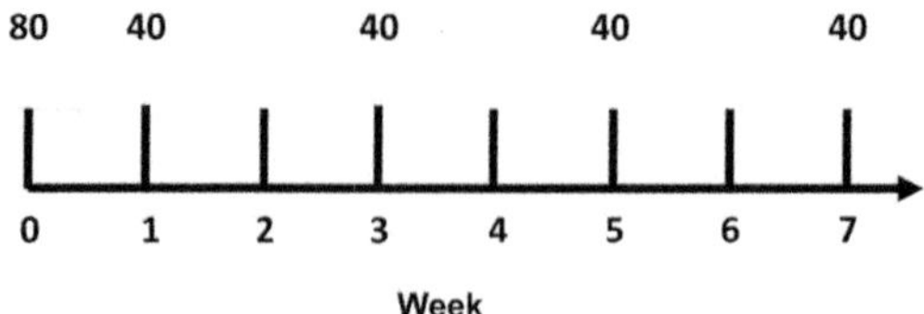

Fig. 10.1 Adalimumab dosing regimen for psoriasis: 80-mg loading dose at baseline, followed by 40 mg the next week and 40 mg EOW thereafter.

FDA approval. REVEAL and CHAMPION, phase 3 pivotal trials on the drug label, investigated the efficacy and safety profiles of adalimumab versus placebo (in controlled and interrupted therapy), and adalimumab versus placebo versus methotrexate (MTX), respectively (Table 10.1).

REVEAL

REVEAL was a 52-week randomized, controlled trial that enrolled 1212 patients from 81 sites across North America.[7] Adalimumab efficacy was assessed by 2 primary end points, achievement of Psoriasis Area Severity Index (PASI) -75 at week 16, and percentage of patients who lost an adequate response between weeks 33 and 52. The study population consisted of 53% of patients with moderate psoriasis, and 47% of patients with severe/very severe psoriasis by Physician's Global Assessment (PGA).

The study was divided into 3 periods: A, B, and C (Fig. 10.2). During period A (weeks 0–15), patients were randomized 2:1 to receive standard recommended dosing of adalimumab or matched placebo dosing. Patients who achieved PASI-75 by week 16 were continued on to period B, whereas those who did not were eligible for a separate Open-Label Extension (OLE) study. During period B, the blind nature of the study was maintained by giving placebo-treated patients 2 injections of 40 mg adalimumab, and adalimumab-treated patients 2 injections of placebo. Then, all patients received 40 mg adalimumab EOW (weeks 16–33). Patients who achieved PASI-75 by week 33 were eligible to continue on to period C (weeks 34–52) to investigate whether adequate response would be lost with interrupted therapy (patients who achieved PASI-50 to PASI-75 response were eligible for the OLE study). Patients originally in the active therapy group from period A were rerandomized in a 1:1 ratio to receive adalimumab or placebo in order to assess for loss of response from weeks 33 to 52. Loss of response was defined as less than PASI-50 response after week 33 (relative to baseline score) and at least a 6-point increase in PASI score from week 33.

At week 16, 71% of adalimumab-treated patients from period A achieved PASI-75, compared with 7% of placebo-treated patients ($P<.001$). Differences in PASI scores occurred by the first study visit at week 4, with mean PASI improvements of 52% versus 9% for placebo-treated patients ($P<.001$). By week 16, 45% and 20% of adalimumab-treated patients had achieved PASI-90 and -100 scores, respectively, in comparison to 2% and 1% of placebo-treated patients ($P<.001$).

The percentage of patients who lost adequate response after stopping adalimumab treatment was 28%, greater than the 5% who lost adequate response despite continuing adalimumab. In addition, loss of response occurred in a significantly shorter time period in patients stopping therapy.

REVEAL demonstrated rapid efficacy of adalimumab in psoriasis and that continuous treatment is more efficacious than interrupted treatment in maintaining adequate response (Fig. 10.3).

Open-Label Extension Study from REVEAL

Patients from REVEAL and 3 other clinical trials were given the option to receive adalimumab therapy in a 3-year OLE trial.[8] This trial aimed to determine additional long-term efficacy and safety data of continuous adalimumab therapy. By doing so, it surpassed the limitations of past trials, such as short duration of study (<1 year), the use of dosages not recommended by the FDA, and the exclusion of patients with less than a PASI-75 response.

Patients could enter this study in 1 of 4 groups: A through D. Group A consisted of patients with less than PASI-75 response at week 16 of REVEAL. Group B consisted of patients who had between PASI-50 and PASI-75 response at week 33 of REVEAL. Group C consisted of patients who received adalimumab during period C of REVEAL. Finally, group D consisted of patients who had initially received placebo during period A and then received adalimumab in period B of the OLE study. Patients with less than PASI-50 response at week 33 and patients who were rerandomized to receive placebo in period C of REVEAL were excluded from this study.

The patients in groups A–D were scheduled to receive uninterrupted treatment with 40 mg SC adalimumab EOW for a minimum of 108 weeks, or until dose escalation. Dose escalation to 40 mg weekly was permitted for patients who did not achieve PASI-50 by week 24 of the OLE study. During this time, patients were permitted to continue shampoos, emollients, and corticosteroids on the palms/soles/inframammary areas,

TABLE 10.1
Summary of phase 3 pivotal trials

	REVEAL	CHAMPION	ADEPT
Eligibility criteria	• Age ≥18 y • Diagnosis of psoriasis for ≥6 mo with stable plaque psoriasis for ≥2 mo • ≥10% BSA • PASI score of ≥12 • PGA of at least moderate severity at the baseline visit	• Age ≥18 y • ≥10% BSA involvement • PASI score ≥10, diagnosis of plaque psoriasis for ≥1 y • Stable plaques for ≥2 mo • All patients were TNF-inhibitor naïve and MTX naïve	• Age ≥18 y • Diagnosis of moderately to severely active PsA • Active psoriatic skin lesions or a documented history of psoriasis • All patients were required to have a history of inadequate response or intolerance to nonsteroidal anti-inflammatory drug therapy for PsA
Washout periods/ exclusion criteria	• 2 wk for topical therapies and UVB phototherapy • 4 wk for UVA phototherapy and nonbiologic systemic therapies • 6 wk for efalizumab • 12 wk for any other biologic therapies	• 2 wk for topical therapies and phototherapy • 4 wk for nonbiologic systemic therapies • 12 wk for biologic therapies	(Exclusion Criteria) • Treatment w/in 4 wk of baseline w/ cyclosporine, tacrolimus, disease-modifying anti-rheumatic drugs other than MTX, or oral retinoids • Topical psoriasis treatments w/in 2 wk of baseline (excluding medicated shampoos or low-potency topical steroids) • Concurrent treatment w/ MTX >30 mg/wk and/or corticosteroids in prednisone-equivalent dosage of >10 mg/d • History of anti-TNF therapy
Results	• By week 16, 71% of adalimumab and 7% of placebo-treated patients achieved PASI-75 • By week 52, 28% of patients rerandomized to the placebo group lost adequate response (<PASI-50) in comparison to 5% of adalimumab-treated patients	• By week 16, 79.6% of adalimumab, 35.5% of MTX, and 18.9% of placebo-treated patients achieved PASI-75 • More adalimumab-treated patients (16.7%) than MTX-treated patients (7.3%) or placebo-treated patients (1.9%) achieved complete disease clearance • Adalimumab response was rapid, with a 57% mean PASI improvement by week 4	• By week 24, 59% of adalimumab and 1% of placebo-treated patients achieved PASI-75

and groin, as long as it was not within 24 hours of a study visit. Phototherapy and other systemic therapies were not permitted.

Adalimumab efficacy was well maintained for up to 3 years of continuous therapy in those with sustained PASI-75 responses in the first 33 weeks of therapy (Table 10.2). Efficacy was best maintained in those who achieved PASI-100.

Comparative Study of Adalimumab Versus Methotrexate Versus Placebo in Patients with Psoriasis

Efficacy and safety results from the randomized, controlled comparative study of adalimumab versus MTX versus placebo in patients with psoriasis (CHAMPION) demonstrated the superiority of adalimumab to placebo, and the noninferiority

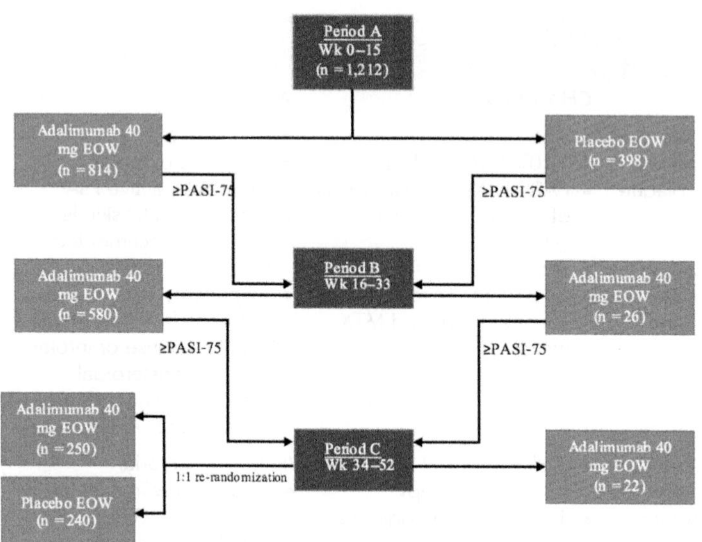

Fig. 10.2 REVEAL study design. Study design describing 3 different treatment periods (period A, period B, and period C). Patients achieving PASI-75 response or greater were continued on to period B, and patients achieving PASI-75 response or greater from period B were continued on to period C. Patients from period A achieving less than PASI-75 response and period B achieving greater than PASI-50 response but less than PASI-75 response were eligible to enter into an OLE study.

of adalimumab to MTX, a widely used systemic treatment.[9]

The study enrolled 271 patients from 28 different sites across Europe and Canada and randomized them in a 2:2:1 ratio to receive either adalimumab, MTX, or placebo for 16 weeks. Adalimumab dosing was SC injection of 80 mg at week 0, and 40 mg EOW. Oral MTX was dosed at 7.5 mg at week 0, increased to 10 mg/wk at week 2, and finally, to 15 mg/wk at week 4. Patients who achieved PASI-50 by week 8 were maintained on the 15 mg/wk dose, and those who did not were increased to 20 mg/wk. Any patient not achieving PASI-50 by week 12 was increased to a maximum study dose of 25 mg/wk. The primary method of assessing efficacy between the 2 agents and placebo was by the proportion of patients that achieved PASI-75 in 16 weeks.

The baseline mean PASI score for the patients in this study was 19.7, and mean body surface area (BSA) coverage was 32.1%. At 16 weeks, 79.6% of patients receiving adalimumab achieved PASI-75 versus 35.5% of patients receiving MTX and 18.9% of patients receiving placebo (Fig. 10.4). PASI-100 was achieved by 16.7% of adalimumab patients, 7.3% of MTX patients, and 1.9% of placebo patients. Response to adalimumab therapy was rapid, indicated by a 57% improvement in PASI score by week 4 of follow-up.

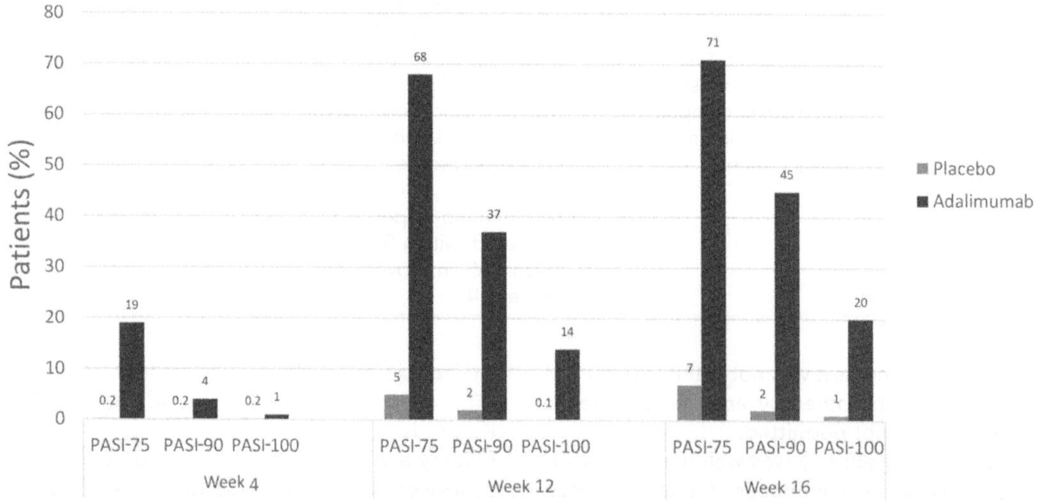

Fig. 10.3 REVEAL efficacy data. Efficacy outcomes after 4, 12, and 16 weeks of treatment with either placebo or adalimumab 40 mg EOW (after baseline dose of 80 mg), defined as percentage of psoriasis patients who met specified PASI response criteria for improvement (PASI-75, -90, -100).

TABLE 10.2
Efficacy information from open-label extension study

Group	PASI-75 Rate	Additional Efficacy Information
A	79% (week 160)	40% mean percentage improvement after 3 y of continuous therapy
B	70% (week 165)	44% mean percentage improvement after 3 y of continuous therapy
C	76% (week 160)	93% mean percentage improvement after 33 wk of therapy PASI-75/90/100 response rates after 160 wk was 76%/50%/31%
D	89% (week 160)	73% mean percentage improvement after 24 wk of therapy PASI-75 response rates at weeks 64/100/160 were 78%/88%/89%

Adalimumab was more effective than MTX and placebo and rapidly improved symptoms. The CHAMPION trial was the first time a biologic agent was compared head to head with MTX for psoriasis.

Efficacy in Psoriatic Arthritis

The ADEPT trial was a pivotal, double-blinded, randomized, placebo-controlled trial designed to evaluate safety and efficacy of adalimumab therapy for moderate-to-severe PsA.[1]

The 315 study patients were divided based on history of MTX use and degree of psoriasis (<3% or ≥3% BSA involvement) and randomized in a 1:1 ratio to receive SC injections of either placebo or 40 mg adalimumab EOW. Primary efficacy endpoints were American College of Rheumatology (ACR) 20 response score at week 12 and any change in the modified total Sharp score of radiographic structural damage of the hands and feet at week 24 from baseline. An important secondary efficacy end point was the improvement of cutaneous psoriasis as assessed by achievement of PASI-50 and PASI-75.

At week 12, ACR20 was achieved by 58% in the adalimumab group and 14% in the placebo group (Fig. 10.5). ACR20, -50, and -70 responses did not differ between patients taking adalimumab in combination with MTX and patients taking adalimumab alone. Radiographs of patients receiving adalimumab indicated inhibition of structural changes as well, with a change in modified total sharp score of −0.2 for adalimumab patients and 1.0 for placebo patients at week 24.

The initial degree of psoriasis was similar between the placebo and adalimumab groups.

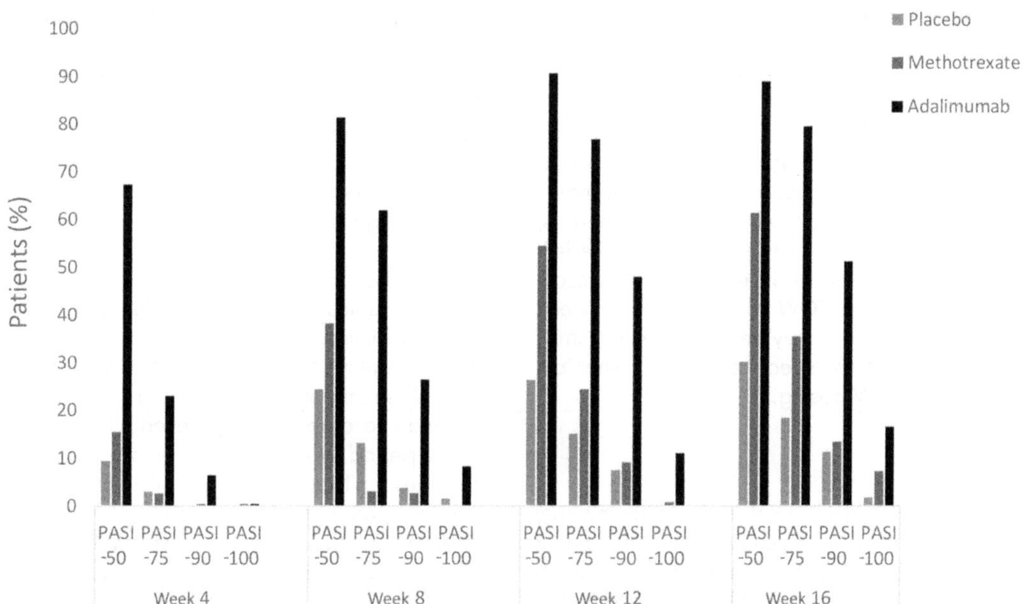

Fig. 10.4 Efficacy data of CHAMPION trial. Efficacy outcomes after 4, 8, 12, and 16 weeks of treatment with either placebo, MTX (7.5 mg at week 0, 10 mg/wk at week 2, 15 mg/wk at week 4, and escalated according to response thereafter), or adalimumab 40 mg EOW (after baseline 80-mg dose), defined as percentage of psoriasis patients who met specified PASI response criteria for improvement (PASI-50, -75, -90, -100).

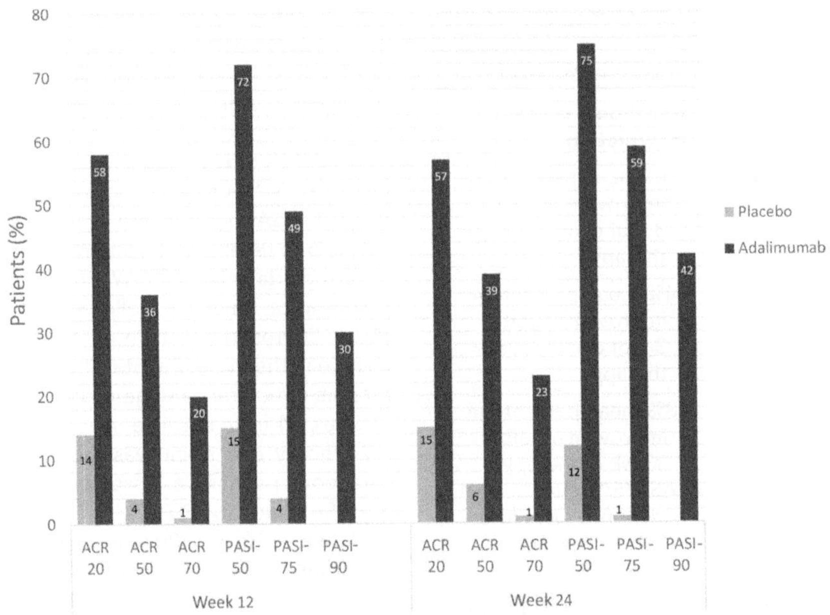

Fig. 10.5 Efficacy data from ADEPT. Efficacy outcomes after 12 and 24 weeks of treatment with either placebo or adalimumab 40 mg EOW, defined as percentage of PsA patients who met specified ACR response criteria for improvement (ACR20, -50, -70) and specified PASI response criteria for improvement (PASI-50, -75, -90).

PASI-75 was achieved by 59% for adalimumab and 1% of placebo patients at week 24 (n = 69).

This trial demonstrated significant improvement in the joint and skin manifestations of PsA and cutaneous psoriasis, resulting in the breakthrough of adalimumab as a potential first-line therapy for these conditions.

Expert Recommendations on Adalimumab Efficacy

Clearance of skin lesions is better maintained with uninterrupted administration of adalimumab injections, although rebound does not commonly occur upon discontinuation of therapy. There is, however, loss of efficacy after the restart of adalimumab therapy.[7] Studies investigating dose escalation from 40 mg EOW to 40 mg every week showed that this may only be beneficial in a small fraction of patients, specifically those who lost response to EOW dosing.[10]

SAFETY

Adalimumab is a well-tolerated drug with minimal side effects in most patients. Given the role of TNF in host defense, the most common concern with adalimumab is the risk of infection and malignancy. Serious infections include the reactivation of tuberculosis (TB), bacterial sepsis, invasive fungal infections, and infections due to opportunistic pathogens. Concerns for malignancy include lymphoma and nonmelanoma skin cancer (NMSC).

The most common adverse reactions in placebo-controlled clinical trials with adalimumab were injection site reaction, seen in 20% of patients receiving active therapy versus 14% of patients receiving placebo. These reactions (erythema, itching, hemorrhage, pain, or swelling) were generally mild-to-moderate and did not require discontinuation of the drug. Other common adverse reactions include mild-to-moderate infection, such as upper respiratory infection, or sinusitis, headache, or rash. Adalimumab is pregnancy category B.[11]

Risk of Infection and Malignancy

Multiple studies have examined the risks of infection and malignancy associated with the use of biologic agents. The PSOLAR (Psoriasis Longitudinal Assessment and Registry) registry was designed to detect adverse events (AEs) over a 6-year period in psoriasis patients using various therapies.[12] The registry enrolled patients on various treatments; the patients were not randomized to the different treatments. Serious infection rates were higher with adalimumab and infliximab in comparison to non-MTX and nonbiologic therapies; the risk of serious infections associated with ustekinumab and etanercept was not increased compared with non-MTX and nonbiologic treatment.

The SABER (Safety Assessment of Biologic Therapy) study, which combined data on patients with autoimmune disease (RA, inflammatory bowel disease, psoriasis, PsA, and ankylosing spondylitis) from 4 large US databases, found no increased risk with TNF inhibitor therapy as a group for hospitalization for serious infections, compared with initiation of nonbiologic medications.[13] The study also examined the incidence of cancer following TNF inhibitor therapy and found no increase in the incidence of solid cancer compared with disease-specific alternative therapy for all immune-mediated diseases.[14] For diseases and cancer types wherein there was a sufficient number of events to estimate risk, no significantly increased risk was detected for lymphoma, leukemia, or NMSC.

ESPRIT 5-year Analysis

The ESPRIT surveillance registry is an ongoing, 10-year observational after-marketing registry designed to prospectively evaluate the long-term safety and efficacy of adalimumab therapy. Five-year results were recently published in July 2015, showing no new safety signals from previous trials.[15]

Eligibility criteria included patients 18 years of age or older with a diagnosis of chronic plaque psoriasis, who initiated adalimumab within 4 weeks of registry entry, initiated adalimumab without being off the drug for more than 70 consecutive days, or participated in a "feeder trial" (adalimumab clinical trial) without being off the drug for more than 70 days after completion of the study. The registry consisted of 2 populations: the "all-treated population" (received at least 1 dose of adalimumab during the registry) and the "new prescription" population (all--treated population patients that received first dose within 4 weeks of registry entry). Patients could continue on concomitant psoriasis therapy with the exception of anakinra, abatacept, or another biologic agent.

Patients were exposed to adalimumab for 13,639 patient-years (PY) during the registry and 19,242 years total (Table 10.3). Over the course of the 5 years, discontinuation rates were 10.6% and 13.1% for the all-treated and new prescription populations, respectively, with the most common reason for discontinuation being loss to follow-up. The rate of serious treatment- emergent adverse events (TEAE) was 4.3/100 PY of total adalimumab exposure, with the most serious TEAE being infection (1/100 PY). Myocardial infarction (MI) was the most common event leading to death (<0.1 Event/100 PY).

Five-year results of this registry showed decreasing rates of serious TEAEs and infections with increased adalimumab exposure, similar to another 5-year registry of psoriasis patients treated with etanercept.[16]

REVEAL

Safety and AE data in the REVEAL trial were separately investigated for the 2 groups: patients in period A (adalimumab-treated and placebo), and the all-adalimumab group (patients who received at least 1 dose of adalimumab throughout the study duration; Table 10.4).

During period A, there was a greater incidence of any AE at all as well as nonserious infectious AEs in the adalimumab-treated group. There were a comparable number of serious AEs, serious infections, and malignancies between the 2 groups (1.8% for both).

In the all-adalimumab group (patients that received at least 1 dose of adalimumab during study duration), infections were the most common serious AE (higher frequency of soft tissue infection such as cellulitis, abscess). One case of TB was reported, in a patient who prematurely discontinued isoniazid prophylaxis without notifying his physician. There were no reported cases of lymphoma, demyelinating syndrome, lupuslike syndrome, or rebound on discontinuation.

Open-Label Extension Trial

In comparison to the safety and AE data from REVEAL, the OLE trial had a similar rate of serious infections and a lower rate of AEs leading to discontinuation of adalimumab therapy (see Table 10.4).

There were 5 cases of candidiasis infection and 2 cases of TB reported. The first TB case was in a 40-year old man who was noncompliant with latent TB therapy, and the second case was in a 36-year old man who had a negative purified protein derivative (PPD) and normal chest radiograph.

Two treatment-emergent deaths (75-year-old man with coronary artery disease and 47-year-old man with unknown cause of death) and 2 other deaths after analysis of adalimumab exposure (68-year old man with MI, 61-year-old woman with an unknown cause of death) were reported.

There were no cases of lymphoma, demyelinating disorder, or lupuslike syndrome reported.

Comparative Study of Adalimumab Versus Methotrexate Versus Placebo in Patients with Psoriasis

Safety and AE assessments in the CHAMPION trial were continued up until 70 days after the

TABLE 10.3
Incidence rates of treatment-emergent adverse events from ESPRIT registry

	<1 y (PY = 493.4) (N = 953)	1–3 y (PY = 3999.9) (N = 2029)	3–5 y (PY = 8506.6) (N = 2109)	>5 y (PY = 6242.9) (N = 968)	Overall Event Rate (Total PY = 19,242.8) (N = 6059)
TEAEs					
Any	280 (56.7)	612 (15.3)	988 (11.6)	2393 (38.3)	4273 (22.2)
Leading to death	8 (1.6)	10 (0.3)	7 (<0.1)	2 (<0.1)	27 (0.1)
Serious TEAEs					
Any	116 (23.5)	219 (5.5)	325 (3.8)	167 (2.7)	827 (4.3)
Serious infection	30 (6.1)	58 (1.5)	64 (0.8)	36 (0.6)	188 (1.0)
≥20 events overall					
Cellulitis	8 (1.6)	9 (0.2)	4 (<0.1)	5 (<0.1)	26 (0.1)
Pneumonia	4 (0.8)	5 (0.1)	9 (0.1)	6 (0.1)	24 (0.1)
MI	5 (1.0)	4 (0.1)	8 (0.1)	3 (<0.1)	20 (0.1)
SCC	0	2 (0.1)	11 (0.1)	7 (0.1)	20 (0.1)
TEAEs leading to drug discontinuation					
Any	149 (30.2)	125 (3.1)	100 (1.2)	14 (0.2)	388 (2.0)
≥5 events overall					
MI	3 (0.6)	3 (<0.1)	1 (<0.1)	1 (<0.1)	8 (<0.1)
Drug hypersensitivity	4 (0.8)	0	1 (<0.1)	0	5 (<0.1)
Bronchitis	1 (0.2)	5 (0.1)	1 (<0.1)	0	7 (<0.1)
Cellulitis	3 (0.6)	3 (<0.1)	1 (<0.1)	0	7 (<0.1)
Pneumonia	2 (0.4)	5 (0.1)	4 (<0.1)	0	11 (0.1)
Arthralgia	2 (0.4)	2 (<0.1)	1 (<0.1)	0	5 (<0.1)
Headache	4 (0.8)	2 (<0.1)	0	0	6 (<0.1)
Psoriasis	13 (2.6)	17 (0.4)	8 (<0.1)	1 (<0.1)	39 (0.2)

Special interest TEAEs					
Cardiovascular					
Cerebrovascular accident	2 (0.4)	5 (0.1)	10	9 (0.1)	26 (0.1)
CHF	2 (0.4)	3 (<0.1)	6	1 (<0.1)	12 (<0.1)
MI	5 (1.0)	4 (0.1)	8	3 (<0.1)	20 (0.1)
Malignancies					
Overall	15 (3.0)	33 (0.8)	76	54 (0.9)	178 (0.9)
Lymphoma	0	0	2	0	2 (<0.1)
Hepatosplenic T-cell lymphoma	0	0	0	0	0
NMSC	4 (0.8)	15 (0.4)	50	43 (0.7)	112 (0.6)
Leukemia	0	0	0	0	0
Melanoma	4 (0.8)	1 (<0.1)	3	2 (<0.1)	10 (<0.1)
Other	7 (1.4)	17 (0.4)	21	10 (0.2)	55 (0.3)
Infection-related					
Infection	69 (14.0)	215 (5.4)	337 (4.0)	864 (13.8)	1485 (7.7)
Oral candidiasis	0	5 (0.1)	0	3 (<0.1)	8 (<0.1)
Opportunistic	0	0	1 (<0.1)	0	1 (<0.1)
Active TB	0	2 (<0.1)	1 (<0.1)	0	3 (<0.1)
Latent TB	1 (0.2)	7 (0.2)	4 (<0.1)	3 (<0.1)	15 (<0.1)

The value in parentheses is a percentage.
Abbreviation: PY, patient years.

TABLE 10.4
Safety data from REVEAL and open-label extension trials

Adverse Event	Period A Placebo 120.7 PY	Period A Adalimumab 250.2 PY	All-Adalimumab Group 540.5 PY	Open-Label Extension 2043.8 PY
Any	498 (4.13)	1155 (4.62)	2157 (3.99)	5009 (245.1)
Serious AE	7 (0.06)	17 (0.07)	33 (0.06)	149 (7.3)
Serious infectious AE	4 (0.03)	7 (0.03)	12 (0.02)	30 (1.5)
Infectious	106 (0.88)	315 (1.26)	650 (1.20)	N/A
Leading to withdrawal	15 (0.12)	18 (0.07)	42 (0.08)	96 (4.7)
Special interest				
TB	0	0	1 (0.002)	2
Opportunistic infection	0	0	1 (0.002)	5
CHF	0	1 (0.004)	1 (0.002)	6
Allergic reaction	0	1 (0.004)	1 (0.002)	12
Injection-site reaction	26 (0.215)	69 (0.276)	92 (0.170)	N/A
Malignancies	1 (0.008)	2 (0.008)	2 (0.004)	15
NMSC	1 (0.008)	4 (0.016)	7 (0.013)	17
Lymphoma	0	0	0	0
Lupuslike syndrome	0	0	0	0
Demyelinating disorder	0	0	0	0

last treatment. Seventy-nine (73.8%) patients in the adalimumab-treated group, 89 (80.9%) patients in the MTX-treated group, and 49 (79.2%) patients in the placebo group reported AEs. There were no serious infections reported during this study, and no significant differences were seen in infection rates between the groups.

Serious AEs varied between groups. In the adalimumab-treated patients, there was 1 case of pancreatitis and 1 case of an ovarian cyst enlargement. In the MTX-treated group, there was 1 case of hepatitis, secondary to MTX use. There was 1 case of calculus of the right uteropelvic junction in the placebo-treated group.

Eight patients discontinued the study due to AEs: 1 adalimumab patient due to elevated aminotransferase concentration, 6 MTX patients (due to upper abdominal pain, retrobulbar optic neuritis, hepatitis, and 3 cases of abnormal liver function tests [LFTs]), and 1 placebo patient due to elevated hepatic enzyme concentration. There were no reported cases of TB or deaths during this study.

Summary on Adalimumab Safety Concerns

Based on these safety data, dermatologists should watch for serious infections such as TB and opportunistic infections, hepatitis B reactivation, and NMSC.

PRECAUTIONS

Special attention should be given to patient populations with a history of TB, malignancy, demyelinating disorders, congestive heart failure (CHF), and certain other conditions, given the role of TNF in such disease pathogenesis.

Infection

Patients using adalimumab are at increased risk for serious infection (bacterial, viral, fungal, and parasitic). Risk is increased with concomitant use of MTX, corticosteroids, and other immunosuppressants, or in patients with underlying predisposing medical conditions. The use of adalimumab with concomitant abatacept and anakinra is not recommended, because RA patients had an increased risk of serious infection with such therapy.[3,17]

Adalimumab should be withheld in patients requiring antibiotics, discontinued in those with serious or opportunistic infections, and should not be initiated in patients with active infection (systemic or localized). Risks and benefits should be discussed before initiating therapy in patients with recurrent/chronic infection, and careful monitoring should take place.[3,18,19]

Tuberculosis

Patients receiving adalimumab therapy are at increased risk for the development of TB or reactivation of latent TB (pulmonary and extrapulmonary TB). Patients should be evaluated based on risk factors for TB and screened for latent TB before initiation and during therapy. A PPD screen with 5-mm or greater induration is considered positive, even in those with a history of BCG vaccination.[20]

TB treatment should be given to any patients with a history of active or latent TB, in whom completion of a treatment course cannot be confirmed as well as in patients with risk factors for TB infection but a negative screen. Adalimumab therapy can be initiated after 1 to 2 months of latent TB treatment, although reactivation of TB remains a possibility despite prophylactic treatment. A TB expert should be consulted in the case of any questions or hesitations.[3]

Opportunistic infections

Opportunistic infections, such as aspergillosis, blastomycosis, candidiasis, histoplasmosis, legionellosis, listeriosis, coccidioidomycosis, cryptococccosis, and pneumocystis, are more likely to present in this population and may present with disseminated rather than localized infection. If the symptomatic patient resides or travels to regions of endemic mycoses, it is important to consider empiric antifungal therapy while waiting on a diagnostic workup. Consider that antigen and antibody testing may be negative in patients with active histoplasmosis.[3,19]

Malignancy

An increased incidence rate for melanoma and NMSC has been shown in psoriasis patients using adalimumab.[21] This rate is associated with the use of high-dose psoralen and UV-A light, cyclosporine, MTX, and immunosuppressants for NMSC.[22] Patients with a personal history of malignancy should take special precaution.

Although there have been resolved cases of lymphoma reported in patients stopping other TNF inhibitors (etanercept, infliximab),[23] there is not sufficient evidence to suggest an increased rate of lymphoma in psoriasis patients using adalimumab. There is, however, a general increased risk of Hodgkin lymphoma and cutaneous T-cell lymphoma in psoriasis patients.[24,25]

Hepatitis B

TNF is thought to promote viral clearance in hepatitis B.[19] If a patient receiving adalimumab therapy develops hepatitis B virus (HBV) reactivation, therapy should be stopped immediately and antiviral therapy should ensue.[3]

Patients should be monitored for signs and symptoms of HBV infection during and for 6 months after stopping therapy.[26] These signs and symptoms includes LFTs, hepatitis B surface antigen, hepatitis B e antigen, and HBV DNA counts in patients at risk for reactivation.[26] No definitive information is available regarding treating HBV carriers with antiviral therapy along with adalimumab, or regarding resuming adalimumab therapy after the control of reactivated HBV infection.

Multiple Sclerosis and Demyelinating Disorders

TNF inhibitors have been associated with new onset or exacerbation of central nervous system demyelinating disorders (multiple sclerosis [MS], optic neuritis) and peripheral demyelinating diseases, such as Guillian-Barré syndrome.[19,27] Adalimumab should not be initiated in patients with a history of MS (including in a first-degree relative, given the increased risk)[28,29] or other demyelinating disorders. Associated neurologic symptoms have been reported to resolve with termination of therapy.[27]

Congestive Heart Failure

Although the role of TNF in CHF is much debated, 2 randomized, controlled trials, RENAISSANCE/ RECOVER (Randomised Etanercept North AmerIcan Strategy to Study Antagonism of CytokinEs/ Research into Etanercept CytOkine Antagonism in VentriculaR dysfunction trial) and ATTACH (anti-TNF Therapy Against Congestive Heart Failure),[30,31] have shown trends toward a worse CHF prognosis that was dose dependent with other TNF inhibitors. Adalimumab should be withdrawn with new-onset or worsening symptoms in patients with pre-existing CHF. Patients diagnosed with class 3 or 4 CHF or ejection fraction less than 50% should avoid adalimumab use, and patients diagnosed with class 1 or 2 CHF should undergo echocardiographic testing before initiating an anti-TNF drug.[19,32,33]

Drug-induced Lupus

Adalimumab therapy can lead to autoantibody formation, although few of these patients develop clinical symptoms. The development of antinuclear antibodies (ANAs) and anti-double-stranded DNA antibodies with initiation of anti-TNF therapy may be a marker for forthcoming treatment failure.[34]

According to 1 study, 19% of adalimumab-treated patients formed autoantibodies.[35] If a patient experiences signs and symptoms of a lupuslike syndrome, the dermatologist should assess circulating ANAs and discontinue therapy.[19]

Blood Dyscrasias

Isolated cases of aplastic anemia, pancytopenia, isolated leukopenia, and thrombocytopenia have been reported with TNF inhibitor use.[36,37] Patients experiencing pallor, easy bruising, bleeding, or persistent fever should seek immediate attention. Adalimumab therapy should be discontinued with significant hematologic abnormalities.[3,19]

Hypersensitivity Reactions

There have been rare reported cases of anaphylaxis, angioneurotic edema, allergic rash, fixed drug reactions, urticarial reactions, and nonspecified drug reactions. Immediately discontinue adalimumab therapy if this occurs and start appropriate therapy.[3]

MONITORING

The information presented is primarily based on psoriasis guidelines from the American Academy of Dermatology (AAD).[19]

A thorough history and physical examination should be taken before initiation of adalimumab therapy, including TB exposure, chronic/recurrent infections, malignancy, neurologic and cardiac history, and a thorough review of systems. Routine follow-up examinations should adequately monitor patients for side effects and AEs.[38]

Aside from baseline TB test, annual monitoring for TB, and a baseline hepatitis profile, routine laboratory testing beyond that for concomitant therapies or comorbidities is generally not supported.[39] The highest grade US Preventive Services Task Force evidence for screening studies is grade B for TB testing (interferon-γ release assay is preferred over tuberculin skin testing), and HBV/hepatitis B virus screening is supported only by grade C evidence.[40] The AAD recommends baseline PPD, LFTs, and complete blood count (CBC). For ongoing monitoring, the AAD recommends yearly PPD and periodic LFTs, CBC, history, and physical examinations (Table 10.5).[19]

The Centers for Disease Control and Prevention recommends TB testing before the therapy initiation as well.[41] Positive skin test findings should be followed with a chest radiograph—if negative, patients should be treated for latent TB (6–9 months of 300 mg isoniazid daily and/or 4 months of 600 mg daily rifampicin),[20] and if positive, patients should receive therapy for active TB. Biologic therapy may be started after 1 to 2 months of prophylactic treatment if the patient is adherent to and tolerating the prophylactic regimen.[42] If a patient has a positive PPD because of prior BCG vaccination, blood tests can be obtained measuring interferon production on stimulation with TB antigens that are not present in BCG. Most guidelines perform annual TB skin testing in patients receiving adalimumab to screen for the TB reactivation, especially in those at risk (ie, health care workers, travelers to endemic areas).

TABLE 10.5
Monitoring recommendations from the American Academy of Dermatology

	Monitoring
History and physical	Baseline and routine
CBC	Baseline and periodically
LFTs	Baseline and periodically
TB skin test	Baseline and annually after
Hepatitis profile	Baseline

Data from Menter A, Gottlieb A, Feldman SR, et al. Guidelines of care for the management of psoriasis and psoriatic arthritis: Section 1. Overview of psoriasis and guidelines of care for the treatment of psoriasis with biologics. J Am Acad Dermatol 2008;58(5):840.

The authors of this section recommend initial baseline monitoring that includes a QuantiFERON-TB Gold (QFT), LFTs, CBC, and hepatitis B and hepatitis C profile. QFT should be repeated annually.

VACCINATIONS

Because of the possibility that biologic agents may impair the body's immunologic response to vaccinations, administration of vaccinations should be carefully considered in patients receiving biologic therapy (Table 10.6). Live vaccines (measles, mumps, and rubella [MMR], varicella, zoster, intranasal influenza, and so forth) are contraindicated within 1 month of treatment.[43] However, scientifically based/standardized recommendations for administering biologically inactive or recombinant vaccines to patients on biologic agents are lacking. Non-live vaccinations may have the potential to achieve adequate immune response, although antibody titers may not achieve optimal levels and may decrease more rapidly if given during biologic therapy.

It is preferable to complete all age-appropriate immunizations according to current immunization guidelines before initiating biologic therapy. The production of antibodies from the vaccine generally occurs in the 2-week period from primary immunization, but could take more than 6 weeks to

TABLE 10.6
Vaccination recommendations from the National Psoriasis Foundation

Vaccination	Before Therapy	During Therapy
Live vaccines (MMR, varicella, herpes zoster, intranasal influenza, oral typhoid, yellow fever, oral polio, smallpox, BCG, rotavirus)	Contraindicated within 1 mo	Contraindicated
Influenza	Vaccinate with inactivated or live	Yearly immunization with inactivated vaccine
Chicken pox	If negative serology, vaccinate	Contraindicated
Zoster	Before therapy: 1 dose for adults ≥50 y	Contraindicated
Human papillomavirus	Unvaccinated males/female patients up to age 26	Same
Hepatitis A	Vaccinate if high risk (diabetes, liver disease, intravenous drug users, homosexual males, and so forth)	Same; consider obtaining postvaccination serology
Hepatitis B	Serology, risk factor assessment; offer vaccination if necessary	High-dose vaccine Consider obtaining serology postvaccination
Pneumococcal	Pneumococcal polysaccharide vaccine (PPSV23) vaccine recommended	Pneumococcal conjugate vaccine followed by PPSV23 if not given prior
Haemophilus influenzae type b	Vaccinate if unvaccinated	Same
MMR	Vaccinate if negative, or seronegative to any component	Contraindicated
Tetanus-diphtheria/diphtheria-tetanus-acellular pertussis (TD/TDAP)	Booster every 10 y and high-risk wounds Offer before therapy, substitute 1 dose with TDAP	Same
Meningococcal	Assess risk factors, vaccinate if high risk (asplenia, complement deficient, group living)	Same
Poliomyelitis	Assess risk factors, vaccinate if high risk (health care worker, laboratory worker)	Same

Data from Lebwohl M, Bagel J, Gelfand JM, et al. From the Medical Board of the National Psoriasis Foundation: monitoring and vaccinations in patients treated with biologics for psoriasis. J Am Acad Dermatol 2008;58(1):94–105; and Wine-Lee L, Keller SC, Wilck MB, et al. From the Medical Board of the National Psoriasis Foundation: vaccination in adult patients on systemic therapy for psoriasis. J Am Acad Dermatol 2013;69(6):1003–13.

peak. A period of 4 times the half-life of adalimumab (8 weeks) has been suggested to allow for the return of the immune system to its baseline before vaccination with live vaccines.

TUMOR NECROSIS FACTOR INHIBITOR THERAPY AND CARDIOVASCULAR RISK REDUCTION

Recent evidence suggests that TNF inhibitor therapy has the potential to reduce cardiovascular risk by lowering systemic inflammation. A retrospective study at Kaiser Permanente Southern California concluded that TNF inhibitor use was associated with a significant reduction in MI risk (50%) and incidence (55%) compared with topical treatments for psoriasis,[44] and a 5-year Danish follow-up study found that patients treated with TNF inhibitors had a significant reduction in cardiovascular risk compared with other therapies (interleukin-12/-23, cyclosporine, retinoids).[45] However, 1 study reported no reduced MI risk in psoriasis patients receiving systemic psoriasis therapy (including TNF inhibitor therapy)[46]; thus, further investigation is warranted to determine the potential for risk reduction.

SUMMARY

The effectiveness of adalimumab for the treatment of moderate-to-severe plaque psoriasis has been demonstrated in multiple studies. It should be considered as a first-line therapy in patients who are candidates for systemic therapy or phototherapy, given its superiority to MTX and its effectiveness in those failing etanercept therapy.[47] The response to adalimumab therapy is varied, and continuous therapy is more likely to provide optimal clearance of psoriatic skin lesions. There is a lack of consistent evidence-based guidelines for monitoring of patients using adalimumab, and based on clinical experience, the authors of this section recommend annual screening solely for TB. CBC and chemistry screens can be monitored annually or only at baseline.

REFERENCES

1. den Broeder A, van de Putte L, Rau R, et al. A single dose, placebo controlled study of the fully human anti-tumor necrosis factor-alpha antibody adalimumab (D2E7) in patients with rheumatoid arthritis. J Rheumatol 2002;29(11):2288–98.
2. Levin EC, Debbaneh M, Koo J, et al. Biologic therapy in erythrodermic and pustular psoriasis. J Drugs Dermatol 2014;13(3):342–54.
3. Safety Information—Humira (adalimumab) injection. Available at: http://www.fda.gov/Safety/MedWatch/SafetyInformation/ucm194134.htm. Accessed October 12, 2015.
4. Gilbert KE, Manalo IF, Wu JJ. Efficacy and safety of etanercept and adalimumab with and without a loading dose for psoriasis: a systematic review. J Am Acad Dermatol 2015;73(2):329–31.
5. Kivitz A, Cohen S, Dowd JE, et al. Clinical assessment of pain, tolerability, and preference of an autoinjection pen versus a prefilled syringe for patient self-administration of the fully human, monoclonal antibody adalimumab: the TOUCH trial. Clin Ther 2006;28(10):1619–29.
6. Mease PJ. Adalimumab in the treatment of arthritis. Ther Clin Risk Manag 2007;3(1):133–48.
7. Menter A, Tyring SK, Gordon K, et al. Adalimumab therapy for moderate to severe psoriasis: a randomized, controlled phase III trial. J Am Acad Dermatol 2008;58(1):106–15.
8. Gordon K, Papp K, Poulin Y, et al. Long-term efficacy and safety of adalimumab in patients with moderate to severe psoriasis treated continuously over 3 years: results from an open-label extension study for patients from REVEAL. J Am Acad Dermatol 2012;66(2):241–51.
9. Saurat J-H, Stingl G, Dubertret L, et al. Efficacy and safety results from the randomized controlled comparative study of adalimumab vs. methotrexate vs. placebo in patients with psoriasis (CHAMPION). Br J Dermatol 2008;158(3):558–66.
10. Leonardi C, Sobell JM, Crowley JJ, et al. Efficacy, safety and medication cost implications of adalimumab 40 mg weekly dosing in patients with psoriasis with suboptimal response to 40 mg every other week dosing: results from an open-label study. Br J Dermatol 2012;167(3):658–67.
11. HUMIRA (adalimumab) [Package Insert]. Abbott Laboratories. Available at: http://www.accessdata.fda.gov/drugsatfda_docs/label/2002/adalabb123102LB.htm. Accessed December 12, 2015.
12. Kalb RE, Fiorentino DF, Lebwohl MG, et al. Risk of serious infection with biologic and systemic treatment of psoriasis: results from the Psoriasis Longitudinal Assessment and Registry (PSOLAR). JAMA Dermatol 2015;151(9):961–9.
13. Haynes K, Beukelman T, Curtis JR, et al. Tumor necrosis factor α inhibitor therapy and cancer risk in chronic immune-mediated diseases. Arthritis Rheum 2013;65(1):48–58.
14. Grijalva CG, Chen L, Delzell E, et al. Initiation of tumor necrosis factor-α antagonists and the risk of hospitalization for infection in patients with autoimmune diseases. JAMA 2011;306(21):2331–9.
15. Menter A, Thaçi D, Papp KA, et al. Five-year analysis from the ESPRIT 10-year postmarketing surveillance registry of adalimumab treatment for moderate to severe psoriasis. J Am Acad Dermatol 2015;73(3):410–9.e6.
16. Kimball AB, Rothman KJ, Kricorian G, et al. OBSERVE-5: observational postmarketing safety surveillance registry of etanercept for the treatment of psoriasis final 5-year results. J Am Acad Dermatol 2015;72(1):115–22.
17. Genovese MC, Cohen S, Moreland L, et al. Combination therapy with etanercept and anakinra in the treatment of patients with rheumatoid arthritis who have been treated unsuccessfully with methotrexate. Arthritis Rheum 2004;50(5):1412–9.
18. Bresnihan B, Cunnane G. Infection complications associated with the use of biologic agents. Rheum Dis Clin North Am 2003;29(1):185–202.
19. Menter A, Gottlieb A, Feldman SR, et al. Guidelines of care for the management of psoriasis and psoriatic arthritis: section 1. Overview of psoriasis and guidelines of care for the treatment of psoriasis with biologics. J Am Acad Dermatol 2008;58(5):826–50.
20. Targeted tuberculin testing and treatment of latent tuberculosis infection. American Thoracic Society. MMWR Recomm Rep 2000;49(RR-6):1–51.

21. Burmester GR, Panaccione R, Gordon KB, et al. Adalimumab: long-term safety in 23 458 patients from global clinical trials in rheumatoid arthritis, juvenile idiopathic arthritis, ankylosing spondylitis, psoriatic arthritis, psoriasis and Crohn's disease. Ann Rheum Dis 2013;72(4):517–24.
22. Paul CF, Ho VC, McGeown C, et al. Risk of malignancies in psoriasis patients treated with cyclosporine: a 5 y cohort study. J Invest Dermatol 2003;120(2):211–6.
23. Brown SL, Greene MH, Gershon SK, et al. Tumor necrosis factor antagonist therapy and lymphoma development: twenty-six cases reported to the Food and Drug Administration. Arthritis Rheum 2002;46(12):3151–8.
24. Gelfand JM, Berlin J, Van Voorhees A, et al. Lymphoma rates are low but increased in patients with psoriasis: results from a population-based cohort study in the United Kingdom. Arch Dermatol 2003; 139(11):1425–9.
25. Gelfand JM, Shin DB, Neimann AL, et al. The risk of lymphoma in patients with psoriasis. J Invest Dermatol 2006;126(10):2194–201.
26. Motaparthi K, Stanisic V, Van Voorhees AS, et al, Medical Board of the National Psoriasis Foundation. From the Medical Board of the National Psoriasis Foundation: recommendations for screening for hepatitis B infection prior to initiating anti-tumor necrosis factor-alfa inhibitors or other immunosuppressive agents in patients with psoriasis. J Am Acad Dermatol 2014;70(1):178–86.
27. Mohan N, Edwards ET, Cupps TR, et al. Demyelination occurring during anti-tumor necrosis factor alpha therapy for inflammatory arthritides. Arthritis Rheum 2001;44(12):2862–9.
28. Barcellos LF, Kamdar BB, Ramsay PP, et al. Clustering of autoimmune diseases in families with a high-risk for multiple sclerosis: a descriptive study. Lancet Neurol 2006;5(11):924–31.
29. Dyment DA, Sadovnick AD, Willer CJ, et al. An extended genome scan in 442 Canadian multiple sclerosis-affected sibships: a report from the Canadian Collaborative Study Group. Hum Mol Genet 2004;13(10):1005–15.
30. Coletta AP, Clark AL, Banarjee P, et al. Clinical trials update: RENEWAL (RENAISSANCE and RECOVER) and ATTACH. Eur J Heart Fail 2002; 4(4):559–61.
31. Chung ES, Packer M, Lo KH, et al, Anti-TNF Therapy Against Congestive Heart Failure Investigators. Randomized, double-blind, placebo-controlled, pilot trial of infliximab, a chimeric monoclonal antibody to tumor necrosis factor-alpha, in patients with moderate-to-severe heart failure: results of the anti-TNF Therapy Against Congestive Heart Failure (ATTACH) trial. Circulation 2003;107(25): 3133–40.
32. Desai SB, Furst DE. Problems encountered during anti-tumour necrosis factor therapy. Best Pract Res Clin Rheumatol 2006;20(4):757–90.
33. Khanna D, McMahon M, Furst DE. Safety of tumour necrosis factor-alpha antagonists. Drug Saf 2004; 27(5):307–24.
34. Pink AE, Fonia A, Allen MH, et al. Antinuclear antibodies associate with loss of response to antitumour necrosis factor-alpha therapy in psoriasis: a retrospective, observational study. Br J Dermatol 2010;162(4):780–5.
35. Bardazzi F, Odorici G, Virdi A, et al. Autoantibodies in psoriatic patients treated with anti-TNF-α therapy. J Dtsch Dermatol Ges 2014;12(5):401–6.
36. Kuruvilla J, Leitch HA, Vickars LM, et al. Aplastic anemia following administration of a tumor necrosis factor-alpha inhibitor. Eur J Haematol 2003;71(5): 396–8.
37. Vidal F, Fontova R, Richart C. Severe neutropenia and thrombocytopenia associated with infliximab. Ann Intern Med 2003;139(3). W–W63.
38. Lebwohl M, Bagel J, Gelfand JM, et al. From the Medical Board of the National Psoriasis Foundation: monitoring and vaccinations in patients treated with biologics for psoriasis. J Am Acad Dermatol 2008;58(1):94–105.
39. van Lümig PPM, Driessen RJB, Roelofs-Thijssen MA, et al. Relevance of laboratory investigations in monitoring patients with psoriasis on etanercept or adalimumab. Br J Dermatol 2011; 165(2):375–82.
40. Ahn CS, Dothard EH, Garner ML, et al. To test or not to test? An updated evidence-based assessment of the value of screening and monitoring tests when using systemic biologic agents to treat psoriasis and psoriatic arthritis. J Am Acad Dermatol 2015; 73(3):420–8.e1.
41. CDC—Tuberculosis (TB). Available at: http://www.cdc.gov/tb/?404;http://www.cdc.gov:80/tb/pubs/LTBI/pdf/TargetedLTBI05.pdf. Accessed December 12, 2015.
42. Doherty SD, Van Voorhees A, Lebwohl MG, et al. National Psoriasis Foundation consensus statement on screening for latent tuberculosis infection in patients with psoriasis treated with systemic and biologic agents. J Am Acad Dermatol 2008;59(2): 209–17.
43. Wine-Lee L, Keller SC, Wilck MB, et al. From the Medical Board of the National Psoriasis Foundation: vaccination in adult patients on systemic therapy for psoriasis. J Am Acad Dermatol 2013;69(6): 1003–13.
44. Wu JJ, Poon K-YT, Channual JC, et al. Association between tumor necrosis factor inhibitor therapy and myocardial infarction risk in patients with psoriasis. Arch Dermatol 2012; 148(11):1244–50.

45. Ahlehoff O, Skov L, Gislason G, et al. Cardiovascular outcomes and systemic anti-inflammatory drugs in patients with severe psoriasis: 5-year follow-up of a Danish nationwide cohort. J Eur Acad Dermatol Venereol 2015;29(6):1128–34.
46. Abuabara K, Lee H, Kimball AB. The effect of systemic psoriasis therapies on the incidence of myocardial infarction: a cohort study. Br J Dermatol 2011;165(5):1066–73.
47. Bissonnette R, Bolduc C, Poulin Y, et al. Efficacy and safety of adalimumab in patients with plaque psoriasis who have shown an unsatisfactory response to etanercept. J Am Acad Dermatol 2010;63(2):228–34.

CHAPTER 11

Ustekinumab

John K. Nia, MD, Mark G. Lebwohl, MD

KEYWORDS

• Ustekinumab • Stelara • Psoriasis • Interleukin-12 • Interleukin-23 • PASI

KEY POINTS

- Ustekinumab is a human immunoglobulin G_{κ} monoclonal antibody that binds to the p40 protein subunit shared by interleukin-12 (IL-12) and IL-23 cytokines.
- Ustekinumab is safe and efficacious for the treatment of moderate-to-severe plaque psoriasis and psoriatic arthritis.
- Efficacy, tolerability, ease of use, and long dosing intervals contribute to patient satisfaction and adherence.

INTRODUCTION

It can be argued that psoriasis is the most successfully treated immune-mediated disease and a promising example of the impact of translational research.[1] Improved understanding of the pathophysiology of psoriasis in the late twentieth and early twenty-first century facilitated the evolution of treatments from nonspecific, immunosuppressive medications to novel targeted therapies.[2] Several biologic agents have been developed for the treatment of psoriasis over the past decade. Biologics act with greater target specificity and generally have not demonstrated end-organ toxicities more commonly observed with other effective systemic agents. Although concern over adverse events (AEs; infections and malignancy) exists with some biological therapies, studies have shown that the risks are minimal and benefits are well documented.[3–6] Targeted therapies, such as tumor necrosis factor (TNF)-α inhibitors, have considerably enhanced the treatment of moderate-to-severe plaque psoriasis and improved overall quality of life in psoriasis patients.[7–13]

Ustekinumab is a human, monoclonal antibody that binds to the shared p40 subunit of interleukin (IL)-12 and IL-23. It was US Food and Drug Administration approved for the treatment of moderate-to-severe plaque psoriasis in 2009 and has proven to be a safe and efficacious treatment.[14] Recommended dosing occurs at weeks 0, 4, and every 12 weeks thereafter (Fig. 11.1). Infrequent dosing, high efficacy, and tolerability could positively affect adherence in psoriasis patients, who, in the past, have not treated their disease adequately.

MECHANISM OF ACTION

Although monoclonal antibodies directed against TNFs proved to be effective in treating psoriasis, more specific targets were sought. Ustekinumab is a human immunoglobulin G_{κ} (IgG_{κ}) monoclonal antibody that binds to the p40 protein subunit shared by IL-12 and IL-23 cytokines, preventing their interactions with the heterodimeric IL-12 receptor subunit. IL-12 and IL-23 are naturally occurring cytokines involved in inflammatory and immune responses. In transgenic mice, the overexpression of IL-12 has been linked to the development of inflammatory skin lesions; not surprisingly, lesional skin in psoriasis patients has demonstrated increased expression of IL-12 compared with nonlesional skin.[15]

IL-12 and IL-23 are produced primarily by antigenic stimulation of dendritic cells and macrophages.[16] IL-12 is composed of a p35 and a p40 subunit, the latter being largely expressed in psoriatic lesional skin; its receptor is made up of IL-12RB1 and IL-12R2 subunits. Binding of IL-12 to its receptor causes activation of a JAK-STAT signaling pathway, causing T cells to be assigned to the Th1 pathway and downstream secretion of its effector interferon-γ (IFN-γ).[17]

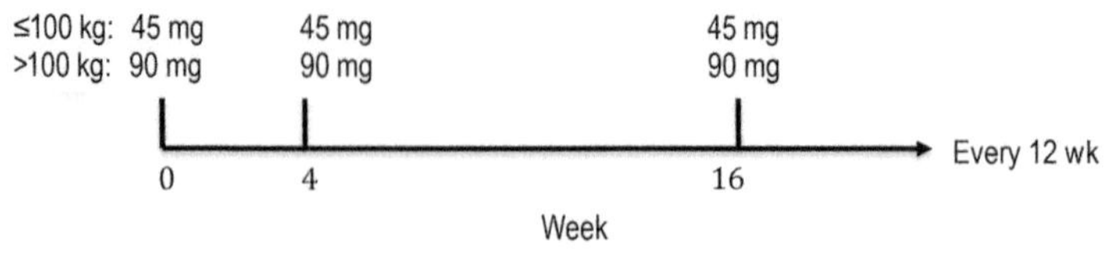

Fig. 11.1 Ustekinumab dosing regimen for psoriasis.

IL-23 is composed of p19 and p40 subunits (both largely expressed in lesional skin). It binds to a receptor made of the IL-12RB1 and IL-23R subunits.[18] Similar to IL-12, binding of the p40 subunit with IL-12RB1 and the p19 subunit with IL-23R signals through JAK-STAT signaling, activating STAT3 and causing a Th17-driven response.[19]

Ustekinumab blocks IL-12 and IL-23 from binding to the IL-12Rβ1 receptor chain of IL-12 (IL-12Rβ1/β2) and IL-23 (IL-12Rβ1/23R) receptor complexes on the surface of natural killer and T cells. In vitro models showed ustekinumab equally disrupted the action of IL-12 and IL-23, blocking STAT 3,4 phosphorylation and ultimately IFN-γ, IL-22, and IL-17 production.[20]

PHARMACOKINETICS

Similar to endogenous IgG, ustekinumab has an approximate half-life of 3 weeks.[20] Peak serum concentration of ustekinumab occurred at approximately 13.5 days after a 45-mg dose and 7 days after a 90-mg dose.[21] Steady-state drug concentrations were achieved by week 28. Ustekinumab is metabolized much the same as human IgG. An Fc receptor binds to IgG and carries it across the cell membrane to be degraded within the cell.[22]

EFFICACY

Compared with conventional therapies, many biologics have exhibited increased efficacy, and ustekinumab is not an exception. Efficacy in psoriasis patients is measured by improvement in Psoriasis Area Severity Index (PASI), body surface area (BSA), Physician Global Assessment (PGA), and dermatology-related quality of life. Ustekinumab has demonstrated short- and long-term efficacy in the treatment of moderate-to-severe psoriasis and remains among the best evaluated biologic in the treatment of psoriasis.[4,6,14,15,23–31] Two landmark, phase III, prospective, long-term extension studies, PHOENIX 1[25] and PHOENIX 2,[4] observed efficacy, measured by clinical response, and safety of ustekinumab in psoriasis patients for up to 5 years.[4,25]

PHOENIX 1 was a multicenter, randomized, double-blinded, placebo-controlled trial that studied 766 patients receiving ustekinumab 45 mg, ustekinumab 90 mg, or placebo in a 1:1:1 ratio. Dosing occurred at weeks 0, 4 and every 12 weeks thereafter, with limited flexibility. Patients initially treated with placebo were rerandomized to receive ustekinumab 45 mg or 90 mg at week 12. The primary efficacy endpoint was the proportion of patients experiencing a 75% improvement from baseline PASI (PASI-75) score at week 12. Patients initially assigned to ustekinumab, who had achieved PASI-75 at weeks 12 and 28, were rerandomized at week 40 to continue on ustekinumab every 12 weeks, or switched to placebo. Patients randomized to placebo at week 40 were placed back on treatment when they lost 50% of PASI improvement (Fig. 11.2).

For many, improvement began within 2 weeks of their first dose. Approximately 67% of patients receiving ustekinumab 45 mg ($P<.0001$) and 66% of patients receiving ustekinumab 90 mg ($P<.0001$) achieved PASI-75 at week 12. Three percent of placebo-treated patients achieved PASI-75 at week 12. Furthermore, roughly 60% of patients receiving ustekinumab 45 mg and ustekinumab 90 mg were deemed clear or almost clear by the physician at week 12. By week 28, 50% of patients achieved 90% reduction from their baseline PASI score (PASI-90), a new clinical standard for efficacy.[32]

Patients initially assigned to ustekinumab, who had achieved PASI-75 at weeks 12 and 28, were rerandomized at week 40 to continue on ustekinumab every 12 weeks, or switched to placebo. Patients randomized to placebo at week 40 were placed back on treatment when they lost 50% of PASI improvement. Importantly, rebound psoriasis was not reported in patients withdrawn from treatment. The median time to loss of PASI-75 was approximately 15 weeks, and 85% of patients reinitiated on treatment saw a PASI-75 within 12 weeks of restarting treatment. Efficacy of therapeutics in psoriasis was also measured by patient-reported outcomes. At week 12, 50% of patients reported that psoriasis had little to no effect on patient's quality of life. These results were sustained for patients continued on therapy

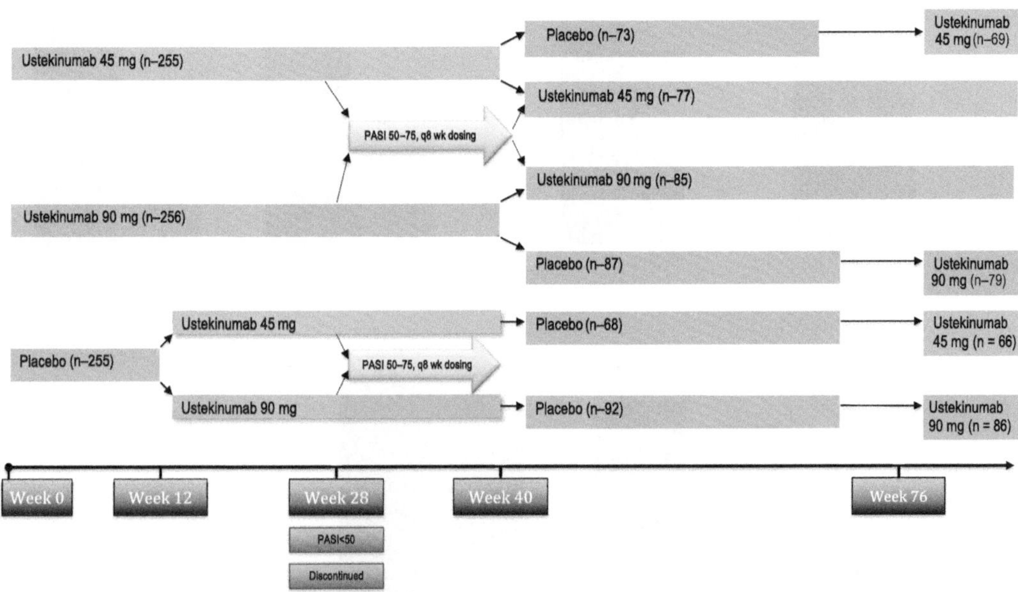

Fig. 11.2 PHOENIX 1 study design—patients were randomized in a 1:1:1 ratio to receive the standard dosage of ustekinumab 45 mg, 90 mg, or placebo. At week 12, patients receiving placebo were then placed on ustekinumab. At week 28, patients with PASI less than 50 were discontinued; patients with PASI-50 to 75 increased dosage frequency to every 8 weeks, and patients with PASI ≥75 continued ustekinumab every 12 weeks. At week 40, patients initially receiving placebo were switched back to placebo, whereas those receiving ustekinumab every 12 weeks were rerandomized to either placebo or ustekinumab every 12 weeks. Patients receiving placebo were placed back on ustekinumab at loss of therapeutic effect. Patients continued to be followed for 5 years.

and worsened for patients when treatment was withheld.

The PHOENIX 2 study enrolled 1230 patients and had the same study design as PHOENIX I through the first 28 weeks; however, it sought to answer whether dosing intensification would improve response in partial responders. Partial responders, defined as patients obtaining greater than 50% PASI improvement and less than 75% PASI improvement, were rerandomized at week 28 to receive every-8-week dosing or continue on every-12-week dosing. Week 12 data were similar to that in PHOENIX 1, with ustekinumab performing superior to placebo, with a PASI-75 of 63.1% and 72% in the 45-mg and 90-mg groups, respectively.

In the portion of patients treated with ustekinumab 45 mg, 22% were partial responders compared with 15.8% receiving 90 mg. Data through 1 year revealed increasing dosing frequency to every 8 weeks in patients receiving 45 mg of ustekinumab did not result in greater efficacy compared with continuing treatment every 12 weeks. However, dosing ustekinumab 90 mg every 8 weeks resulted in a high PASI-75 rate. This finding prompted investigators to allow more dosing flexibility in the long-term extension phase. Patients receiving 45 mg every 12 weeks were able to increase dose 45 mg every 8 weeks and then to 90 mg every 8 weeks. Similarly, patients receiving 45 mg every 8 weeks could increase frequency to 90 mg every 8 weeks; and patients who were receiving 90 mg every 12 weeks could increase their dose to every 8 weeks.

Most patients receiving ustekinumab maintained their clinical response over time. The long-term extension phase of PHOENIX 1 demonstrated in the overall population that 63.4% of patients receiving 45 mg ustekinumab and 72% of patients receiving 90 mg ustekinumab maintained a PASI-75 after 5 years. Comparably, high levels of clinical response were maintained over 244 weeks in patients studied in the PHOENIX 2 study; 76.5% (ustekinumab 45 mg) and 78.6% (ustekinumab 90 mg) of patients achieved a PASI-75, and 50.0% (ustekinumab 45 mg) and 55.5% (ustekinumab 90) attained PASI-90. Notably, improved response was observed following dosing adjustments, allowing clinicians to customize treatment for their patients. Ustekinumab was also noted to improve nail psoriasis until up to 1 year of treatment in those receiving maintenance treatment (Fig. 11.3).[33]

Several randomized, controlled trials have compared efficacy of ustekinumab against other systemic and biologic agents.[6,24,34–40] The Active Comparator (CNTO1275/Enbrel) Psoriasis Trial (ACCEPT)[41] study was a direct comparator study establishing greater efficacy of ustekinumab

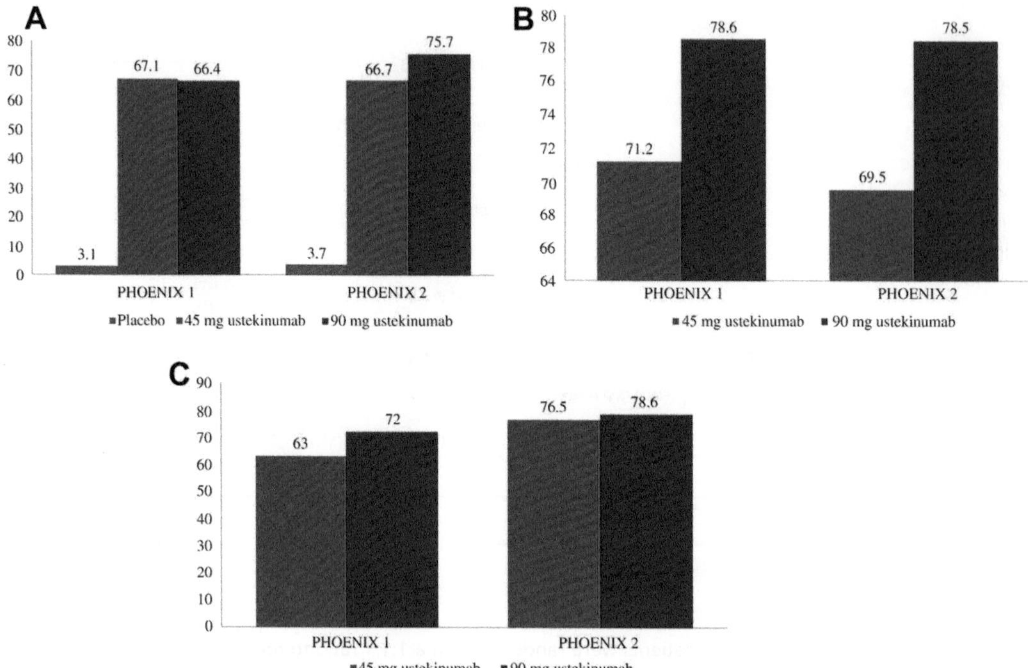

Fig. 11.3 (*A*) Week 12 PASI-75 rates in the overall population, PHOENIX 1 and PHOENIX 2. (*B*) Week 28 PASI-75 rates in the overall population, PHOENIX 1 and PHOENIX 2. (*C*) Week 244 PASI-75 rates in the overall population, PHOENIX 1 and PHOENIX 2.

over etanercept. The Psoriasis Longitudinal Assessment and Registry (PSOLAR)[40] is a prospective observational study (sponsored by Janssen Biotech) comparing the safety and efficacy of 3 TNF inhibitors (adalimumab, infliximab, etanercept) with ustekinumab. At 6 and 12 months, comparisons of percentage decrease in BSA, PGA, and patient-reported outcomes showed ustekinumab to be more effective than the TNF inhibitors. At 12 months, 59.2% of patients receiving ustekinumab achieved a PGA of clear or almost clear, compared with 56.5%, 42.0%, and 57.6% for adalimumab, infliximab, and etanercept, respectively. The mean improvement of BSA from baseline for patients treated with ustekinumab after 1 year was 16.3%. Patients treated with infliximab saw a decrease of 17.6% BSA after 1 year, whereas patients on etanercept and adalimumab saw less significant decreases of 13.8% and 12.3%, respectively. The mean improvement in dermatology quality-of-life index from baseline was 7.5 for ustekinumab, compared with 6.9, 5.4, and 4.9 for infliximab, etanercept, and adalimumab, respectively.

FACTORS EFFECTING DECREASED EFFICACY

Although ustekinumab has demonstrated efficacy for psoriasis, there remains a portion of patients who have shown insufficient response.[42] It is unclear what is responsible for the lack of response; however, heavier patients are notoriously difficult to treat, and there are well-documented effects of body mass index on disease incidence, severity, and response to biologic treatment.[43] PHOENIX 2 investigators noted patients who needed increased dosing in ustekinumab were heavier, had more severe psoriasis, and were more likely to have comorbidities.[4,25] The highest incidence of dosing adjustments was observed among patients weighing greater than 100 kg who were originally randomized to 45 mg. Clinical and pharmacokinetic data support a 90-mg dose in patients (>100 kg); lower serum concentrations were noted in heavier patients at each dose.[44] Per the package insert, the recommended administration for patients weighing less than or equal to 100 kg (220 lbs) is 45 mg initially and 4 weeks later, followed by 45 mg every 12 weeks. For patients weighing greater than 100 kg, the recommended dose is 90 mg initially and 4 weeks later, followed by 90 mg every 12 weeks.[21]

In the PHOENIX 2 study, partial responders were more likely to have failed treatment with at least 1 conventional systemic or biological agent compared with nonresponders.[4] In some clinical trials, patients with prior TNF inhibitor use had worse PGA and percentage BSA responses compared with biologic-naïve patients.[40,42]

PSOLAR reinforced the effect of weight on response to biologic therapy; patients with lower weight experienced superior results compared with heavier patients. Disease severity correlated with larger decreases in BSA but a lower PGA response. PSOLAR demonstrated patients with prior TNF inhibitor use had less of a response compared with bionaïve patients, whereas prior ustekinumab use had no effect on response.[40]

EFFICACY IN PALMOPLANTAR PSORIASIS

Palmar plantar psoriasis (PPP) is a disabling and disfiguring form of psoriasis characterized by the presence of plaques with and without sterile pustules and fissures on the palms and soles in conjunction with psoriatic plaques in the typical distribution.[45] PPP is associated with a higher degree of pain and an increased morbidity compared with psoriasis patients without palm and sole involvement.[46] It is also notoriously difficult to treat using previous conventional therapies.

In an open-label, 24-week study to evaluate the safety and efficacy of ustekinumab in patients with moderate-to-severe PPP, 20 subjects received either 45 mg (patients weighing ≤100 kg), or 90 mg (patients weighing >100 kg), of ustekinumab subcutaneously at weeks 0, 4, and 16. After 16 weeks of treatment with ustekinumab, 7 of 20 subjects achieved clinical clearance (defined as a Palm-Sole PGA of clear or almost clear). After 16 weeks of treatment, 6 of 9 subjects who received 90 mg of ustekinumab achieved clinical clearance, compared with only 1 of 11 subjects who received 45 mg.[47]

EFFICACY IN PEDIATRIC PSORIASIS

Ustekinumab has been shown to be safe and effective in treatment of pediatric psoriasis. The CADMUS trial is a phase 3, multicenter, double-blinded, placebo-controlled study of 110 male and female patients aged 12 to 17 years old.[48] Patients were randomly assigned to receive a standard dose adjusted by weight (0.75 mg/kg [<60 kg], 45 mg [60–100 kg], 90 mg [>100 kg]), a half-standard dose (0.375 mg/kg [<60 kg], 22.5 mg [60–100 kg], 45 mg [<100 kg]) at weeks 0, 4, followed by every 12 weeks, or placebo at week 0 and 4 with crossover to standard or half-standard dosing at week 12.

The results of this study were apparent very quickly. By week 4, approximately one-third of patients in each ustekinumab group were clear or almost clear. At week 12, 67.6% of patients receiving the half-standard dose and 69.4% of patients receiving the standard dose achieved a PGA of 0 or 1, and 54.1% of patients receiving the half-standard dose and 61.1% of those receiving the full dose achieved PASI-90. In time points beyond week 12, clinical response was more favorable in the standard dose compared with the half-standard dose. Pharmacokinetic and efficacy date for the dose adjustment of 0.75 mg/kg was appropriate for patients weighing less than 60 kg. Adverse events in this study were similar across treatment groups, with no observed dose effect.[48]

EFFICACY IN PSORIATIC ARTHRITIS

IL-12, IL-23, and IL-17 play a pivotal role in the synovial changes seen in psoriatic arthritis.[49] Treatment modalities involved nonsteroidal anti-inflammatory drugs, disease modifying antirheumatic drugs, and TNF inhibitors. Several studies assessed the efficacy and safety of ustekinumab in patients with psoriatic arthritis.[50–52] Clinical response in psoriatic arthritis is measured by a 20% improvement in baseline from the American College of Rheumatology (ACR20). In 1 phase 3, international, placebo-controlled trial to assess the efficacy and safety of ustekinumab in patients with psoriatic arthritis, patients were randomized to receive ustekinumab 45 mg, 90 mg, or placebo in a 1:1:1 ratio, and 50% of patients receiving ustekinumab also received methotrexate.[52] ACR20 responses were significantly higher in patients treated with ustekinumab as were improvements in skin disease, dactylitis, enthesitis, and disease activity as measured by C-reactive peptide. Ustekinumab proved to be effective independent of methotrexate use.

Another phase 3 randomized, controlled study assessed patients previously treated with a TNF inhibitor.[51] Investigators reinforced that ustekinumab was effective in treating psoriatic arthritis in patients already exposed to TNF inhibitor, although not as effective as those who were bionaïve. These 2 studies continued for 2 years and showed clinical and radiographic evidence that ustekinumab is safe and effective in psoriatic arthritis.[50]

SAFETY

Ustekinumab has been the foremost biologic evaluated for safety in patients with psoriasis.[4,53,54] The PHOENIX 1, PHOENIX 2, and ACCEPT trials are the preeminent sources of long-term safety data collected for patients treated with ustekinumab. Investigators found no statistically significant difference in overall

AEs between ustekinumab- and placebo-treated patients. Most reported AEs were nasopharyngitis, upper respiratory infections, headaches, and arthralgias. More than 5 years in the PHOENIX 1 and 2 trials, there was no evidence of cumulative end-organ toxicity. There was a low incidence of autoantibodies to ustekinumab. One ustekinumab-treated patient developed reversible posterior encephalopathy syndrome; however, there were no reported cases of demyelinating disease.[55]

Theoretically, a blockade of the actions of IL-12 and IL-23 could predispose a person to viral, bacterial, and fungal infections.[56,57] Rates of infections and serious infections were comparable during the placebo-controlled portions of randomized, controlled trials, and rates of serious infections in ustekinumab-treated patients were comparable to those expected in patients with psoriasis treated with conventional systemic drugs.[58] Although patients on TNF inhibitors are at increased risk for reactivation of latent tuberculosis (TB) reactivation, ustekinumab does not appear to increase this risk.[4,58]

In placebo-controlled periods, rates of infections, serious infections, and malignancies were comparable with those of patients receiving placebo.[58] Rates of malignancies other than nonmelanoma skin cancer in ustekinumab-treated patients were consistent with rates expected in the general population, suggesting that ustekinumab does not increase rate of malignancy.[58] Of more than 12,000 patients (40,388 patient-years) observed in PSOLAR, overall incidence rates for malignancy (0.68/100 patient-years), serious infection (1.6/100 patient years), and mortality (0.93/100 patient years) were significantly lower when compared with other biologics.[59] Most common reported types of serious infections were pneumonia and cellulitis. PSOLAR demonstrated a higher risk of serious infections with adalimumab and infliximab compared with nonbiologic treatment, while also observing no increased risk of serious infections with ustekinumab or etanercept.[60]

Early studies exhibited a higher risk of major adverse cardiovascular events (MACEs) in patients receiving anti-IL-12/23 antibodies compared with those in placebo groups. Concern over a possible link between ustekinumab and MACEs prompted an in-depth investigation. PSOLAR found ustekinumab to have a significantly lower rate of MACEs (0.33/100 patient-years) compared with other biologics.[61] The risk of MACEs in patients treated with anti-IL-12/23 biological was evaluated in 2 large meta-analysis studies that came to conflicting conclusions.[62,63] Reich and colleagues[64] analyzed 3000 patients on ustekinumab and found no increase in MACEs compared with patients in the general or psoriasis populations.

MONITORING

The information presented is primarily based on psoriasis guidelines from the American Academy of Dermatology (AAD).[65]

A thorough history and physical examination should be taken before initiation of ustekinumab therapy, including TB exposure, chronic/recurrent infections, malignancy, neurologic and cardiac history, and a thorough review of systems. Routine follow-up examinations should adequately monitor patients for side effects and AEs.[48]

Aside from baseline TB test, annual monitoring for TB, and a baseline hepatitis profile, routine laboratory testing beyond that for concomitant therapies or comorbidities is generally not supported.[66] The highest grade US Preventive Services Task Force evidence for screening studies is grade B for TB testing (interferon-γ release assay is preferred over tuberculin skin testing), and hepatitis B virus/hepatitis C virus screening is supported only by grade C evidence.[60] The AAD recommends baseline PPD, liver function tests (LFTs), and complete blood count (CBC). For ongoing monitoring, the AAD recommends yearly PPD and periodic LFTs, CBC, history, and physical examinations (Table 11.1).[65]

The Centers for Disease Control and Prevention (CDC) recommends TB testing before the therapy initiation as well.[67] Positive skin test findings should be followed with a chest radiograph—if negative, patients should be treated for latent TB (6–9 months of 300 mg isoniazid daily and/or

TABLE 11.1
Monitoring recommendations from the American Academy of Dermatology

Monitoring	
History and physical	Baseline and routine
CBC	Baseline and periodically
LFTs	Baseline and periodically
TB skin test	Baseline and annually after
Hepatitis B serology	Not specified

Data from Menter A, Gottlieb A, Feldman SR, et al. Guidelines of care for the management of psoriasis and psoriatic arthritis: section 1. Overview of psoriasis and guidelines of care for the treatment of psoriasis with biologics. J Am Acad Dermatol 2008;58(5):838.

4 months of 600 mg daily rifampicin),[68] and if positive, patients should receive therapy for active TB. Biologic therapy may be started after 1 to 2 months of prophylactic treatment if the patient is adherent to and tolerating the prophylactic regimen.[69] If a patient has a positive PPD because of prior BCG vaccination, blood tests can be obtained measuring IFN production on stimulation with TB antigens that are not present in BCG. Most guidelines perform annual TB skin testing in patients receiving ustekinumab to screen for the TB reactivation, especially in those at risk (ie, health care workers, travelers to endemic areas).

The authors of this section recommend initial baseline monitoring that includes a QuantiFERON-TB Gold (QFT), LFTs, CBC, and hepatitis B and hepatitis C profile. QFT should be repeated annually.

TABLE 11.2
Vaccination recommendations from the National Psoriasis Foundation

Vaccination	Before Therapy	During Therapy
Live vaccines (measles, mumps, and rubella [MMR], varicella, herpes zoster, intranasal influenza, oral typhoid, yellow fever, oral polio, smallpox, BCG, rotavirus)	Contraindicated within 1 mo	Contraindicated
Influenza	Vaccinate with inactivated or live	Yearly immunization with inactivated vaccine
Chicken pox	If negative serology, vaccinate	Contraindicated
Zoster	Before therapy: 1 dose for adults >50 y	Contraindicated
Human papillomavirus	Unvaccinated males/female patients up to age 26	Same
Hepatitis A	Vaccinate if high risk (diabetes, liver disease, intravenous drug users, homosexual men, and so forth)	Same; consider obtaining postvaccination serology
Hepatitis B	Serology, risk factor assessment. Offer vaccination if necessary	High-dose vaccine, consider obtaining serology postvaccination
Pneumococcal	Pneumococcal polysaccharide vaccine (PPSV23) vaccine recommended	Pneumococcal conjugate vaccine followed by PPSV23 if not given prior
MMR	Vaccinate if negative, or seronegative to any component	Contraindicated
Tetanus-diphtheria/diphtheria-tetanus-acellular pertussis (TD/TDAP)	Booster every 10 y and high-risk wounds offer before therapy, substitute 1 dose with TDAP	Same
Meningococcal	Assess risk factors, vaccinate if high risk (asplenia, complement deficient, group living)	Same
Poliomyelitis	Assess risk factors, vaccinate if high risk (health care worker, laboratory worker)	Same
Haemophilus influenzae type b	Vaccinate if unvaccinated	Same

Data from Lebwohl M, Bagel J, Gelfand JM, et al. From the Medical Board of the National Psoriasis Foundation: monitoring and vaccinations in patients treated with biologics for psoriasis. J Am Acad Dermatol 2008;58(1):99; and Wine-Lee L, Keller SC, Wilck MB, et al. From the Medical Board of the National Psoriasis Foundation: vaccination in adult patients on systemic therapy for psoriasis. J Am Acad Dermatol 2013;69(6):1003–13.

VACCINATIONS

Patients should receive all immunizations appropriate for age as recommended by current immunization guidelines. Per the package insert, patients undergoing treatment with ustekinumab should not receive any live vaccines. If a patient requires immunization with a live vaccine, ustekinumab should be stopped for 6 months before and 2 weeks after vaccination. Multiple studies and case reports have linked ustekinumab with duration and severity of herpes zoster; thus, vaccination should be considered before initiation of therapy.[70] Brodmerkel and colleagues[71] found long-term treatment with ustekinumab does not compromise the immune response to T-cell-dependent/-independent vaccines in psoriasis patients. Inactivated vaccines are safe; however, it is not certain to confer immunity while on ustekinumab. The pneumococcal and annual inactivated influenza vaccines are recommended and may be taken during therapy.[21] A summary of vaccination recommendations by the National Psoriasis Foundation can be found in Table 11.2.

SUMMARY AND RECOMMENDATIONS

Ustekinumab is a highly efficacious and safe therapy recommended for the treatment of moderate-to-severe psoriasis. This molecule is directed against the p40 component of IL-12 and IL-23 and is thus more targeted than earlier biologic therapies; consequently, it would be expected to suppress less of the immune system. Indeed, individuals born with IL-12Rβ1 deficiency are susceptible to mycobacterial and salmonella infections but not to other opportunistic infections.[72,73] In clinical studies and in practice, there has not been an increase in these infections nor have there been any other signals of immunosuppression in patients treated with ustekinumab.

Dosing as infrequently as every 12 weeks is a major advantage over all of the currently available injected or oral psoriasis therapies and may be the reason that a high proportion of patients treated with ustekinumab continue the therapy.[74] Ustekinumab can be used as a first-line agent in treating psoriasis and psoriatic arthritis. Efficacy, tolerability, ease of use, and long dosing intervals contribute to patient satisfaction and adherence.

REFERENCES

1. Lebwohl M. Biologics for psoriasis: a translational research success story. J Invest Dermatol 2015; 135(5):1205–7.
2. Bartlett BL, Tyring SK. Ustekinumab for chronic plaque psoriasis. Lancet 2008;371(9625):1639–40.
3. Bongartz T, Sutton AJ, Sweeting MJ, et al. Anti-TNF antibody therapy in rheumatoid arthritis and the risk of serious infections and malignancies: systematic review and meta-analysis of rare harmful effects in randomized controlled trials. JAMA 2006;295(19): 2275–85.
4. Langley RG, Lebwohl M, Krueger GG, et al. Long-term efficacy and safety of ustekinumab, with and without dosing adjustment, in patients with moderate-to-severe psoriasis: results from the PHOENIX 2 study through 5 years of follow-up. Br J Dermatol 2015;172(5):1371–83.
5. Hochberg MC, Lebwohl MG, Plevy SE, et al. The benefit/risk profile of TNF-blocking agents: findings of a consensus panel. Semin Arthritis Rheum 2005; 34(6):819–36.
6. Thaci D, Blauvelt A, Reich K, et al. Secukinumab is superior to ustekinumab in clearing skin of subjects with moderate to severe plaque psoriasis: CLEAR, a randomized controlled trial. J Am Acad Dermatol 2015;73(3):400–9.
7. Gottlieb AB, Langley RG, Strober BE, et al. A randomized, double-blind, placebo-controlled study to evaluate the addition of methotrexate to etanercept in patients with moderate to severe plaque psoriasis. Br J Dermatol 2012;167(3): 649–57.
8. Menter A, Tyring SK, Gordon K, et al. Adalimumab therapy for moderate to severe psoriasis: a randomized, controlled phase III trial. J Am Acad Dermatol 2008;58(1):106–15.
9. Papp K, Okun M, Vender R. Adalimumab in the treatment of psoriasis: pooled efficacy and safety results from three pivotal studies. J Cutan Med Surg 2009;13(Suppl 2):S58–66.
10. Revicki D, Willian MK, Saurat JH, et al. Impact of adalimumab treatment on health-related quality of life and other patient-reported outcomes: results from a 16-week randomized controlled trial in patients with moderate to severe plaque psoriasis. Br J Dermatol 2008;158(3):549–57.
11. Saurat JH, Stingl G, Dubertret L, et al. Efficacy and safety results from the randomized controlled comparative study of adalimumab vs. methotrexate vs. placebo in patients with psoriasis (CHAMPION). Br J Dermatol 2008;158(3):558–66.
12. Tyring S, Gottlieb A, Papp K, et al. Etanercept and clinical outcomes, fatigue, and depression in psoriasis: double-blind placebo-controlled randomised phase III trial. Lancet 2006;367(9504):29–35.
13. Revicki DA, Willian MK, Menter A, et al. Relationship between clinical response to therapy and health-related quality of life outcomes in patients with moderate to severe plaque psoriasis. Dermatology 2008;216(3):260–70.

14. Kimball AB, Gordon KB, Fakharzadeh S, et al. Long-term efficacy of ustekinumab in patients with moderate-to-severe psoriasis: results from the PHOENIX 1 trial through up to 3 years. Br J Dermatol 2012;166(4):861–72.
15. Famenini S, Wu JJ. The efficacy of ustekinumab in psoriasis. J Drugs Dermatol 2013;12(3):317–20.
16. Benson JM, Peritt D, Scallon BJ, et al. Discovery and mechanism of ustekinumab: a human monoclonal antibody targeting interleukin-12 and interleukin-23 for treatment of immune-mediated disorders. MAbs 2011;3(6):535–45.
17. Harden JL, Krueger JG, Bowcock AM. The immunogenetics of psoriasis: a comprehensive review. J Autoimmun 2015;64:66–73.
18. Oppmann B, Lesley R, Blom B, et al. Novel p19 protein engages IL-12p40 to form a cytokine, IL-23, with biological activities similar as well as distinct from IL-12. Immunity 2000;13(5):715–25.
19. Kagami S, Rizzo HL, Lee JJ, et al. Circulating Th17, Th22, and Th1 cells are increased in psoriasis. J Invest Dermatol 2010;130(5):1373–83.
20. Benson JM, Sachs CW, Treacy G, et al. Therapeutic targeting of the IL-12/23 pathways: generation and characterization of ustekinumab. Nat Biotechnol 2011;29(7):615–24.
21. Stelara [package insert]. Horsham, PA: Janssen Biotech, Inc; 2014.
22. Ghetie V, Ward ES. Transcytosis and catabolism of antibody. Immunol Res 2002;25(2):97–113.
23. Abuabara K, Wan J, Troxel AB, et al. Variation in dermatologist beliefs about the safety and effectiveness of treatments for moderate to severe psoriasis. J Am Acad Dermatol 2013;68(2):262–9.
24. Griffiths CE, Strober BE, van de Kerkhof P, et al. Comparison of ustekinumab and etanercept for moderate-to-severe psoriasis. N Engl J Med 2010;362(2):118–28.
25. Kimball AB, Papp KA, Wasfi Y, et al. Long-term efficacy of ustekinumab in patients with moderate-to-severe psoriasis treated for up to 5 years in the PHOENIX 1 study. J Eur Acad Dermatol Venereol 2013;27(12):1535–45.
26. Leonardi CL, Kimball AB, Papp KA, et al. Efficacy and safety of ustekinumab, a human interleukin-12/23 monoclonal antibody, in patients with psoriasis: 76-week results from a randomised, double-blind, placebo-controlled trial (PHOENIX 1). Lancet 2008;371(9625):1665–74.
27. Papp KA, Langley RG, Lebwohl M, et al. Efficacy and safety of ustekinumab, a human interleukin-12/23 monoclonal antibody, in patients with psoriasis: 52-week results from a randomised, double-blind, placebo-controlled trial (PHOENIX 2). Lancet 2008;371(9625):1675–84.
28. Scherl EJ, Kumar S, Warren RU. Review of the safety and efficacy of ustekinumab. Therap Adv Gastroenterol 2010;3(5):321–8.
29. Gottlieb AB, Cooper KD, McCormick TS, et al. A phase 1, double-blind, placebo-controlled study evaluating single subcutaneous administrations of a human interleukin-12/23 monoclonal antibody in subjects with plaque psoriasis. Curr Med Res Opin 2007;23(5):1081–92.
30. Kauffman CL, Aria N, Toichi E, et al. A phase I study evaluating the safety, pharmacokinetics, and clinical response of a human IL-12 p40 antibody in subjects with plaque psoriasis. J Invest Dermatol 2004;123(6):1037–44.
31. Krueger GG, Langley RG, Leonardi C, et al. A human interleukin-12/23 monoclonal antibody for the treatment of psoriasis. N Engl J Med 2007;356(6):580–92.
32. Puig L. PASI90 response: the new standard in therapeutic efficacy for psoriasis. J Eur Acad Dermatol Venereol 2015;29(4):645–8.
33. Rich P, Bourcier M, Sofen H, et al. Ustekinumab improves nail disease in patients with moderate-to-severe psoriasis: results from PHOENIX 1. Br J Dermatol 2014;170(2):398–407.
34. Lin VW, Ringold S, Devine EB. Comparison of ustekinumab with other biological agents for the treatment of moderate to severe plaque psoriasis: a bayesian network meta-analysis. Arch Dermatol 2012;148(12):1403–10.
35. Lucka TC, Pathirana D, Sammain A, et al. Efficacy of systemic therapies for moderate-to-severe psoriasis: a systematic review and meta-analysis of long-term treatment. J Eur Acad Dermatol Venereol 2012;26(11):1331–44.
36. Reich K, Burden AD, Eaton JN, et al. Efficacy of biologics in the treatment of moderate to severe psoriasis: a network meta-analysis of randomized controlled trials. Br J Dermatol 2012;166(1):179–88.
37. Galvan-Banqueri M, Marin Gil R, Santos Ramos B, et al. Biological treatments for moderate-to-severe psoriasis: indirect comparison. J Clin Pharm Ther 2013;38(2):121–30.
38. Schmitt J, Rosumeck S, Thomaschewski G, et al. Efficacy and safety of systemic treatments for moderate-to-severe psoriasis: meta-analysis of randomized controlled trials. Br J Dermatol 2014;170(2):274–303.
39. Lebwohl M, Strober B, Menter A, et al. Phase 3 studies comparing brodalumab with ustekinumab in psoriasis. N Engl J Med 2015;373(14):1318–28.
40. Strober BE, Bissonnette R, Fiorentino D, et al. Comparative effectiveness of biologic agents for the treatment of psoriasis in a real-world setting: results from a large, prospective, observational study (psoriasis longitudinal assessment and

registry [PSOLAR]). J Am Acad Dermatol 2016;74(5):851–61.e4.
41. Young MS, Horn EJ, Cather JC. The ACCEPT study: ustekinumab versus etanercept in moderate-to-severe psoriasis patients. Expert Rev Clin Immunol 2011;7(1):9–13.
42. Umezawa Y, Saeki H, Nakagawa H. Some clinical factors affecting quality of the response to ustekinumab for psoriasis. J Dermatol 2014;41(8):690–6.
43. Puig L. Obesity and psoriasis: body weight and body mass index influence the response to biological treatment. J Eur Acad Dermatol Venereol 2011;25(9):1007–11.
44. Lebwohl M, Yeilding N, Szapary P, et al. Impact of weight on the efficacy and safety of ustekinumab in patients with moderate to severe psoriasis: rationale for dosing recommendations. J Am Acad Dermatol 2010;63(4):571–9.
45. Morales-Munera C, Vilarrasa E, Puig L. Efficacy of ustekinumab in refractory palmoplantar pustular psoriasis. Br J Dermatol 2013;168(4):820–4.
46. Pettey AA, Balkrishnan R, Rapp SR, et al. Patients with palmoplantar psoriasis have more physical disability and discomfort than patients with other forms of psoriasis: implications for clinical practice. J Am Acad Dermatol 2003;49(2):271–5.
47. Au SC, Goldminz AM, Kim N, et al. Investigator-initiated, open-label trial of ustekinumab for the treatment of moderate-to-severe palmoplantar psoriasis. J Dermatolog Treat 2013;24(3):179–87.
48. Landells I, Marano C, Hsu MC, et al. Ustekinumab in adolescent patients age 12 to 17 years with moderate-to-severe plaque psoriasis: results of the randomized phase 3 CADMUS study. J Am Acad Dermatol 2015;73(4):594–603.
49. Gottlieb A, Menter A, Mendelsohn A, et al. Ustekinumab, a human interleukin 12/23 monoclonal antibody, for psoriatic arthritis: randomised, double-blind, placebo-controlled, crossover trial. Lancet 2009;373(9664):633–40.
50. Kavanaugh A, Ritchlin C, Rahman P, et al. Ustekinumab, an anti-IL-12/23 p40 monoclonal antibody, inhibits radiographic progression in patients with active psoriatic arthritis: results of an integrated analysis of radiographic data from the phase 3, multicentre, randomised, double-blind, placebo-controlled PSUMMIT-1 and PSUMMIT-2 trials. Ann Rheum Dis 2014;73(6):1000–6.
51. Ritchlin C, Rahman P, Kavanaugh A, et al. Efficacy and safety of the anti-IL-12/23 p40 monoclonal antibody, ustekinumab, in patients with active psoriatic arthritis despite conventional non-biological and biological anti-tumour necrosis factor therapy: 6-month and 1-year results of the phase 3, multicentre, double-blind, placebo-controlled, randomised PSUMMIT 2 trial. Ann Rheum Dis 2014;73(6):990–9.
52. McInnes IB, Kavanaugh A, Gottlieb AB, et al. Efficacy and safety of ustekinumab in patients with active psoriatic arthritis: 1 year results of the phase 3, multicentre, double-blind, placebo-controlled PSUMMIT 1 trial. Lancet 2013;382(9894):780–9.
53. Correr CJ, Rotta I, Teles Tde S, et al. Efficacy and safety of biologics in the treatment of moderate to severe psoriasis: a comprehensive meta-analysis of randomized controlled trials. Cad Saude Publica 2013;29(Suppl 1):S17–31.
54. Nast A, Jacobs A, Rosumeck S, et al. Efficacy and safety of systemic long-term treatments for moderate-to-severe psoriasis: a systematic review and meta-analysis. J Invest Dermatol 2015;135(11):2641–8.
55. Lebwohl M, Leonardi C, Griffiths CE, et al. Long-term safety experience of ustekinumab in patients with moderate-to-severe psoriasis (part I of II): results from analyses of general safety parameters from pooled phase 2 and 3 clinical trials. J Am Acad Dermatol 2012;66(5):731–41.
56. Filipe-Santos O, Bustamante J, Chapgier A, et al. Inborn errors of IL-12/23- and IFN-gamma-mediated immunity: molecular, cellular, and clinical features. Semin Immunol 2006;18(6):347–61.
57. Puel A, Cypowyj S, Bustamante J, et al. Chronic mucocutaneous candidiasis in humans with inborn errors of interleukin-17 immunity. Science 2011;332(6025):65–8.
58. Gordon KB, Papp KA, Langley RG, et al. Long-term safety experience of ustekinumab in patients with moderate to severe psoriasis (part II of II): results from analyses of infections and malignancy from pooled phase II and III clinical trials. J Am Acad Dermatol 2012;66(5):742–51.
59. Papp K, Gottlieb AB, Naldi L, et al. Safety surveillance for ustekinumab and other psoriasis treatments from the psoriasis longitudinal assessment and registry (PSOLAR). J Drugs Dermatol 2015;14(7):706–14.
60. Ahn CS, Dothard EH, Garner ML, et al. To test or not to test? An updated evidence-based assessment of the value of screening and monitoring tests when using systemic biologic agents to treat psoriasis and psoriatic arthritis. J Am Acad Dermatol 2015;73(3):420–8.e1.
61. Bigby M. The use of anti-interleukin-12/23 agents and major adverse cardiovascular events. Arch Dermatol 2012;148(6):753–4.
62. Tzellos T, Kyrgidis A, Trigoni A, et al. Association of anti-IL-12/23 biologic agents ustekinumab and briakinumab with major adverse cardiovascular events. J Eur Acad Dermatol Venereol 2013;27(12):1586–7.
63. Ryan C, Leonardi CL, Krueger JG, et al. Association between biologic therapies for chronic plaque psoriasis and cardiovascular events: a meta-analysis of

randomized controlled trials. JAMA 2011;306(8):864–71.

64. Reich K, Langley RG, Lebwohl M, et al. Cardiovascular safety of ustekinumab in patients with moderate to severe psoriasis: results of integrated analyses of data from phase II and III clinical studies. Br J Dermatol 2011;164(4):862–72.
65. Menter A, Gottlieb A, Feldman SR, et al. Guidelines of care for the management of psoriasis and psoriatic arthritis: section 1. Overview of psoriasis and guidelines of care for the treatment of psoriasis with biologics. J Am Acad Dermatol 2008;58(5):826–50.
66. van Lümig PP, Driessen RJ, Roelofs-Thijssen MA, et al. Relevance of laboratory investigations in monitoring patients with psoriasis on etanercept or adalimumab. Br J Dermatol 2011;165(2):375–82.
67. CDC - Tuberculosis (TB) [Internet]. Available at: http://www.cdc.gov/tb/?404;http://www.cdc.gov:80/tb/pubs/LTBI/pdf/TargetedLTBI05.pdf. Accessed February 1, 2016.
68. Targeted tuberculin testing and treatment of latent tuberculosis infection. American Thoracic Society. MMWR Recomm Rep 2000;49(RR-6):1–51.
69. Doherty SD, Van Voorhees A, Lebwohl MG, et al. National Psoriasis Foundation consensus statement on screening for latent tuberculosis infection in patients with psoriasis treated with systemic and biologic agents. J Am Acad Dermatol 2008;59(2):209–17.
70. Kalb RE, Fiorentino DF, Lebwohl MG, et al. Risk of serious infection with biologic and systemic treatment of psoriasis: results from the psoriasis longitudinal assessment and registry (PSOLAR). JAMA Dermatol 2015;151(9):961–9.
71. Brodmerkel C, Wadman E, Langley RG, et al. Immune response to pneumococcus and tetanus toxoid in patients with moderate-to-severe psoriasis following long-term ustekinumab use. J Drugs Dermatol 2013;12(10):1122–9.
72. Fieschi C, Dupuis S, Catherinot E, et al. Low penetrance, broad resistance, and favorable outcome of interleukin 12 receptor beta1 deficiency: medical and immunological implications. J Exp Med 2003;197(4):527–35.
73. de Beaucoudrey L, Samarina A, Bustamante J, et al. Revisiting human IL-12Rβ1 deficiency: a survey of 141 patients from 30 countries. Medicine 2010;89(6):381–402.
74. Cao Z, Carter C, Wilson KL, et al. Ustekinumab dosing, persistence, and discontinuation patterns in patients with moderate-to-severe psoriasis. J Dermatolog Treat 2015;26(2):113–20.

CHAPTER 12

Secukinumab

Elaine J. Lin, MD, Shivani P. Reddy, BS, Vidhi V. Shah, BA,
Jashin J. Wu, MD

KEYWORDS

• Secukinumab • Cosentyx • Interleukin-17A • Monoclonal antibody • ERASURE • FIXTURE • JUNCTURE • FEATURE

KEY POINTS

- Secukinumab is a first-in-class human monoclonal antibody against interleukin-17A.
- Secukinumab has been demonstrated in clinical studies to be significantly more efficacious in the treatment of plaque psoriasis in comparison to etanercept and ustekinumab.
- The most common side effects attributable to secukinumab are monilial infections.
- Secukinumab is now US Food and Drug Administration–approved for the treatment of psoriatic arthritis and ankylosing spondylitis.

INTRODUCTION

Secukinumab is a first-in-class human monoclonal antibody against interleukin-17A (IL-17A). The evolving literature on the role of immune cells and inflammatory mediators in the pathogenesis of psoriasis has advanced therapeutic efficacy tremendously in the last 20 years. Early clinical studies of T-cell–targeted therapies, such as those involving cyclosporine, indicated an integral role of T cells in the pathogenesis of psoriasis.[1] Focus of research has recently been directed toward Th17 cells, a subset of T cells producing the cytokine IL-17A. On January 21, 2015, the US Food and Drug Administration (FDA) approved secukinumab for the treatment of adult patients with moderate-to-severe plaque psoriasis who are candidates for systemic therapy or phototherapy.

Secukinumab is manufactured by Novartis Pharmaceuticals under the trade name of Cosentyx. Administered through subcutaneous injections, there are 3 different devices: secukinumab lyophilized powder in single-use vials reconstituted with sterile water for injection (reconstitution done by health care provider only), prefilled syringes (PFSs), and autoinjector/pens (Sensoready Pen). All forms administer a single dose of 150 mg of secukinumab and are to be stored in a refrigerator, between 2°C and 8°C (36°F and 46°F). The recommended dose and regimen are a 300-mg subcutaneous injection at weeks 0, 1, 2, 3, and 4 followed by maintenance dosing of 300 mg every 4 weeks thereafter (Fig. 12.1). Dosing at 150 mg, secukinumab can be used in some patients. Injection sites should be alternated, and bruised, red, scaly, hard, or psoriatic skin should be avoided. Recommended sites include front of thighs, lower abdomen (except 2 inches around the navel), and upper outer arms.[2]

Following a subcutaneous injection of secukinumab, 55%–77% reaches systemic circulation. Peak serum concentrations are reached in approximately 6 days after administration, and steady-state concentrations are reached by week 24 when following the every 4-week dosing regimen. At 1 and 2 weeks after a single 300-mg dose, secukinumab concentrations in interstitial fluid in lesional and nonlesional skin of plaque psoriasis patients ranged from 27% to 40% of serum concentrations. The mean half-life of secukinumab ranges from 22 to 31 days.[2]

MECHANISM OF ACTION

Secukinumab is a recombinant, high-affinity, fully human immunoglobulin 1/kappa monoclonal antibody that selectively binds to and neutralizes IL-17A. IL-17A is a naturally occurring proinflammatory cytokine that has been associated with several chronic inflammatory diseases and plays a key role in the pathogenesis of plaque psoriasis.[3] Sources of IL-17A found in psoriatic skin include Th17 cells, mast cells, and

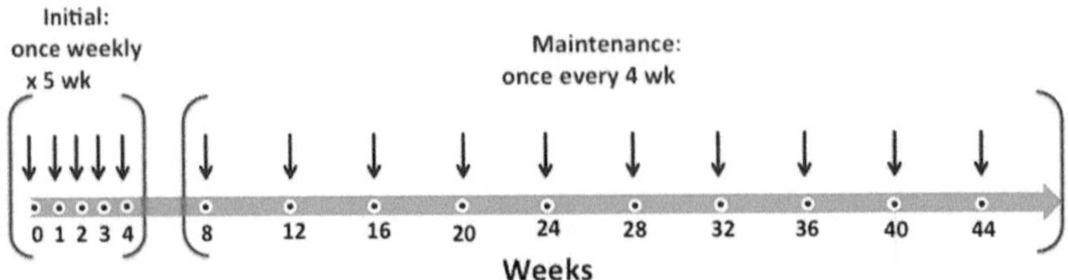

Fig. 12.1 Recommended initial and maintenance dosing schedule of secukinumab.

neutrophils. IL-17A upregulates the expression of inflammatory-related genes in target cells, including endothelial cells, fibroblasts, and epithelial cells, including keratinocytes, and causes the release of cytokines, chemokines, antimicrobial peptides, and other mediators that help sustain inflammation in the skin.[3,4]

Psoriatic lesions are thought to have higher expression of Th17 and IL-17A, which activate keratinocytes, leading to aberrant differentiation and proliferation and the production of keratinocyte-derived angiogenic and chemoattractant factors. Further recruitment of inflammatory cells and synergy of inflammatory cytokines set up a positive feedback loop for inflammation and keratinocyte-mediated psoriatic epidermal changes.[5] These changes include acanthosis, hyperkeratosis, and parakeratosis. At therapeutic levels, secukinumab intercepts disease pathogenesis, leading to normalization of skin histology and achievement of clear to almost clear skin for most psoriatic patients.

EFFICACY

Secukinumab has been proven to be a highly efficacious treatment in subjects with moderate-to-severe plaque psoriasis with the most pronounced effects seen with a 300-mg dose.[6] Clinically meaningful and statistically significant improvement based on coprimary endpoints of Psoriasis Area Severity Index (PASI) -75 response and Investigator Global Assessment for clear to almost clear skin (IGA 0/1) at week 12 was produced by 4 phase III double-blind, randomized, placebo-controlled trials (ERASURE, FIXTURE, JUNCTURE, and FEATURE) that evaluated 2-dose regimens using either 300 mg or 150 mg of secukinumab compared with placebo (Table 12.1).[6–8]

Enrolled subjects were 18 years of age or older with plaque psoriasis diagnosed at least 6 months before randomization who had a minimum body surface area (BSA) involvement of 10%, an IGA score 3 or greater, and a PASI score 12 or greater and who were candidates for phototherapy or systemic therapy. Exclusion criteria included forms of psoriasis other than chronic-plaque type, ongoing use of certain psoriasis treatments, active or ongoing inflammatory disease or chronic or recurrent infectious disease, evidence of tuberculosis (TB), history of human immunodeficiency virus infection, hepatitis B or C, underlying immunocompromising conditions, lymphoproliferative diseases, malignancy or history of malignancy within the past 5 years, significant medical problems, pregnant or nursing women, and women of child-bearing potential not using effective contraception during the study. Across all 4 studies, enrolled patients were characterized as 79% biologic-naïve, 45% nonbiologic failures, 8% biologic failures, 6% anti-tumor necrosis factor (TNF) failures, and 2% IL-12/23 inhibitor failures. However, median baseline PASI score,[9,10] baseline IGA score range (moderate to severe), median baseline BSA (≥27), and median Dermatology Life Quality Index score[11–13] of patients were generally consistent across all treatment groups.[2]

ERASURE AND FIXTURE

The ERASURE trial enrolled 738 patients, whom were randomized into the secukinumab 150 mg, secukinumab 300 mg, or placebo arm. Each group received their respective doses at weeks 0, 1, 2, 3, and 4 followed by a dose every 4 weeks until week 48. The FIXTURE trial evaluated 1308 patients, whom were randomized into similar arms to the ERASURE trial with similar dosing schedules, but with the addition of an etanercept arm. Patients randomized to etanercept received 50-mg doses twice per week for 12 weeks followed by 50 mg every week. In both trials, patients in the placebo group who were nonresponders at week 12 were crossed over to receive secukinumab in either the 150-mg or the 300-mg dose at weeks 12, 13,14, 15, and 16 followed by the same dose every 4 weeks. Each study consisted of a 12-week induction period (baseline to week 12) and a 40-week maintenance period (weeks 12–52).

TABLE 12.1
Psoriasis Area Severity Index-75, -90, -100, Investigator Global Assessment 0/1 response rates at week 12 in 4 phase III clinical trials on secukinumab

	ERASURE (n = 738)			FIXTURE (n = 1306)			
	300 mg Secukinumab (%) (n = 245)	**150 mg Secukinumab (%) (n = 244)**	**Placebo (%) (n = 246)**	**300 mg Secukinumab (%) (n = 323)**	**150 mg Secukinumab (%) (n = 327)**	**Etanercept (%) (n = 323)**	**Placebo (%) (n = 324)**
IGA 0/1	65.3[a]	51.2[a]	2.4	62.5[a,b]	51.1[a,b]	27.2	2.8
PASI-75	81.6[a]	71.6[a]	4.5	77.1[a,b]	67.0[a,b]	44	4.9
PASI-90	59.2[a]	39.1[a]	1.2	54.2[a,b]	41.9[a,b]	20.7	1.5
PASI-100	28.6[a]	12.8[a]	0.8	24.1[b]	14.4[b]	4.3	0
	FEATURE			**JUNCTURE**			
	300 mg Secukinumab (%) (n = 59)	**150 mg Secukinumab (%) (n = 59)**	**Placebo (%) (n = 59)**	**300 mg Secukinumab (%) (n = 60)**	**150 mg Secukinumab (%) (n = 61)**	**Placebo (%) (n = 61)**	
IGA 0/1	69.0[a]	52.5[a]	0	73.3[a]	53.3[a]	0	
PASI-75	75.9[a]	69.5[a]	0	86.7[a]	71.7[a]	3.3	
PASI-90	60.3[a]	45.8[a]	0	55.0[a]	40.0[a]	0	
PASI-100	43.1[a]	8.5	0	26.7	16.7	0	

[a] *P*<.001 for the comparison with placebo.
[b] *P*<.001 for the comparison with etanercept.

In the ERASURE study, 81.6% and 71.6% of subjects, respectively, achieved a PASI-75 response, and 65.3% and 51.2%, respectively, achieved an IGA 0/1 response, at week 12. These values were significantly higher in comparison to placebo; 4.5% and 2.4% of the placebo group achieved a respective PASI-75 or IGA 0/1 response at week 12 (*P*<.001 for each comparison of secukinumab vs placebo) (see Table 12.1).[6]

In the FIXTURE study, 77.1% and 67.0% of subjects, respectively, achieved a PASI-75 response, and 65.3% and 51.2%, respectively, achieved an IGA 0/1 response, at week 12. These values were significantly higher in comparison to etanercept and to placebo; 44.0% and 27.2% of the etanercept group and 4.9% and 2.8% of the placebo group achieved a respective PASI-75 and IGA 0/1 response at week 12 (*P*<.001 for each comparison of secukinumab vs etanercept and secukinumab vs placebo) (see Table 12.1).[6]

In both trials, continued treatment through week 52 was associated with sustained high response rates (PASI-75 response in 81%–84% for 300 mg, and 72%–82% for 150 mg at week 52) in most patients (Table 12.2).[6]

FEATURE AND JUNCTURE

The FEATURE and JUNCTURE studies evaluated the safety, tolerability, and usability of administering secukinumab with a PFS or an autoinjector pen, respectively, and have also demonstrated the superior efficacy of secukinumab to placebo at week 12.[7,8] The FEATURE and JUNCTURE studies enrolled 177 and 182 patients, respectively. Patients in each trial were randomized into the secukinumab 150 mg, secukinumab 300 mg, or placebo arm and received their respective doses at weeks 0, 1, 2, 3, and 4 followed by a dose every 4 weeks.

In FEATURE, treatment with secukinumab 300 and 150 mg via the PFS resulted in 75.9% and 69.5% of subjects, respectively, achieving a PASI-75 response, and 69.0% and 52.5%, respectively, achieving an IGA 0/1 response, at week 12. These values were significantly higher in comparison to placebo; 0% of the placebo group achieved a PASI-75 or IGA 0/1 response at week 12 (*P*<.001 for each comparison of secukinumab vs placebo). Usability of PFS was demonstrated by most subjects successfully following the steps in the instructions for use for self-injection via the PFS and the absence of critical hazard incidents. In addition, acceptability of the PFS was evaluated at baseline and at week 12 by Self-Injection Assessment Questionnaire domains, which included feelings about injections, self-confidence, and satisfaction with self-injection. Scores for all 3 domains remained high from baseline to week 12 in all groups, indicating that self-injections with PFS was acceptable to subjects before the first injection and remained highly acceptable up to week 12.

In JUNCTURE, treatment with secukinumab 300 and 150 mg via the autoinjector pen resulted in 86.7% and 71.7% of subjects, respectively, achieving a PASI-75 response, and 73.3% and 53.3%, respectively, achieving an IGA 0/1 response, at week 12. These values were significantly higher in comparison to placebo; 3.3% and 0% of the placebo group achieved a PASI-75 or IGA 0/1 response at week 12, respectively (*P*<.001 for each comparison of secukinumab vs placebo). Usability was evaluated in a similar fashion to the FEATURE trial and demonstrated high subject-reported injection tolerability, ease of use, absence of critical use-related hazards, and acceptability that was high at baseline and remained high up to week 12.

In all 4 studies, coprimary endpoints (PASI-75 response and IGA 0/1 response at week 12) and key secondary endpoints (ie, PASI-90 response at week 12) were met by both dosage arms of secukinumab with significantly higher proportions of patients compared with the placebo or etanercept (FIXTURE only) arm (Fig. 12.2). Efficacy is dose dependent as evidenced by consistently better responses across all efficacy end points with the 300-mg versus the 150-mg regimen in each of the 4 trials. Onset of efficacy was observed early during the course of therapy; a 50% reduction in mean PASI from baseline was achieved by week 3 in the 300-mg group and by week 4 in the 150-mg group across all 4 trials.[6–8] With regards to a maintenance regimen of secukinumab, recent evidence (SCULPTURE study) indicates that regular 4-week interval dosing is more efficacious than a re-treatment-as-needed regimen in maintaining long-term psoriasis control.[2]

In comparison to other biologic agents, FIXTURE demonstrated the superior efficacy of both doses of secukinumab over etanercept. The secukinumab 300-mg and 150-mg regimen arms achieved a respective 33% and 23% higher PASI-75 response rate compared with the etanercept arm at week 12 as well as a respective 12% and 10% higher PASI-75 response rate at week 52 (Fig. 12.3).[6] The CLEAR trial, a prospective double-blind study, showed that secukinumab (79.0%) was superior to ustekinumab (57.6%) in achieving PASI-90 at week 16 for moderate-to-severe plaque psoriasis (*P*<.0001).[14] As a secondary endpoint, PASI-100 response at week 16 was significantly greater with secukinumab (44.3%)

TABLE 12.2
Psoriasis Area Severity Index-75 and Investigator Global Assessment 0/1 response rates from week 12 to week 52 in ERASURE and FIXTURE trials

	ERASURE			FIXTURE			
	300 mg Secukinumab (%) (n = 245)	**150 mg Secukinumab (%) (n = 244)**	**Placebo**	**300 mg Secukinumab (%) (n = 323)**	**150 mg Secukinumab (%) (n = 327)**	**Etanercept (%) (n = 323)**	**Placebo**
IGA 0/1 from wk 12 to wk 52	74.4	59.2	NE	79.7	67.7	56.8	NE
PASI-75 from wk 12 to wk 52	80.5	72.4	NE	84.3	82.2	72.5	NE

Abbreviation: NE, not evaluated.

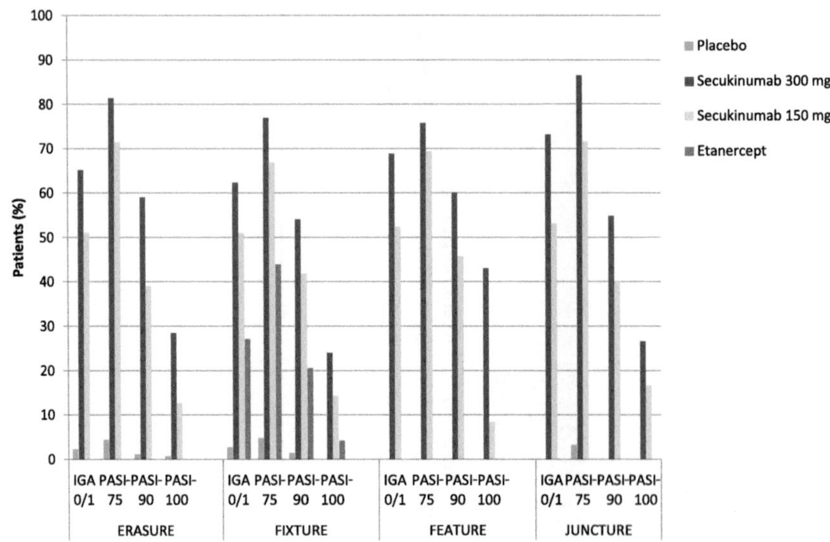

Fig. 12.2 PASI-75, PASI-90, PASI-100, IGA 0/1 response rates at week 12 in 4 phase III clinical trials on secukinumab.

than ustekinumab (28.4%) (*P*<.0001) (Fig. 12.4).[14] Secukinumab is the only biologic agent to show greater efficacy than an IL-12/23 inhibitor and TNF inhibitor for the treatment of moderate-to-severe plaque psoriasis. These results are crucial to consider clinically because they provide head-to-head comparisons that may guide the choice of appropriate treatment.

Secukinumab was FDA approved for psoriatic arthritis (PsA) in January 2016. In FUTURE 2, a randomized double-blind phase 3 trial, subcutaneous secukinumab 300 mg and 150 mg were found to significantly improve signs and symptoms of PsA versus placebo.[11] Patients with PsA were randomized to receive secukinumab 300 mg (n = 100), 150 mg (n = 100), 75 mg (n = 99), or placebo (n = 98). Secukinumab or placebo was given at weeks 0, 1, 2, 3, and 4, and then every 4 weeks thereafter. American College of Rheumatology 20 response rates at week 24 were 54%, 51%, 29%, and 15% of patients assigned to secukinumab 300 mg (*P*<.0001),

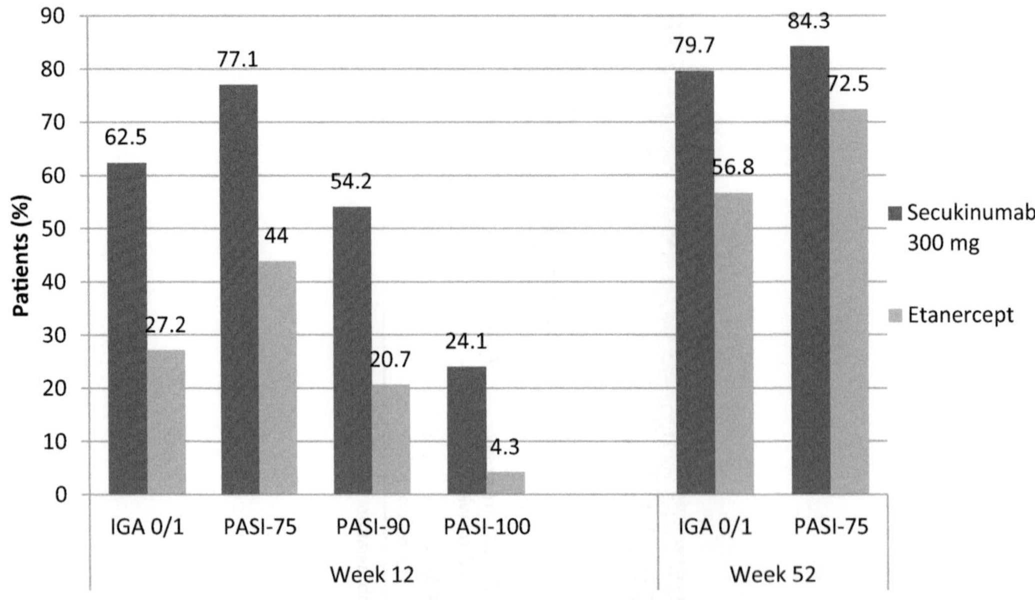

Fig. 12.3 FIXTURE trial: efficacy end points comparing secukinumab and etanercept.

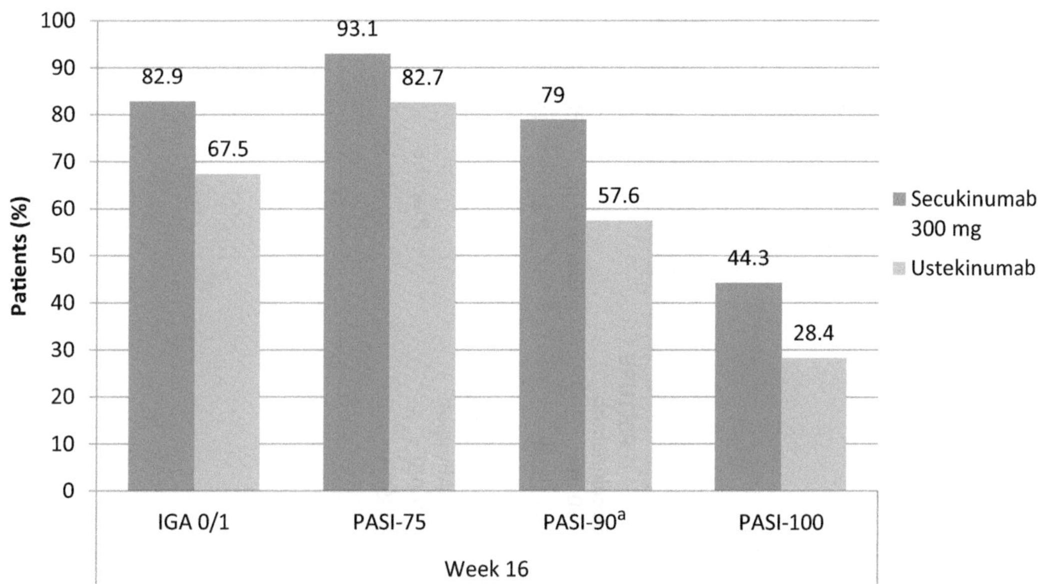

Fig. 12.4 CLEAR trial: efficacy end points comparing secukinumab and ustekinumab. [a] Primary endpoint.

150 mg (*P*<.0001), 75 mg (*P* = .0399), and placebo arms, respectively.

For patients with PsA and concomitant moderate-to-severe plaque psoriasis, dosing and administration should follow the schedule for plaque psoriasis outlined above. The recommended dose for PsA is a 150-mg subcutaneous injection at weeks 0, 1, 2, 3, and 4 followed by 150 mg every 4 weeks thereafter. Dosage at 300 mg can be considered if there is no improvement.[2]

SAFETY

All 4 phase III clinical trials (ERASURE, FIXTURE, JUNCTURE, and FEATURE) evaluated the safety of secukinumab in comparison to placebo up to 12 weeks after treatment initiation (Tables 12.3 and 12.4).[6–8] Although it was not stated to be significant, secukinumab at both doses had a higher rate of at least 1 adverse event (AE) than placebo, which was driven by mainly nonserious upper respiratory tract infections. Some of the most common AE reported over the 12-week induction period across all 4 trials were nasopharyngitis, diarrhea, and upper respiratory tract infection.[2,6–8]

In regards to serious adverse events (SAEs), secukinumab had slightly, but not significantly, higher proportions compared with placebo in the ERASURE and FIXTURE trials over the induction period. However, this difference was only observed in the first 12 weeks and did not translate into a higher risk over the 52-week treatment course. The safety of secukinumab is evidenced by comparable exposure-adjusted incidence rates of SAEs across all secukinumab dosing groups and placebo over 52 weeks (Table 12.5).[6] Notably, secukinumab demonstrates comparable safety to etanercept over 52 weeks of treatment.

Preclinical data suggest that IL-17 is important in the mucosal defense against *Candida*, thus making infection with this fungus a possible side effect to secukinumab use. Indeed, *Candida* infections were found to be more common, although without mention of statistical significance, with secukinumab than with etanercept during the 52-week treatment period. In the 300-mg and 150-mg secukinumab groups, 4.7% and 2.3% reported mild-to-moderate *Candida* infection, respectively, whereas 1.2% of the etanercept group reported mild-to-severe infection.[6] Notably, there were no cases of chronic or systemic candidiasis; all cases were responsive to standard treatment and did not lead to treatment discontinuation.

Neutropenia was also noted in clinical trials, although most cases were transient and reversible and showed no indication of dose-related effects. Rates of serious infection, malignancy, unspecified tumors, and major adverse cardiovascular events, and discontinuations due to AE were all very low. During the entire 52-week period, ERASURE reported 1 subject (0.3 events per 100 patient-years) and 5 subjects (1.7 events per 100 patient-years) who developed benign or malignant neoplasms in the 300-mg and 150-mg secukinumab groups, respectively, compared with 1 subject (1.5 events per 100 patient-years) in the placebo group. FIXTURE reported only 1 subject

TABLE 12.3
Summary of adverse events reported through week 12 in 4 clinical trials

	ERASURE			FIXTURE			
	Secukinumab 300 mg	**Secukinumab 150 mg**	**Placebo**	**Secukinumab 300 mg**	**Secukinumab 150 mg**	**Etanercept**	**Placebo**
Subjects with any AE, n (%)	135 (55.1)	148 (60.4)	116 (47)	181 (55.5)	191 (58.4)	186 (57.6)	163 (49.8)
	JUNCTURE			**FEATURE**			
	Secukinumab 300 mg	**Secukinumab 150 mg**	**Placebo**	**Secukinumab 300 mg**	**Secukinumab 150 mg**	**Placebo**	
Subjects with any AE, n (%)	42 (70.0)	39 (63.9)	33 (54.1)	30 (50.8)	34 (57.6)	28 (47.5)	

TABLE 12.4
Summary of adverse reactions reported through week 12 in ERASURE, FIXTURE, FEATURE, and JUNCTURE trials

Adverse Reaction	Secukinumab 300 mg (N = 691) n (%)	Secukinumab 150 mg (N = 692) n (%)	Placebo (N = 694) n (%)
Nasopharyngitis[a]	79 (11.4)	85 (12.3)	60 (8.6)
Headache	45 (6.5)	38 (5.5)	63 (9.1)
Diarrhea[a]	28 (4.1)	18 (2.3)	10 (1.4)
Pruritus[b]	22 (3.2)	21 (3.0)	18 (2.6)
Upper respiratory tract infection[a]	17 (2.5)	22 (3.2)	5 (0.7)
Rhinitis[a]	10 (1.4)	10 (1.4)	5 (0.7)
Oral herpes[a]	9 (1.3)	1 (0.1)	2 (0.3)
Pharyngitis[a]	8 (1.2)	7 (1.0)	0 (0)
Urticaria[a]	4 (0.6)	8 (1.2)	1 (0.1)
Rhinorrhea[a]	8 (1.2)	2 (0.3)	1 (0.1)

[a] Occurred at a rate higher in secukinumab group than placebo.
[b] Data from FEATURE trial missing.

(0.2 events per 100 patient-years) in the 300-mg secukinumab group who developed a benign or malignant neoplasm in the 52-week period. No serious opportunistic infections while on secukinumab or secukinumab-related deaths have been reported.

All therapeutic protein products pose a risk of immunogenicity. Treatment-emergent antisecukinumab antibodies while using secukinumab were detected in a total of 6 subjects across all 4 clinical trials. Although 1 patient's antibodies were classified as neutralizing, none of antibodies were associated with AE or loss of efficacy (defined as an increase in PASI score by 6 points from the minimum PASI score achieved on treatment).[6–8]

PRECAUTIONS

Infections

Caution should be exercised when considering secukinumab in patients with chronic infection or history of recurrent infection. Although infections occurred at higher rates with secukinumab compared with placebo in the induction period of clinical trials, they were largely attributed to common infections: nasopharyngitis (11.4% vs 8.6%), upper respiratory tract infections (2.5% vs 0.7%), and mucocutaneous infections with *Candida* (1.2% vs 0.3%).[2] Of note, the studies did not mention statistical significance of any of these values. In the ERASURE/FIXTURE trials, serious infections in long-term treatment were not consistently shown to be more common in secukinumab than placebo.[12] Patients should seek medical advice if signs and symptoms of infection occur. In the event of serious infection, discontinue secukinumab and closely monitor patients until infection resolves.

Tuberculosis

As is the case with all immunosuppressant agents in the treatment of plaque psoriasis, secukinumab is contraindicated in patients with active TB. All patients should be evaluated for TB before treatment. Patients with latent TB and a history of latent or active TB in whom adequacy of treatment

TABLE 12.5
Rates of nonfatal serious adverse events during 52-week treatment period in ERASURE/FIXTURE trials

	Treatment Arm			
Trial	Secukinumab 300 mg (Incidence Rate per 100 Subject-Years)	Secukinumab 150 mg (Incidence Rate per 100 Subject-Years)	Etanercept (Incidence Rate per 100 Subject-Years)	Placebo (Incidence Rate per 100 Subject-Years)
ERASURE	6.3	6.4	—	7.4
FIXTURE	6.8	6.0	7.0	8.3

cannot be confirmed should initiate appropriate anti-TB therapy before initiation of secukinumab. Although observational and focused studies are needed to further evaluate the full range of side effects of secukinumab, there are currently no reports of reactivated latent TB in any psoriasis trial.

Crohn Disease

Although currently not an absolute contraindication, caution must be taken with patients with a history of Crohn disease and initiating secukinumab therapy as studies have suggested potential worsening of the disease. A phase II study showed that blockade of IL-17A in Crohn patients was not only ineffective for disease treatment but also exacerbated disease for some patients.[13] In this study, 39 patients with Crohn disease were treated with secukinumab, of which at least 4 were suspected to have drug-related worsening of Crohn disease.[13] In the FIXTURE study, 1 patient developed a new diagnosis of Crohn disease while on the 150-mg secukinumab regimen.[12] Patients who receive secukinumab and have active Crohn disease should be monitored closely.

Hypersensitivity Reactions

Secukinumab-associated anaphylaxis and urticarial reactions have been reported in clinical trials.[2] If serious hypersensitivity reactions ensue, the drug should be discontinued immediately and appropriate therapy initiated. The removable cap of the Sensoready Pen and the Cosentyx PFS contain latex and, therefore, should not be handled by latex-allergic patients.

Pregnancy

Secukinumab is pregnancy category B and should only be used if the potential benefit to the mother outweighs the potential risk to the fetus. Excretion of secukinumab in human milk and the safety and effectiveness of secukinumab in the pediatric population have not been evaluated.[2]

MONITORING

To date, no formal guidelines have been set on safety monitoring in patients receiving secukinumab. The information presented is primarily based on psoriasis guidelines from the American Academy of Dermatology (AAD).[15]

A thorough history and physical examination should be taken before initiation of secukinumab therapy, including TB exposure, chronic/recurrent infections, malignancy, neurologic and cardiac history, and a thorough review of systems. Routine follow-up examinations should adequately monitor patients for side effects and AEs.[16]

Aside from baseline TB test, annual monitoring for TB, and a baseline hepatitis profile, routine laboratory testing beyond that for concomitant therapies or comorbidities is generally not supported.[17] The highest grade US Preventive Services Task Force evidence for screening studies is grade B for TB testing (interferon-γ release assay is preferred over tuberculin skin testing), and hepatitis B virus/hepatitis C virus (HBV/HCV) screening is supported only by grade C evidence.[18] The AAD recommends baseline purified protein derivative (PPD) skin test, liver function tests (LFTs), and complete blood count (CBC). For ongoing monitoring, the AAD recommends yearly PPD and periodic LFTs, CBC, history, and physical examinations (Table 12.6).[15]

The Centers for Disease Control and Prevention recommends TB testing before the therapy initiation as well.[19] Positive skin test findings should be followed with a chest radiograph—if negative, patients should be treated for latent TB (6–9 months of 300 mg isoniazid daily and/or 4 months of 600 mg daily rifampicin),[20] and if positive, patients should receive therapy for active TB. Biologic therapy may be started after 1 to 2 months of prophylactic treatment if the patient is adherent to and tolerating the prophylactic regimen.[9] If a patient has a positive PPD due to prior BCG vaccination, blood tests can be obtained measuring interferon production on stimulation with TB antigens that are not present in BCG. Most guidelines perform annual TB skin testing in patients receiving secukinumab to screen for the TB reactivation, especially in those at risk (ie, health care workers, travelers to endemic areas).

The authors of this section recommend initial baseline monitoring that includes a

TABLE 12.6
Monitoring recommendations from the American Academy of Dermatology

	Monitoring
History and physical	Baseline and routine
CBC	Baseline and periodically
LFTs	Baseline and periodically
TB skin test	Baseline and annually after
Hepatitis profile	Not specified

Data from Menter A, Gottlieb A, Feldman SR, et al. Guidelines of care for the management of psoriasis and psoriatic arthritis: section 1. Overview of psoriasis and guidelines of care for the treatment of psoriasis with biologics. J Am Acad Dermatol 2008;58(5):840.

QuantiFERON-TB Gold (QFT), LFTs, CBC, and HBV and HCV profile. QuantiFERON-TB Gold (QFT) should be repeated annually.

Patients specifically taking secukinumab should be monitored for signs and symptoms of inflammatory bowel disease. In addition, if the patient is receiving concomitant CYP456 substrates, particularly those with narrow therapeutic indices, monitoring for therapeutic effect or drug concentration of the CYP450 substrate can be considered.

VACCINATIONS

Because of the possibility that biologic agents may impair the body's immunologic response to vaccinations, administration of vaccinations should be carefully considered in patients receiving biologic therapy (Table 12.7).[16] Live vaccines (measles, mumps, and rubella [MMR], varicella, zoster, intranasal influenza, and so forth) are contraindicated within 1 month of treatment. However, scientifically based/standardized recommendations for administering

TABLE 12.7
Vaccination recommendations for biologic agents from the National Psoriasis Foundation

Vaccination	Before Therapy	During Therapy
Live vaccines (MMR, varicella, herpes zoster, intranasal influenza, oral typhoid, yellow fever, oral polio, smallpox, BCG, rotavirus)	Contraindicated within 1 mo	Contraindicated
Influenza	Vaccinate with inactivated or live	Yearly immunization with inactivated vaccine
Chicken pox	If negative serology, vaccinate	Contraindicated
Zoster	Before therapy: 1 dose for adults ≥50 y	Contraindicated
Human papilloma virus	Unvaccinated male/female patients up to age 26	Same
Hepatitis A	Vaccinate if high risk (diabetes, liver disease, intravenous drug users, homosexual men, and so forth)	Same; consider obtaining postvaccination serology
Hepatitis B	Serology, risk factor assessment. Offer vaccination if necessary	High-dose vaccine Consider obtaining serology postvaccination
Pneumococcal	Pneumococcal polysaccharide vaccine (PPSV23) vaccine recommended	Pneumococcal conjugate vaccine followed by PPSV23 if not given prior
Haemophilus influenzae type b	Vaccinate if unvaccinated	Same
MMR	Vaccinate if negative, or seronegative to any component	Contraindicated
Tetanus-diphtheria/diphtheria-tetanus-acellular pertussis (TD/TDAP)	Booster every 10 y and high-risk wounds Offer before therapy, substitute 1 dose with TDAP	Same
Meningococcal	Assess risk factors, vaccinate if high risk (asplenia, complement deficient, group living)	Same
Poliomyelitis	Assess risk factors, vaccinate if high risk (health care worker, laboratory worker)	Same

From Lebwohl M, Bagel J, Gelfand JM, et al. From the Medical Board of the National Psoriasis Foundation: monitoring and vaccinations in patients treated with biologics for psoriasis. J Am Acad Dermatol 2008;58(1):99; with permission.

biologically inactive or recombinant vaccines to patients on biologic agents are lacking. Non-live vaccinations may have the potential to achieve adequate immune response, although antibody titers may not achieve optimal levels and may decrease more rapidly if given during biologic therapy.

It is preferable to complete all age-appropriate immunizations according to current immunization guidelines before initiating biologic therapy. The production of antibodies from the vaccine generally occurs in the 2-week period from primary immunization, but could take more than 6 weeks to peak.

Specific to secukinumab, non-live vaccinations are allowable during the course of treatment but may not elicit an adequate immune response sufficient to prevent disease.[2] However, a study demonstrated that healthy subjects who were vaccinated with inactivated trivalent subunit influenza virus and conjugate group C meningococcal vaccine 2 weeks after a 150-mg secukinumab dose were able to achieve protective antibody levels (measured 1 month after vaccination) comparable to individuals who did not receive secukinumab before vaccination.[10]

SUMMARY AND RECOMMENDATIONS

Although secukinumab has been demonstrated to have superior efficacy to ustekinumab and etanercept, efficacy is not the only important facet to be considered when choosing an appropriate therapeutic agent. Other important considerations are length of drug survival, efficacy in PsA, and frequency of dosing schedule. Because of the lack of prospective and observational studies, it is difficult to evaluate the persistence of efficacy and the real-world utility of secukinumab. Secukinumab is FDA approved for the treatment of PsA, which offers an additional reason for its use. In addition, patient compliance may interfere with medication adherence, because secukinumab is dosed more frequently (2 shots every 4 weeks) than other medications with similar efficacy (ie, ustekinumab, 1 shot dosed every 12 weeks).

Overall, emerging evidence of the efficacy of secukinumab in the treatment of psoriasis and its relatively good safety profile make secukinumab a welcomed new therapeutic agent. With any novel agent, prospective registry data, data from after-marketing surveillance, and accumulation of related literature will be needed to ascertain the safety and long-term efficacy of secukinumab.

REFERENCES

1. Ellis CN, Gorsulowsky DC, Hamilton TA, et al. Cyclosporine improves psoriasis in a double-blind study. JAMA 1986;256(22):3110–6.
2. Cosentyx [package insert]. East Hanover (NJ): Novartis Pharmaceuticals Corporation; 2016. Available at: http://www.pharma.us.novartis.com/product/pi/pdf/cosentyx.pdf. Accessed February 21, 2016.
3. Miossec P, Kolls JK. Targeting IL-17 and TH17 cells in chronic inflammation. Nat Rev Drug Discov 2012;11(10):763–76.
4. Kirkham BW, Kavanaugh A, Reich K. Interleukin-17A: a unique pathway in immune-mediated diseases: psoriasis, psoriatic arthritis and rheumatoid arthritis. Immunology 2014;141(2):133–42.
5. Martin DA, Towne JE, Kricorian G, et al. The emerging role of IL-17 in the pathogenesis of psoriasis: preclinical and clinical findings. J Invest Dermatol 2013;133(1):17–26.
6. Langley RG, Elewski BE, Lebwohl M, et al. Secukinumab in plaque psoriasis–results of two phase 3 trials. N Engl J Med 2014;371(4):326–38.
7. Paul C, Lacour JP, Tedremets L, et al. Efficacy, safety and usability of secukinumab administration by autoinjector/pen in psoriasis: a randomized, controlled trial (JUNCTURE). J Eur Acad Dermatol Venereol 2015;29(6):1082–90.
8. Blauvelt A, Prinz JC, Gottlieb AB, et al. Secukinumab administration by pre-filled syringe: efficacy, safety and usability results from a randomized controlled trial in psoriasis (FEATURE). Br J Dermatol 2015;172(2):484–93.
9. Doherty SD, Van Voorhees A, Lebwohl MG, et al. National Psoriasis Foundation consensus statement on screening for latent tuberculosis infection in patients with psoriasis treated with systemic and biologic agents. J Am Acad Dermatol 2008;59(2):209–17.
10. Chioato A, Noseda E, Stevens M, et al. Treatment with the interleukin-17A-blocking antibody secukinumab does not interfere with the efficacy of influenza and meningococcal vaccinations in healthy subjects: results of an open-label, parallel-group, randomized single-center study. Clin Vaccine Immunol 2012;19(10):1597–602.
11. McInnes IB, Mease PJ, Kirkham B, et al. Secukinumab, a human anti-interleukin-17A monoclonal antibody, in patients with psoriatic arthritis (FUTURE 2): a randomised, double-blind, placebo-controlled, phase 3 trial. Lancet 2015;386(9999):1137–46.
12. Langley RG, Elewski BE, Lebwohl M, et al. Supplementary appendix to secukinumab in plaque psoriasis—results of two phase three trials. N Engl J Med 2014;371(4):326–38.

13. Hueber W, Sands BE, Lewitzky S, et al. Secukinumab, a human anti-IL-17A monoclonal antibody, for moderate to severe Crohn's disease: unexpected results of a randomised, double-blind placebo-controlled trial. Gut 2012;61(12):1693–700.
14. Thaci D, Blauvelt A, Reich K, et al. Secukinumab is superior to ustekinumab in clearing skin of subjects with moderate to severe plaque psoriasis: CLEAR, a randomized controlled trial. J Am Acad Dermatol 2015;73(3):400–9.
15. Menter A, Gottlieb A, Feldman SR, et al. Guidelines of care for the management of psoriasis and psoriatic arthritis: section 1. Overview of psoriasis and guidelines of care for the treatment of psoriasis with biologics. J Am Acad Dermatol 2008;58(5):826–50.
16. Lebwohl M, Bagel J, Gelfand JM, et al. From the Medical Board of the National Psoriasis Foundation: monitoring and vaccinations in patients treated with biologics for psoriasis. J Am Acad Dermatol 2008;58(1):94–105.
17. van Lumig PP, Driessen RJ, Roelofs-Thijssen MA, et al. Relevance of laboratory investigations in monitoring patients with psoriasis on etanercept or adalimumab. Br J Dermatol 2011;165(2):375–82.
18. Ahn CS, Dothard EH, Garner ML, et al. To test or not to test? An updated evidence-based assessment of the value of screening and monitoring tests when using systemic biologic agents to treat psoriasis and psoriatic arthritis. J Am Acad Dermatol 2015;73(3):420–8.e1.
19. CDC - Tuberculosis (TB) [Internet]. Available at: http://www.cdc.gov/tb/?404;http://www.cdc.gov:80/tb/pubs/LTBI/pdf/TargetedLTBI05.pdf. Accessed February 1, 2016.
20. Targeted tuberculin testing and treatment of latent tuberculosis infection. American Thoracic Society. MMWR Recomm Rep 2000;49(RR-6):1–51.

CHAPTER 13

Ixekizumab

Shivani P. Reddy, BS, Vidhi V. Shah, BA, Jashin J. Wu, MD

KEYWORDS

• Ixekizumab • Taltz • Interleukin-17A • Monoclonal antibody • UNCOVER-2 • UNCOVER-3

KEY POINTS

- Ixekizumab is a humanized monoclonal antibody against interleukin-17A.
- Ixekizumab is more efficacious in the treatment of plaque psoriasis in comparison to etanercept and placebo.
- Ixekizumab has led to higher clinical response rates and skin clearance rates in clinical trials than any other agent currently approved by the US Food and Drug Administration for the treatment of psoriasis.
- The most common side effects attributable to ixekizumab are injection-site reactions, upper respiratory tract infections, nausea, and tinea infections.

INTRODUCTION

Ixekizumab, a biologic marketed under the brand name Taltz, was approved in March 2016 for the treatment of moderate-to-severe plaque psoriasis by the US Food and Drug Administration (FDA). Another drug that targets a specific cytokine to reducing inflammation and skin lesions, ixekizumab is 1 of 3 biologic agents, including secukinumab and brodalumab, that targets the interleukin-17 (IL-17) pathway in the pathogenesis of psoriasis.[1]

Ixekizumab currently does not have any other FDA-approved indications other than plaque psoriasis (although it is also effective for psoriatic arthritis).[1,2] The current recommended dosing of ixekizumab is subcutaneous injection of 160 mg at baseline, followed by 80 mg every other week (EOW) until week 12, followed by 80 mg every 4 weeks for maintenance dosing (Fig. 13.1).[1] In comparison to secukinumab and brodalumab, the dosing regimen for ixekizumab is more favorable because there are fewer injections required overall in the loading and maintenance phases (secukinumab requires 10 injections in the loading phase, and brodalumab requires EOW injections in the maintenance phase).[3]

MECHANISM OF ACTION

Ixekinumab is a humanized monoclonal immunoglobulin G4 (IgG4) antibody that targets the IL-17 pathway in the pathogenesis of psoriasis. IL-17 is produced by Th17 cells and functions in the activation/recruitment of neutrophils, blockade of neutrophil apoptosis, release of inflammatory cytokines, and stimulation of psoriasis angiogenesis.[4–7] Th17 cells and IL-17 messenger RNA are increased in psoriasis lesions, and Th17 cells are increased in the blood of psoriasis patients.[8,9] Of the 6 isoforms of IL-17, ixekizumab specifically binds to and inhibits IL-17A, the most potent isoform involved in psoriasis.[10,11]

IL-17A dimerizes with itself to form a homodimer or with IL-17F to form a heterodimer, rendering it functionally active.[12,13] T cells, natural killer cells, mast cells, and neutrophils all produce IL-17A and IL-17F; however, Th17 cells characteristically produce IL-17A.[13] These homodimers and heterodimers bind to and activate the IL-17 cell surface receptors IL-17RA and IL-17RC, triggering the inflammatory cascade that leads to psoriasis lesions.[13]

Other IL-17 blocking agents include secukinumab and brodalumab. Similarly to ixekizumab, secukinumab (IgG1 mAb) targets IL-17A, whereas broadalumab (IgG2 monoclonal antibody [mAb]) is specifically directed against the IL-17 receptor IL-17RA. However, as opposed to secukinumab and broadalumab, which are fully human mAbs, ixekinumab is a humanized mAb. Fully human antibodies are thought to have less immunogenicity, which could in turn imply less risk for loss

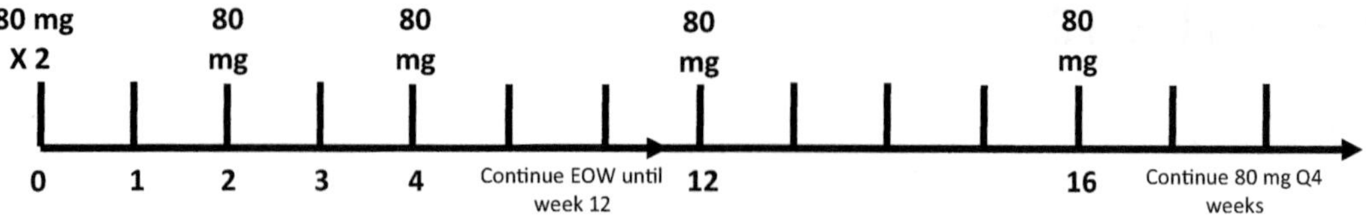

Fig. 13.1 Ixekizumab dosing schedule. Recommended dosing for ixekizumab is a loading dose of 160 mg (two 80-mg injections) at week 0, followed by 80 mg EOW until week 12, followed by 80 mg every 4 weeks thereafter. Available methods of subcutaneous injections include an autoinjector or a prefilled syringe, each containing 1 mL of 80 mg ixekizumab. Self-injection is permitted so long as the dermatologist has carefully explained and evaluated the patient's ability to do so. Patients tend to prefer the pen over the syringe, because it is less painful, more convenient, faster, and safer. Before injection, the solution should be inspected visually for particulate matter and/or discoloration. The medication should be clear and colorless to slightly yellow, and if any variation is present, the solution should be discarded. (*Data from* Eli Lilly and Company, Indianapolis (IN): 2016. Available at: http://pi.lilly.com/us/taltz-uspi.pdf.)

of efficacy, although high-titer antibodies that affect ixekizumab efficacy are uncommon (occurring in only about 2% of treated patients).[14,15]

EFFICACY

Ixekizumab is highly effective in clinical trials, with higher response and clearance rates than other FDA-approved psoriasis treatment agents.[12,16]

Phase 2 Trial and Open-Label Extension Study

A phase 2 double-blinded, multicenter, randomized, dose-ranging study was performed in 142 adults (18 years or greater) with moderate-to-severe plaque psoriasis for at least 6 months. Subjects were required to have a Psoriasis Area Severity Index (PASI) score of at least 12, Physician Global Assessment (PGA) score of at least 3, and a minimum of 10% body surface area (BSA) affected with psoriasis.[17] Patients were randomized to receive subcutaneous injections of placebo or 10 mg, 25 mg, 75 mg, or 150 mg of ixekizumab at weeks 0, 2, 4, 8, 12, and 16. The primary outcome was the proportion of patients achieving 75% improvement in PASI score (PASI-75) at 12 weeks. Secondary assessments included achievement of PASI-90, PASI-100, PGA score, joint-pain visual analogue scale (VAS) to assess psoriatic arthritis joint pain, Nail Psoriasis Severity Index (NAPSI), the Psoriasis Scalp Severity Index (PSSI), an itch VAS, and Dermatology Life Quality Index (DLQI).

By week 12, PASI-75 and PASI-90 were achieved by more patients in the 25-mg, 75-mg, and 150-mg ixekizumab groups, and PASI-100 by more patients in the 75-mg and 150-mg groups (P<.001 for each PASI level and group vs placebo). Statistically significant differences in outcome were seen as early as week 1 in the 75-mg and 100-mg groups, and with more patients achieving PASI-75 as early as week 2 in the 150-mg group as compared with placebo (Table 13.1).

By week 12, there was more improvement in PSSI score in the 25-mg, 75-mg, and 150-mg groups versus placebo. Greater reduction in NAPSI score occurred as early as week 2 versus placebo in the 75-mg group, and greater reduction in joint-pain VAS occurred by week 12 in the 150-mg group. DLQI score and itch severity improved with ixekizumab treatment as well (see Table 13.1).

A 52-week, open-label extension (OLE) study of this trial enrolled patients from the original trial who achieved less than PASI-75 improvement from baseline (Table 13.2).[18] Patients with PASI-75 or greater entered a treatment-free period (weeks 20–32) and were entered into the OLE after falling to less than PASI-75, or at week 32 if PASI-75 was maintained throughout the treatment-free period.[16] The 120 patients who enrolled were scheduled to receive 120 mg of ixekizumab every 4 weeks; 103 patients completed this OLE study until the end. By week 52, 77% of patients achieved PASI-75, 68% PASI-90 response, and 48% PASI-100. Patients who responded to treatment in the original trial continued to maintain high levels of response at week 52 (PASI-75 maintained in 95% of original PASI-75 responders, PASI-90 maintained in 94% of original PASI-90 responders, and PASI-100 maintained in 82% of PASI-100 responders). Response rates were unaffected by dosing group from the original trial.

UNCOVER-2 and UNCOVER-3 Phase 3 Trials

UNCOVER-2 and UNCOVER-3 were both 12-week, prospective, double-blinded, multicenter phase 3 trials in patients age 18 years or

TABLE 13.1
Primary and secondary efficacy endpoint data after 12 weeks of study (Dermatology Life Quality Index score after 8 weeks)

	Placebo	Ixekizumab 10 mg	Ixekizumab 25 mg	Ixekizumab 75 mg	Ixekizumab 100 mg
PASI-75 (% of patients)	8	29	77	83	82
PASI-90 (% of patients)	0	18	50	59	71
PASI-100 (% of patients)	0	0	17	38	39
NAPSI % change (from baseline ± what?)	6.8 ± 41.1	14.3 ± 97.8	−24.0 ± 32.8	−57.1 ± 36.7	−49.3 ± 35.9
PSSI % change (from baseline)	6.8 ± 41.1	−43.4 ± 62.8	−87.1 ± 23.6	−94.8 ± 14.5	−84.8 ± 41.5
Joint-pain VAS score change (from baseline)	4.8 ± 48.2	−5.9 ± 47.6	−17.0 ± 28.1	−18.6 ± 13.4	−39.0 ± 27.5
DLQI score change (at 8 wk)	−2.4 ± 4.4	Not provided	−7.1 ± 6.5	−8.5 ± 5.1	−7.8 ± 5.7

Data from Leonardi C, Matheson R, Zachariae C, et al. Antiinterleukin-17 monoclonal antibody ixekizumab in chronic plaque psoriasis. N Engl J Med 2012;366(13):1190–9.

greater, designed to assess whether ixekizumab every 2 weeks or every 4 weeks was superior to placebo and noninferior or superior to etanercept.[16] Trial patients were required to have a diagnosis of moderate-to-severe plaque psoriasis (defined as >10% BSA, PGA score of 3 or greater, PASI score of 12 or more) for at least 6 months. A total of 1224 patients in UNCOVER-2 and 1346 patients in UNCOVER-3 were randomized in a 2:2:2:1 ratio to receive 1 of 2 dosing schedules of ixekizumab, etanercept, or placebo. These dosing schedules consisted of a 160-mg loading dose of ixekizumab followed by 80 mg every 2 weeks or every 4 weeks, etanercept 50 mg twice weekly, or placebo injections. Primary endpoints of this study were achievement of PASI-75 or greater and static physician global assessment (sPGA) scores of clear or minimal with at least a 2-point reduction from baseline at the start of the 12 weeks. Secondary assessments included sPGA, PASI-90, PASI-100, itch numeric rating scale (NRS), and DLQI.

Both dosing regimens of ixekizumab had greater efficacy than placebo and etanercept at week 12 ($P<.0001$). In addition, greater numbers of ixekizumab-treated patients achieved PASI-75 as early as week 1 as compared with etanercept (UNCOVER-2: $P<.0001$ for 4-week group, $P = .22$ for 2-week group; UNCOVER-3: $P = .35$ for 4-week group, $P = .0003$ for 2-week group). In UNCOVER-2 and UNCOVER-3, complete clearing occurred in 41% and 38% of patients given ixekizumab every 2 weeks, 31% and 35% given ixekizumab every 4 weeks, 0.6% and 0% of patients given placebo, and 5% and 28% of patients given etanercept, respectively. Greater DLQI improvement in patients receiving ixekizumab was observed as soon as week 2 and in greater proportions thereafter compared with placebo and etanercept ($P<.0001$). Greater improvement in itch NRS scores occurred with ixekizumab versus placebo and etanercept ($P<.0001$ for each ixekizumab dose vs placebo or etanercept) (Fig. 13.2, Table 13.3).

Overall, these studies demonstrated that ixekizumab has greater efficacy in the treatment of moderate-to-severe psoriasis than placebo and etanercept. PASI-75 was achieved by 90% of patients by week 12 in patients receiving ixekizumab every 2 weeks, with rapid onset of efficacy.

Efficacy in Other Forms of Psoriasis

A Japanese open-label study of ixekizumab investigated efficacy in erythrodermic psoriasis (EP) and generalized pustular psoriasis (GPP) in addition to moderate-to-severe plaque psoriasis.[19] A total of 78 plaque psoriasis, 8 EP, and 5 GPP patients received standard loading and maintenance doses of ixekizumab. By week 12, PASI-75 and PASI-90 were achieved by 98.7% (77/88) and 83.3% (65/78) of plaque psoriasis patients, 100% (8/8) and 62.5% (5/8) of EP patients, and 80% (4/5) and 60% (3/5) of GPP patients, respectively. Overall, these results emphasize the potential of ixekizumab to treat less common forms of psoriasis.

TABLE 13.2
Safety data from phase 2 trial and open-label extension study

	Placebo (n = 27)	**Ixekizumab 10 mg (n = 28)**	**Ixekizumab 25 mg (n = 30)**	**Ixekizumab 75 mg (n = 29)**	**Ixekizumab 150 mg (n = 28)**	**OLE Study (n = 120)**
Serious AEs	0	0	0	0	0	8.3% (10)
Serious infection	—	—	—	—	—	1.7% (2)
Cardiovascular	—	—	—	—	—	2.5% (3)
Malignancy (rectal cancer)	—	—	—	—	—	0.8% (1)
Hidradenitis suppurativa	—	—	—	—	—	0.8% (1)
AEs	63% (17)	75% (21)	70% (21)	59% (17)	46% (13)	66.7% (80)
Nasopharyngitis	19% (5)	11% (3)	10% (3)	10% (3)	14% (4)	10% (12)
Upper respiratory infection (URI)	4% (1)	4% (1)	10% (3)	3% (1)	4% (1)	7.5% (9)
Sinusitis	—	—	—	—	—	4.2% (5)
Diarrhea	—	—	—	—	—	4.2% (5)
Basal cell carcinoma	—	—	—	—	—	0.8% (1)
Allergy/hypersensitivity	7% (2)	4% (1)	3% (1)	7% (2)	4% (1)	—
Injection-site reaction	0	0	10% (3)	3% (1)	7% (2)	—
Headache	4% (1)	14% (4)	13% (4)	3% (1)	4% (1)	—

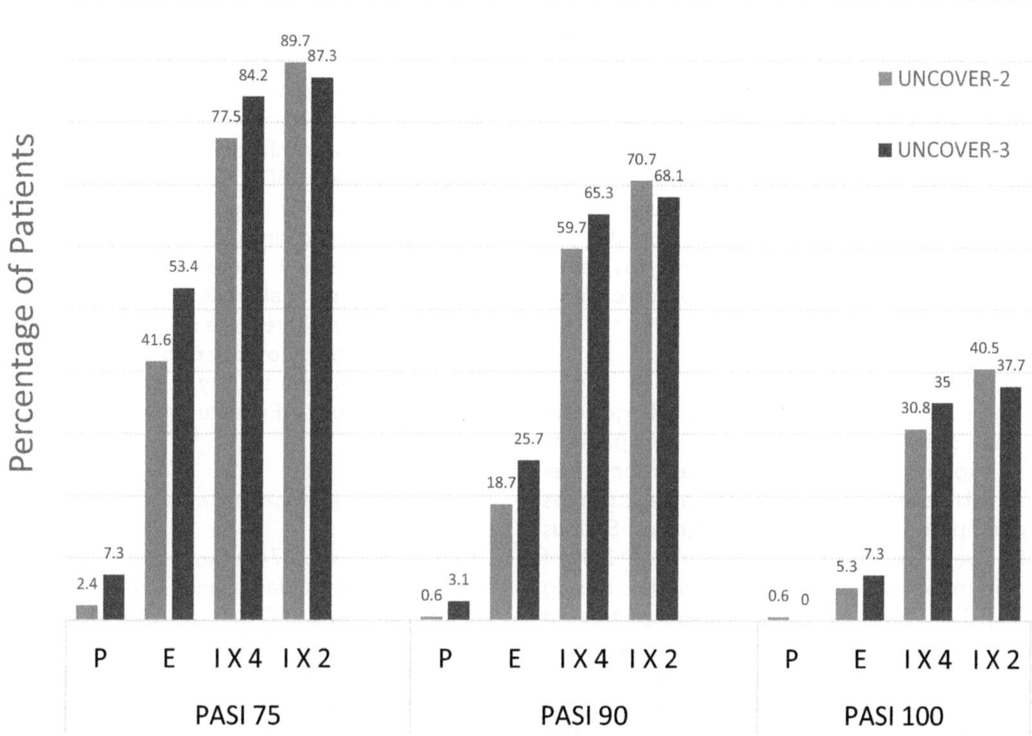

Fig. 13.2 Clinical responses from UNCOVER-2 and UNCOVER-3 after 12 weeks. E, etanercept; IX2, ixekizumab every 2 weeks; IX4, ixekizumab every 4 weeks; P, placebo.

SAFETY

Phase 2 Trial and OLE Study

In the 12-week phase 2 trial, adverse events (AEs) were reported in 63% of patients in both the ixekizumab groups and the placebo groups.[17] No serious AEs, including death, or major cardiovascular events were reported, although the study duration and size were not long or large enough to adequately detect such events. The most common AEs reported were nasopharyngitis, upper respiratory infection, injection-site reaction, and headache; however, there were no dose-related trends in the incidence or severity of these events.

In the 52-week OLE study, the exposure-adjusted incidence rates were 0.47 per patient-year for AEs and 0.06 per patient-year for serious AEs.[18] Adverse events were reported in 67%

TABLE 13.3
Safety data from UNCOVER-2 and UNCOVER-3

	Ixekizumab 2-wk Group (n = 734)	Ixekizumab 4-wk Group (n = 729)	Etanercept (n = 739)	Placebo (n = 360)
Serious AE	2% (14)	2% (14)	2% (14)	2% (7)
Infection	26% (190)	26% (191)	22% (159)	21% (74)
Adverse events	58% (424)	58% (419)	54% (399)	44% (160)
Nasopharyngitis	8% (61)	8% (58)	7% (55)	8% (28)
URI	4% (27)	3% (24)	5% (34)	3% (12)
Injection site reaction	10% (76)	9% (62)	11% (80)	1% (4)
Pruritus	2% (14)	2% (16)	1% (8)	1% (5)
Headache	5% (33)	5% (34)	4% (31)	2% (8)
Arthralgia	3% (20)	3% (18)	2% (17)	2% (8)

(n = 80) of patients. There was 1 reported case of a thalamic infarction as determined by clinical signs and symptoms (no imaging reported). Serious AEs were reported in 8% (n = 10) of patients, the most notable being 1 patient with rectal cancer and 1 patient with depression and suicide attempt. There were no cases of major cardiac events, tuberculosis (TB), invasive fungal infection, or deaths. The safety data from this trial are limited by the lack of a control group as well as possible bias toward OLE retention of patients without safety concerns.

UNCOVER-2 and UNCOVER 3

In the combined data from these 2 large-scale phase 3 trials, the percentage of patients who experienced an AE was higher in both ixekizumab dosing groups and etanercept groups as compared with the placebo group. Serious AEs were reported in 1.9% (n = 28) of ixekizumab-treated patients (both dosing groups), 1.9% (n = 14) of etanercept-treated patients, and 1.9% (n = 7) of placebo patients.[16] The most common AEs were nasopharyngitis, upper respiratory tract infection, injection-site reactions/erythema/pain, pruritus, headache, and arthralgia.

Overall, infections were more frequent with ixekizumab treatment than etanercept or placebo, although less than 1% of these were severe. There were 14 reported cases of mucocutaneous *Candida* infection in ixekizumab-treated patients, 5 cases in etanercept-treated patients, and 2 cases in placebo patients. There were no reported cases of TB. Less than 4% of patients experienced allergic or hypersensitivity reactions, but these were more frequent in ixekizumab-treated patients (n = 50, 3% of patients) as opposed to etanercept (n = 18, 2% of patients) or placebo (n = 7, 2% of patients). Most of these hypersensitivity cases were mild in severity, with the exception of 1 case of leukocytoclastic vasculitis that progressed to a serious AE resulting in a hospital admission.

Major adverse cardiovascular events included 1 myocardial infarction in an etanercept-treated patient, 1 cerebral embolism in an ixekizumab-treated patient (every 4 weeks), and 1 acute myocardial infarction in a placebo patient.

Overall, the safety profiles from these phase 3 trials at week 12 were comparable to the phase 2 trials at week 20 and comparable with etanercept. Most AEs were mild to moderate in severity, and there were no clear discrepancies in rates of serious infection, malignancy, or major cardiovascular events as compared with placebo. The safety data from this trial are limited by its short duration; however, longer-term studies are currently ongoing (UNCOVER-1, UNCOVER-2, UNCOVER-3).

Summary and Additional Safety Concerns

Warnings and precautions on the FDA label for ixekizumab include infections, TB, and inflammatory bowel disease (IBD).[1] Safety data from clinical trials show that ixekizumab is well tolerated overall. Rates of nasopharyngitis and upper respiratory tract infection were equal among all treatment groups in all trials, including the long-term OLE study. There were no cases of multiple sclerosis or reports of laboratory abnormalities indicating end-organ toxicity in any of the trials, and other serious AEs were limited to isolated cases.

Mucosal inflammation and inflammatory bowel disease

Given the role of IL-17A as an effector cytokine at skin and mucosal surfaces, and its overexpression in intestinal tissue in Crohn disease, it was originally thought that IL-17A inhibition may improve symptoms of Crohn. A study on secukinumab for patients with moderate-to-severe Crohn, however, was terminated prematurely after secukinumab was ineffective and associated with a high number of AEs in comparison to placebo.[20] Blockade of IL-17A may rarely be associated with increased mucosal inflammation.[12,21] The phase 3 trial data on ixekizumab reported 1 case of exacerbated ulcerative colitis in a patient receiving ixekizumab every 2 weeks that required mesalazine dose escalation, and 1 new onset case of Crohn disease in a patient receiving ixekizumab every 2 weeks that had no previous history of chronic gastrointestinal symptoms.[16]

Neutropenia

IL-17 may play a role in the mobilization and homeostasis of neutrophils[22]; thus, IL-17 blockade may be associated with neutropenia in psoriasis patients. In the 12-week phase 2 trial, 2 ixekizumab-treated patients had Common Terminology Criteria for Adverse Events grade 2 neutropenia (1000 to <1500 cells per cubic milliliter) with no concurrent infection.[17] In the OLE study, there was no effect on mean neutrophil count in patients on prolonged ixekizumab treatment, and no cases of neutropenia higher than grade 2.[18] In the combined phase 3 trial data, grade 3 neutropenia (500 to <1000 cells per cubic milliliter) occurred in 2 ixekizumab-treated patients (every 2 weeks), 4 etanercept-treated patients, and 1 placebo-treated patient.[16] Grade 4 neutropenia (<500 cells per cubic milliliter) occurred in 1 patient treated with ixekizumab (every 4 weeks) that normalized at a 2-day retest. None of these patients had a concurrent infection.

Suicide

There have been limited data on a possible association of suicide risk in patients treated with the IL-17 receptor blocker brodalumab; however, there have been no reported cases of suicide in patients treated with ixekizumab.[12] Treatment-emergent depression was reported in 1 placebo patient, 3 etanercept-treated patients, and 5 ixekizumab-treated patients in the phase 3 trials.[16] There were 2 cases of suicide attempt reported in ixekizumab-treated patients: 1 of these patients had a prior history of suicide attempt, and both cases were preceded by important psychological triggers not attributed to ixekizumab.[16]

PRECAUTIONS

Infections

Caution should be exercised when considering ixekizumab in patients with chronic infection or history of recurrent infection.[1] In the event of serious infection, discontinue ixekinumab and closely monitor patients until infection resolves.

Tuberculosis

As is the case with all immunomodulatory agents in the treatment of plaque psoriasis, ixekizumab is contraindicated in patients with active TB.[1] All patients should be evaluated for TB before treatment based on risk factors and screened for latent TB before initiation and during therapy. A purified protein derivative (PPD) screen with 5-mm or greater induration is considered positive, even in those with a history of BCG vaccination.[23] There are currently no reports of reactivated latent TB in any ixekizumab psoriasis clinical trials; thus, additional observational and focused studies are needed to further evaluate the full range of side effects of ixekizumab.

Inflammatory Bowel Disease

Use of ixekizumab in the presence of IBD is not a contraindication, although caution should be taken when initiating therapy in this patient population because studies have suggested potential worsening of the IBD.[1] The phase 3 study showed that blockade of IL-17A was associated with more episodes of Crohn (0.1%) and ulcerative colitis (0.2%) as compared with placebo.[1,16] Although IBD exacerbations were uncommon, the possibility of IBD flares should be considered in patients who receive ixekizumab and have active or past history of IBD.

Hypersensitivity Reactions

Ixekizumab-associated angioedema and urticarial reactions have been reported in clinical trials (≤0.1%); however, there were no anaphylaxis events reported from the UNCOVER trials.[1,17,18] If serious hypersensitivity reactions ensue, the drug should be discontinued immediately and appropriate therapy initiated. The ixekizumab autoinjector and prefilled syringe do not contain latex.[1]

Pregnancy

There is currently no available information regarding ixekizumab use in pregnancy and associated risks. Human forms of IgG cross the placental barrier; thus, ixekizumab may be transmitted from the mother to fetus. However, the authors of this section advise that use in pregnant women, if needed, is not likely to cause a serious medical issue.

MONITORING

The information presented is primarily based on psoriasis guidelines from the American Academy of Dermatology (AAD).[11]

A thorough history and physical examination should be taken before initiation of ixekizumab therapy, including TB exposure, chronic/recurrent infections, malignancy, neurologic and cardiac history, and a thorough review of systems. Routine follow-up examinations should adequately monitor patients for side effects and AEs.[24]

Aside from baseline TB test, annual monitoring for TB, and a baseline hepatitis profile, routine laboratory testing beyond that for concomitant therapies or comorbidities is generally not supported.[25] The highest grade US Preventive Services Task Force evidence for screening studies is grade B for TB testing (interferon-γ [IFN-γ] release assay is preferred over tuberculin skin testing), and hepatitis B virus/ hepatitis C virus screening is supported only by grade C evidence.[26] The AAD recommends baseline PPD, liver function tests (LFTs), and complete blood count (CBC). Periodic history and physical examinations are recommended as well, and yearly PPD and periodic LFTs and CBC can be considered for ongoing monitoring (Tables 13.4 and 13.5).[24]

The Centers for Disease Control and Prevention recommends TB testing before the therapy initiation as well.[23] Positive skin test findings should be followed with a chest radiograph; if negative, patients should be treated for latent TB (6–9 months of 300 mg isoniazid daily and/ or 4 months of 600 mg daily rifampicin),[27] and if positive, patients should receive therapy for

TABLE 13.4
Monitoring recommendations from the American Academy of Dermatology

	Monitoring
History and physical	Baseline and routine
CBC	Baseline and periodically
LFTs	Baseline and periodically
TB skin test	Baseline and annually after
Hepatitis profile	Not specified

active TB. Biologic therapy may be started after 1 to 2 months of prophylactic treatment if the patient is adherent to and tolerating the prophylactic regimen.[28] If a patient has a positive PPD because of prior BCG vaccination, blood tests can be obtained measuring IFN production on stimulation with TB antigens that are not present in BCG. Most guidelines perform annual TB skin testing in patients receiving ixekizumab to screen for the TB reactivation, especially in those at risk (ie, health care workers, travelers to endemic areas).

TABLE 13.5
Vaccination recommendations from the National Psoriasis Foundation

Vaccination	Before Therapy	During Therapy
Live vaccines (MMR, varicella, herpes zoster, intranasal influenza, oral typhoid, yellow fever, oral polio, smallpox, BCG, rotavirus)	Contraindicated within 1 mo	Contraindicated
Influenza	Vaccinate with inactivated or live	Yearly immunization with inactivated vaccine
Chicken pox	If negative serology, vaccinate	Contraindicated
Zoster	Before therapy: 1 dose for adults ≥50 y	Contraindicated
Human papillomavirus	Unvaccinated males/female patients up to age 26	Same
Hepatitis A	Vaccinate if high risk (diabetes, liver disease, intravenous drug users, homosexual men, and so forth)	Same; consider obtaining postvaccination serology
Hepatitis B	Serology, risk factor assessment. Offer vaccination if necessary	High-dose vaccine Consider obtaining serology postvaccination
Pneumococcal	Pneumococcal polysaccharide vaccine (PPSV23) vaccine recommended	Pneumococcal conjugate vaccine followed by PPSV23 if not given prior
H aemophilus influenzae type b	Vaccinate if unvaccinated	Same
MMR	Vaccinate if negative, or seronegative to any component	Contraindicated
Tetanus-diphtheria/diphtheria-tetanus-acellular pertussis (TDAP)	Booster every 10 y and high-risk wounds Offer before therapy, substitute 1 dose with TDAP	Same
Meningococcal	Assess risk factors, vaccinate if high risk (asplenia, complement deficient, group living)	Same
Poliomyelitis	Assess risk factors, vaccinate if high risk (health care worker, laboratory worker)	Same

From Lebwohl M, Bagel J, Gelfand JM, et al. From the Medical Board of the National Psoriasis Foundation: monitoring and vaccinations in patients treated with biologics for psoriasis. J Am Acad Dermatol 2008;58(1):94–105; with permission.

The authors of this section recommend initial baseline monitoring that includes a QuantiFERON-TB Gold (QFT), LFTs, CBC, and hepatitis B and hepatitis C profile. QFT should be repeated annually.

VACCINATIONS

Because of the possibility that biologic agents may impair the body's immunologic response to vaccinations, administration of vaccinations should be carefully considered in patients receiving biologic therapy.[24] Live vaccines (measles, mumps, and rubella [MMR], varicella, zoster, intranasal influenza, and so forth) are contraindicated in patients receiving ixekizumab according to the FDA-approved label; this label seems to be based on lack of evidence of safety for use of live vaccines in this setting rather than on data showing (or even a theoretic risk that) there would be a problem.

Scientifically based/standardized recommendations for administering biologically inactive or recombinant vaccines to patients on biologic agents are lacking. A study conducted on inactivated trivalent subunit influenza virus and conjugate group C meningococcal vaccinations in healthy patients using secukinumab demonstrated that IL-17A blockade does not interfere with the effectiveness of these vaccines, as assessed by levels of antibody protection.[29] However, further studies may be needed in order to confirm vaccine effectiveness with secukinumab and ixekizumab use.

It is preferable to complete all age-appropriate immunizations according to current immunization guidelines before initiating biologic therapy. The production of antibodies from the vaccine generally occurs in the 2-week period from primary immunization, but could take more than 6 weeks to peak.

SUMMARY

Ixekizumab has greater efficacy compared with most FDA-approved agents available to patients with moderate-to-severe psoriasis, based on data from clinical trials.[12] More data are needed from prospective registries, after-marketing surveillance, and additional studies to provide conclusive information and guidelines on efficacy, safety, monitoring, vaccinations, and use in specialized populations. However, ixekizumab does offer significant potential for complete clearance of psoriasis and may become a first-line biologic agent.[12]

REFERENCES

1. Eli Lilly and Company [Internet]. Indianapolis (IN): [publisher unknown]; 2016. Available at: http://pi.lilly.com/us/taltz-uspi.pdf.
2. Lilly's ixekizumab met primary endpoint in a phase 3 study investigating the treatment of psoriatic arthritis (NYSE: LLY). Investor.lilly.com. N.p., 2016. Web. 16 June 2016.
3. Farahnik B, Beroukhim K, Zhu TH, et al. Ixekizumab for the treatment of psoriasis: a review of phase III trials. Dermatol Ther (Heidelb) 2016;6(1):25–37.
4. Blauvelt A. New concepts in the pathogenesis and treatment of psoriasis: key roles for IL-23, IL-17A and TGF-β1. Expert Rev Dermatol 2007; 2(1):69–78.
5. Fitch E, Harper E, Skorcheva I, et al. Pathophysiology of psoriasis: recent advances on IL-23 and Th17 cytokines. Curr Rheumatol Rep 2007;9(6): 461–7.
6. Nestle FO, Kaplan DH, Barker J. Psoriasis. N Engl J Med 2009;361(5):496–509.
7. Lowes MA, Suárez-Fariñas M, Krueger JG. Immunology of psoriasis. Annu Rev Immunol 2014;32: 227–55.
8. Lowes MA, Kikuchi T, Fuentes-Duculan J, et al. Psoriasis vulgaris lesions contain discrete populations of Th1 and Th17 T cells. J Invest Dermatol 2008; 128(5):1207–11.
9. Kagami S, Rizzo HL, Lee JJ, et al. Circulating Th17, Th22, and Th1 cells are increased in psoriasis. J Invest Dermatol 2010;130(5):1373–83.
10. Weaver CT, Hatton RD, Mangan PR, et al. IL-17 family cytokines and the expanding diversity of effector T cell lineages. Annu Rev Immunol 2007; 25:821–52.
11. Krueger JG, Fretzin S, Suárez-Fariñas M, et al. IL-17A is essential for cell activation and inflammatory gene circuits in subjects with psoriasis. J Allergy Clin Immunol 2012;130(1):145–54.e9.
12. Blauvelt A. Ixekizumab: a new anti-IL-17A monoclonal antibody therapy for moderate-to severe plaque psoriasis. Expert Opin Biol Ther 2016; 16(2):255–63.
13. Gaffen SL, Jain R, Garg AV, et al. The IL-23-IL-17 immune axis: from mechanisms to therapeutic testing. Nat Rev Immunol 2014;14(9):585–600.
14. Gao SH, Huang K, Tu H, et al. Monoclonal antibody humanness score and its applications. BMC Biotechnol 2013;13:55.
15. Levin EC, Gupta R, Brown G, et al. Biologic fatigue in psoriasis. J Dermatolog Treat 2014;25(1):78–82.
16. Griffiths CEM, Reich K, Lebwohl M, et al. Comparison of ixekizumab with etanercept or placebo in moderate-to-severe psoriasis (UNCOVER-2 and UNCOVER-3): results from two phase 3 randomised trials. Lancet 2015;386(9993):541–51.

17. Leonardi C, Matheson R, Zachariae C, et al. Anti-interleukin-17 monoclonal antibody ixekizumab in chronic plaque psoriasis. N Engl J Med 2012;366(13):1190–9.
18. Gordon KB, Leonardi CL, Lebwohl M, et al. A 52-week, open-label study of the efficacy and safety of ixekizumab, an anti-interleukin-17A monoclonal antibody, in patients with chronic plaque psoriasis. J Am Acad Dermatol 2014;71(6):1176–82.
19. Saeki H, Nakagawa H, Ishii T, et al. Efficacy and safety of open-label ixekizumab treatment in Japanese patients with moderate-to-severe plaque psoriasis, erythrodermic psoriasis and generalized pustular psoriasis. J Eur Acad Dermatol Venereol 2015;29(6):1148–55.
20. Hueber W, Sands BE, Lewitzky S, et al. Secukinumab, a human anti-IL-17A monoclonal antibody, for moderate to severe Crohn's disease: unexpected results of a randomised, double-blind placebo-controlled trial. Gut 2012;61(12):1693–700.
21. Langley RG, Elewski BE, Lebwohl M, et al. Secukinumab in plaque psoriasis–results of two phase 3 trials. N Engl J Med 2014;371(4):326–38.
22. Kolls JK, Lindén A. Interleukin-17 family members and inflammation. Immunity 2004;21(4):467–76.
23. Centers for Disease Control and Prevention. Guide for primary health care providers: targeted tuberculin testing and treatment of latent tuberculosis infection. Available at: http://www.cdc.gov/tb/?404;http://www.cdc.gov:80/tb/pubs/LTBI/pdf/TargetedLTBI05.pdf. Accessed May 1, 2016.
24. Lebwohl M, Bagel J, Gelfand JM, et al. From the Medical Board of the National Psoriasis Foundation: monitoring and vaccinations in patients treated with biologics for psoriasis. J Am Acad Dermatol 2008;58(1):94–105.
25. van Lümig PPM, Driessen RJB, Roelofs-Thijssen MA, et al. Relevance of laboratory investigations in monitoring patients with psoriasis on etanercept or adalimumab. Br J Dermatol 2011;165(2):375–82.
26. Ahn CS, Dothard EH, Garner ML, et al. To test or not to test? An updated evidence-based assessment of the value of screening and monitoring tests when using systemic biologic agents to treat psoriasis and psoriatic arthritis. J Am Acad Dermatol 2015;73(3):420–8.e1.
27. Targeted tuberculin testing and treatment of latent tuberculosis infection. American Thoracic Society. MMWR Recomm Rep 2000;49(RR-6):1–51.
28. Doherty SD, Van Voorhees A, Lebwohl MG, et al. National Psoriasis Foundation consensus statement on screening for latent tuberculosis infection in patients with psoriasis treated with systemic and biologic agents. J Am Acad Dermatol 2008;59(2):209–17.
29. Chioato A, Noseda E, Stevens M, et al. Treatment with the interleukin-17A-blocking antibody secukinumab does not interfere with the efficacy of influenza and meningococcal vaccinations in healthy subjects: results of an open-label, parallel-group, randomized single-center study. Clin Vaccine Immunol 2012;19(10):1597–602.

CHAPTER 14

Biosimilars

Shivani P. Reddy, BS, Catherine Ni, MD, Jashin J. Wu, MD

KEYWORDS

• Biosimilar • Inflectra • Remsima • CT-P13 • Infliximab-dyyb

KEY POINTS

- Through the Biologics Price Competition and Innovation act, the US Food and Drug Administration (FDA) has defined a biosimilar as a biologic product that is highly similar to the original product notwithstanding minor differences in clinically inactive components.
- Preclinical analytical assessments are used to determine variations in biosimilar agents and are critical for their approval.
- Inflectra (infliximab-dyyb, CT-P13), a recently approved biosimilar by the FDA, is indicated in patients with chronic severe psoriasis when other systemic therapies are medically less appropriate.

INTRODUCTION

The development of biosimilar agents such as tumor necrosis factor (TNF) inhibitors has significant potential to change the standards of psoriasis therapy in forthcoming years. The availability of biologic drugs for the treatment of moderate-to-severe psoriasis has revolutionized psoriasis treatment, and, as the patents for these medications (adalimumab, etanercept, infliximab) are expiring soon, dermatologists can expect increased advocacy for biosimilars.

The development of biosimilars is not the same as developing a generic, in part because biologics are so much more complex than small molecule drugs. Biologics are so complex that no company can duplicate them, not even the originator company. Each batch of an innovator biologic may differ in small ways from other batches. Variation within an innovator product occurs and is acceptable as long as it is not thought to have clinical implications. Similarly, biosimilars are not identical to the innovator product but can be marketed if the differences between the biosimilar and the innovator are sufficiently small that no clinical implications are expected. An extensive array of data is required to demonstrate biosimilarity (more data than are required of batch-to-batch variants in the innovator product).

The Biologics Price Competition and Innovation (BCPI) act was created as a part of the Affordable Care Act in 2010 as an abbreviated licensure pathway for biologic products that were "biosimilar" to, or interchangeable with, the original biologic product.[1] Through the BCPI act, the US Food and Drug Administration (FDA) has defined a biosimilar as a biologic product that is highly similar to the original product notwithstanding minor differences in clinically inactive components. No clinically meaningful differences between the biologic and the biosimilar in terms of safety, purity, and potency can exist. These aspects of the biosimilar drug must be demonstrated through analytical studies, animal studies, and at least 1 clinical study, unless the FDA deems it unnecessary. The biosimilar, however, does not need to demonstrate its independent efficacy and safety for FDA approval, as is typically required for the original biologic off which it is modeled.[1]

The greatest potential for biosimilar agents in the treatment of psoriasis is in association with TNF inhibitors (infliximab, etanercept, and adalimumab); however, many clinical trials investigating these biosimilar agents are currently in the preliminary stages and results have yet to be published. An infliximab biosimilar by the brand name of Inflectra was recently approved in April 2016 by the FDA for the treatment of adult severe plaque psoriasis, adult and pediatric moderately-to-severely active Crohn disease unresponsive to conventional therapy, moderate-to-severe rheumatoid arthritis in combination with methotrexate, active ankylosing spondylitis, and active psoriatic arthritis.

SMALL MOLECULE GENERIC DRUGS

In approving a generic drug, the FDA requires pharmaceutical equivalence to the reference drug (identical amounts of same active drug ingredient in the same dosage form and route of administration), bioequivalence to the reference drug, and adequate labeling and manufacturing.[2] Bioequivalence is generally used to establish similarity between a generic drug and reference drug and is defined as the absence of significant differences in the availability of the active ingredient at the site of drug action.[3] Two drugs are bioequivalent if the 90% confidence intervals (CIs) of pharmacokinetic parameters (maximum concentration, area under the curve) of generic-to-reference drug ratios fall within 80% to 125%. This bioequivalence ensures that the rate and extent of absorption of the generic drug does not differ from the reference drug.[3]

Generic drugs approved by the FDA have the same high-quality, strength, purity, and stability as the reference drug. In addition, the generic manufacturing, packaging, and testing sites must pass the same quality standards as those of brand name drugs.[4]

CREATION OF THE BIOSIMILAR AND ANALYTICAL ASSESSMENTS

The creation of original biologic agents takes place in unique genetically bioengineered cell lines. Companies that produce biosimilar agents do not have access to these specific cell lines and thus use new cell lines to produce biosimilars. This, in addition to the other multiple steps involved in production, induces variations in the biosimilar from the original reference biologic agent, which are determined in preclinical analytical assessments.[5]

The process of creating the biosimilar involves recombinant DNA that encodes the exact same amino acid sequence as the originator biologic. This recombinant DNA is placed within a plasmid and transfected into a new cell line in order to produce the biosimilar protein product, which is then collected and purified. This entire process is tightly optimized and monitored to minimize variation from the reference biologic.[5]

In comparison to the creation of generic small molecule drugs, which are produced by chemical synthesis, the creation of biosimilars occurs within living cells and can involve quaternary folding of structures.[6] Glycosylation, folding, charge, the presence of impurities, and individual amino acid variants can differ and potentially alter the function of the protein product.[7,8] In addition, biosimilars can undergo physical and chemical degradation such as deamidation, cleavage, and aggregation; these changes can make a molecule more likely to be recognized by the body as foreign (Table 14.1).[9]

Preclinical analytical assessments are used to determine these variations and are critical for approval of these biosimilar agents. There are approximately 40 different analytical methods that are used to assess approximately 100 various drug attributes.[5]

Drug companies are required by the FDA to provide information on any manufacturing changes as well as bioanalytical data characterizing each drug batch.[10] Posttranslational modifications are evaluated using mass spectrometry, assessing for glycosylation, phosphorylation, acetylation, sulfation, glycation, and charge.[11,12] If minor changes do exist, however, the FDA

TABLE 14.1
Comparison of characteristics of small molecule drugs, biologic agents, generic small molecule drugs, and biosimilar agents

Small molecule drug	*Biologic agent*
• Chemically synthesized • Low molecular weight (100–1000 Da) • Commonly orally delivered • Less immunogenicity • Same chemical entity from batch to batch	• Produced in living cells • Medium to high molecular weight (18–150 kDa) • Commonly parenterally delivered • Greater immunogenicity • Biologic agents are not identical from batch to batch
Generic small molecule drug	***Biosimilar agent***
• Bioequivalent to reference drug[3] • Same strength, purity, and stability • Demonstrating clinical efficacy and safety is not required for regulatory approval	• Protein backbone is identical; however, there is increased variation from biologic agent due to heterogeneity in posttranslational modifications, degradation, and so forth • Clinical comparative studies are necessary to demonstrate bioequivalence

does not necessarily mandate clinical studies to re-evaluate efficacy.

In addition, functional assays are necessary to compare the biosimilar agent to the biologic agent. Functional assays includes the evaluation of drug binding affinity and avidity to the target and ability to neutralize target cytokines.[13] End product assessments include evaluation of impurities, aggregates, product stability (shelf-life and temperature alterations), and product devices for delivery (autoinjectors and prefilled syringes).[14]

REGULATION

Given the increased complexity in developing biosimilars as compared with generic molecules, they are susceptible to more stringent regulatory pathways to maintain the quality and safety of the drug. The European Medicines Agency (EMA) was the first organization to develop and publish guidelines for biosimilars development,[15] and the FDA has released 7 guidances for the development of biosimilars at present.[16] The FDA recommends a stepwise totality-of-the-evidence approach in assessing biosimilarity demonstration (Fig. 14.1).[17] Both agencies require the primary amino acid sequence, potency, dose, and route of administration of the biosimilar and biologic product to be identical, and any differences in higher-order structure and posttranslational modifications must be minimal and cannot impact safety, efficacy, or immunogenicity.[18,19] In order to demonstrate biosimilarity, 1 phase I trial for pharmacokinetics or a single pivotal phase 3 trial is required for FDA approval.[18,19]

Biosimilar companies have argued that clinical studies should not be required to be repeated with each manufacturing change, especially if companies producing biologics are not required to.[5] The inability to exactly replicate each batch of drug is true for the reference biologic agents as well as for the biosimilars. For example, Schiestl and colleagues[7] analyzed the biochemical fingerprint of etanercept and found that it varied by 20% to 40% in basic variants and degree of glycosylation.

Although the biosimilar regulation pathway differs between various regions of the world, the guidelines for approval and licensing are similar between main organizations (EMA, FDA, and World Health Organization). The stringent analyses of structural and functional components of a biosimilar will help assure quality, efficacy, and safety of this novel therapy.

EXTRAPOLATION

Although biosimilars have primarily been studied in rheumatoid arthritis and ankylosing spondylitis patients, approval has been extended to multiple indications. There is much debate about what clinical and scientific data should be required for approval for extrapolation of indications and whether biosimilars should have to repeat studies that have already been conducted by the original reference biologic.[20]

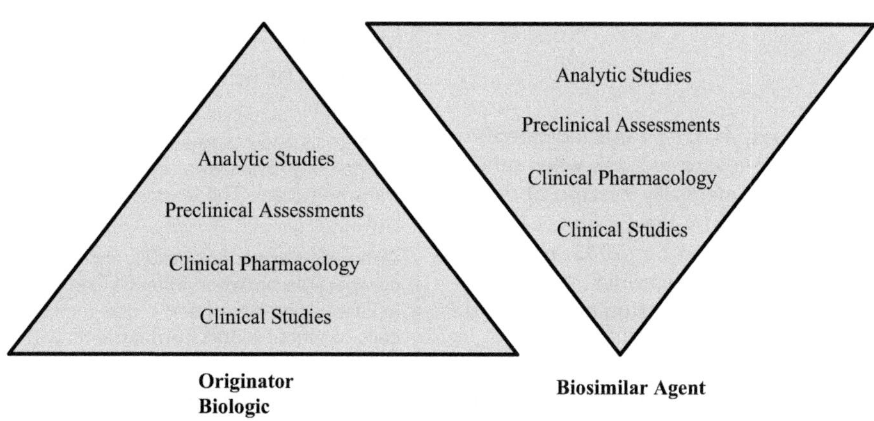

Fig. 14.1 Emphasis of approval steps for biosimilar agents versus originator biologic. The emphasis on different developmental steps to approval of a biosimilar agent is different than that of the originator biologic agent. Analytical studies form the basis for approval of biosimilar agents, whereas clinical studies form the basis for approval of originator biologic agents. (*Data from* US Food and Drug Administration. Scientific considerations in demonstrating biosimilarity to a reference product: guidance for industry. 2015. Available at: http://www.fda.gov/downloads/DrugsGuidanceComplianceRegulatoryInformation/Guidances/UCM291128.pdf. Accessed March 8, 2016.)

There are several issues that the FDA states should be justified scientifically in order to consider extrapolation of indications. The first is that the mechanism of action in the condition of use—including the target/receptor for each activity/function of the biosimilar, binding, dose/concentration response, pattern of molecular signaling on engagement of target receptors, relationship between biosimilar structure and target/receptor interactions, and location and expression of the target/receptors—should be the same. The pharmacokinetics and biodistribution in various patient populations, differences in expected toxicities in each indication and patient population, and any other factors affecting safety and/or effectiveness of the biosimilar in each indication and patient population are all issues that should all be addressed as well.[21]

The EMA and FDA both deemed that when the mechanism of action differs between various indications or is not fully understood, separate clinical trials should be conducted.[19] In obtaining data, the most sensitive patient population and clinical endpoint should be used in order to determine clinically meaningful differences in efficacy and safety.[19] In order to minimize variations in response to biosimilar therapy due to individual patient characteristics, clinicians should give careful attention to comorbidities and concomitant medications and try to keep populations homogenous in order to appropriately attribute differences in response to the biosimilar.[20] These clarifications and precautions are important given that biologic therapies are often approved for multiple diseases with different pathogeneses, as is trying to be done with biosimilars.

INFLECTRA

Inflectra (infliximab-dyyb, CT-P13) is indicated in patients with chronic severe psoriasis when other systemic therapies are medically less appropriate. It was initially approved by the European Medicines Association in September 2013 and marketed under the name Remsima, based on several clinical and nonclinical studies described in this chapter.

The recommended dosing of Inflectra in plaque psoriasis is 5 mg/kg given intravenously at weeks 0, 2, and 6 followed by a maintenance regimen of 5 mg/kg every 8 weeks thereafter. It is contraindicated in patients with moderate-to-severe heart failure (New York Heart Association Class 3 or 4) as well as in patients that have displayed a severe hypersensitivity reaction to infliximab, any inactive components of the product, or murine proteins.[22] The precautions in Inflectra administration are largely similar to those in infliximab administration.

The major measurable physicochemical characteristics and biological activities of infliximab-dyyb and reference infliximab that have been assessed are comparable between the 2 agents (Box 14.1).[23,24]

CLINICAL TRIALS

There are currently no clinical trial data published for biosimilars in psoriasis; however, there are limited data available for infliximab-dyyb in rheumatoid arthritis and ankylosing spondylitis patients. There are 2 registered studies for an adalimumab biosimilar and 1 registered study for an etanercept biosimilar in psoriasis patients.[27]

The PLANETRA study was conducted in 606 patients with rheumatoid arthritis, and the PLANETAS study was conducted in 250 patients with ankylosing spondylitis on the infliximab-dyyb biosimilar to infliximab. The results of these studies

BOX 14.1
Comparable physiochemical attributes of Inflectra (infliximab-dyyb, CT-P13) to infliximab

Amino acid sequences are identical. Fourier-transform infrared spectroscopy and other structural analyses indicate that secondary/tertiary structures are highly comparable.[26]

Binding affinities for TNF and other infliximab ligands are highly similar. Neither binds lymphotoxin.[23,25]

Extent of TNF neutralization was equivalent.[23,25]

Apoptosis and complement-dependent cytotoxicity levels were equivalent in a transmembrane TNF-expressing Jurkat cell line.[23,25]

Antibody-dependent cellular cytotoxicity was comparable between Inflectra and infliximab in vitro, using peripheral blood mononuclear cells or whole blood from patients with CD20.[25]

Deamidation and oxidation profiles are similar. Although some numerical differences in glycosylation exist, overall type and distribution of glycans observed in Inflectra and infliximab are similar.[23,25]

Data from Refs.[23–26]

indicated no clinically relevant differences in efficacy and safety.[26,28]

In the PLANETRA study, patients with inadequate response to methotrexate were randomized 1:1 to receive either infliximab-dyyb or infliximab. After 54 weeks of study, the American College of Rheumatology 20 response in both groups was very similar (infliximab-dyyb 74.7%, reference product 71.3%), as was the safety profile and immunogenicity.[29]

In the PLANETAS study, patients were randomized 1:1 to receive either infliximab-dyyb or infliximab. By week 54 of study, the Assessment of Spondylo Arthritis International Society (ASAS) 20 response (odds ratio [OR] 0.89, 95% CI 0.50, 1.59), ASAS40 response (OR 1.26, 95% CI 0.73, 2.15), and ASAS partial remission rates were comparable between treatment groups. There were no significant differences between treatment groups in adverse events, serious adverse events, infections, and infusion-related reactions.[30]

Two randomized controlled trials of adalimumab biosimilar in 798 psoriasis patients have been completed, and data from these trials are pending.[31,32] One study on ABP 501 enrolled 350 patients and was completed in March 2015, with results yet to be posted. The second study on GP 2017 enrolled 448 patients and is scheduled to be completed in April 2016. One randomized control trial of etanercept biosimilar GP2015 in 546 psoriasis patients was completed in March 2015, but has yet to post study results,[33] and another study of etanercept biosimilar CHS-0214 in 496 psoriasis patients is scheduled to be complete in May 2016 (Table 14.2).[34]

ADDITIONAL CONSIDERATIONS AND SUMMARY

There are several aspects of biosimilar therapy that must be considered before implementation into clinical practice. Given that the current version of the originator biologic product will likely remain on the market, the patient and clinician will have to select between a biologic or biosimilar for treatment, weighing factors such as price, insurance coverage, and immunogenicity if switching between agents.[19] Clinicians will also have to weigh the uncertainty within different batches of the innovator against the possibility of greater variation but more data on biosimilarity with the biosimilar.

The degree of interchangeability between the original biologic and biosimilar is largely unknown (as is the degree of interchangeability between different batches of innovator products), and the FDA has not provided guidance on this. Interchangeability may lead to repeated switching between the biosimilar and reference biologic (which currently happens with different batches of the innovator product), which could lead to increased immunogenicity and potentially compromise the safety and efficacy of either agent (although there will be more data that this does not occur with the use of the biosimilar than is currently available for different batches of the innovator).[19,35,36] The American Academy of Dermatology (AAD) recommends that in order to substitute a biosimilar for a biologic, the biosimilar must have a unique nonproprietary name and be designated as interchangeable by the FDA, the prescribing physician must provide permission for the substitution to the pharmacist, the patient must be informed and educated about the switch, and a permanent record must be made of the switch in the patient's medical record, although the AAD has not recommended this for different batches of the innovator product.[37]

It is important that pharmacovigilance and continuous monitoring ensue following regulatory approval of biosimilars.[19] Adverse events, side effects, and potential risk factors should be identified with increased use of these agents by drug companies and reported accordingly to regulatory agencies.

If a patient does not respond to a biosimilar as expected, it would be important for the clinician to reassess the same way as they would with an altogether different biologic. The patient should not be switched to the original biologic agent, but in cases of poorly responsive disease, the dosage can be modified, concomitant therapy can be added, or an alternative therapy can be given.[38]

The approval of biosimilar therapy for the treatment of psoriasis has some potential to broaden access of biologic-based therapy for patients suffering from this condition as well as other inflammatory disorders. Specifically, biosimilars have potential to lower cost and possibly increase access to patients.[18] Much of the basis for approval of biosimilars is built on preexisting knowledge and experience with the various batches of the reference biologic, and subjecting biosimilar agents to rigorous developmental regulations will facilitate a smoother transition of this therapeutic modality into clinical practice.

TABLE 14.2
Phase 3 clinical trials of biosimilars in psoriasis

Clinical Trial	Dosing	Start Date/ Completion Date	Primary Outcome Measures	Secondary Outcome Measures
NCT01970488 *Study to Compare Efficacy and Safety of ABP 501 and Adalimumab (Humira) in Adults with Moderate to Severe Plaque Psoriasis*	ABP 501: 80 mg at week 1/day 1, and 40 mg subcutaneously (SC) at week 2 and every 2 wk thereafter until week 52 Adalimumab: 80 mg at week 1/day 1, and 40 mg SC EOW thereafter until week 14. At week 16, subjects with a Psoriasis Area and Severity Index (PASI)-50 response remain on study for up to 52 wk; subjects initially randomized to adalimumab rerandomized (1:1) to ABP 501 or adalimumab treatment for weeks 16–48	October 2013/ March 2015	PASI score improvement after 16 wk of treatment	PASI-75 response, sPGA, BSA, AEs, SAEs, laboratory values, vital signs, antidrug antibodies
NCT02016105 *Study to Demonstrate Equivalent Efficacy and to Compare Safety of Biosimilar Adalimumab (GP2017) and Humira (ADACCESS)*	GP2017: 80 mg SC in week 0, followed by 40 mg SC EOW, starting at week 1 and ending at week 51 Adalimumab: 80 mg SC at week 0, followed by 40 mg SC EOW, starting at week 1 and ending at week 51	December 2013/ estimated April 2016	PASI-75 response rate	PASI-50, PASI-90, PASI-100, IGA, health-related quality of life
NCT01891864 *(etanercept) Study to Demonstrate Equivalent Efficacy and to Compare Safety of Biosimilar Etanercept (GP2015) and Enbrel*	GP2015: 50 mg twice weekly for the first 12 wk and 50 mg once weekly thereafter Etanercept: 50 mg twice weekly for the first 12 wk and 50 mg once weekly thereafter	June 2013/ March 2015	PASI-75 response rate after 12 wk	PASI-50, PASI-90, PASI score, injection site reactions, immunogenicity
NCT02134210 *(etanercept) Study to Compare the Efficacy and Safety of CHS-0214 vs Enbrel in Subjects with Chronic Plaque Psoriasis (RaPsOdy)*	CHS-0214: 50 mg SC twice weekly for 12 wk Etanercept: 50 mg SC twice weekly times 12 wk	June 2014/ May 2016	PASI-75 response rate after 12 wk	Not available

Abbreviation: EOW, every other week.

REFERENCES

1. U.S. Food and Drug Administration. Scientific considerations in demonstrating biosimilarity to a reference product: guidance for industry. 2015. Available at: http://www.fda.gov/downloads/DrugsGuidanceComplianceRegulatoryInformation/Guidances/UCM291128.pdf. Accessed March 8, 2016.
2. Research C for DE and. Understanding Generic Drugs - Facts about Generic Drugs [Internet]. 2016. Available at: http://www.fda.gov/Drugs/ResourcesForYou/Consumers/BuyingUsingMedicineSafely/UnderstandingGenericDrugs/ucm167991.htm. Accessed June 21, 2016.
3. CFR - Code of Federal Regulations Title 21 [Internet]. 2016. Available at: http://www.accessdata.fda.gov/scripts/cdrh/cfdocs/cfcfr/CFRSearch.cfm?fr=320.1. Accessed June 21, 2016.
4. Research C for DE and. Understanding Generic Drugs [Internet]. 2016. Available at: http://www.fda.gov/Drugs/ResourcesForYou/Consumers/BuyingUsingMedicineSafely/UnderstandingGenericDrugs/. Accessed June 22, 2016.
5. Blauvelt A, Cohen AD, Puig L. Biosimilars for psoriasis: preclinical analytical assessment to determine similarity. Br J Dermatol 2016;174(2):282–6.
6. Olech E. Biosimilars: rationale and current regulatory landscape. Semin Arthritis Rheum 2016;45(Suppl 5):S1–10.
7. Schiestl M, Stangler T, Torella C, et al. Acceptable changes in quality attributes of glycosylated biopharmaceuticals. Nat Biotechnol 2011;29(4):310–2.
8. Zuperl S, Pristovsek P, Menart V, et al. Chemometric approach in quantification of structural identity/similarity of proteins in biopharmaceuticals. J Chem Inf Model 2007;47(3):737–43.
9. Ryan AM. Frontiers in nonclinical drug development: biosimilars. Vet Pathol 2015;52(2):419–26.
10. Calvo B, Zuñiga L. Therapeutic monoclonal antibodies: strategies and challenges for biosimilars development. Curr Med Chem 2012;19(26):4445–50.
11. Chirino AJ, Mire-Sluis A. Characterizing biological products and assessing comparability following manufacturing changes. Nat Biotechnol 2004;22(11):1383–91.
12. U.S. Department of Health and Human Services. Food and Drug Administration. Reference product exclusivity for biological products filed under section 351(a) of the PHS act. Available at: http://www.fda.gov/downloads/Drugs/GuidanceComplianceRegulatoryInformation/Guidances/UCM407844.pdf. Accessed April 3, 2016.
13. Locatelli F, Roger S. Comparative testing and pharmacovigilance of biosimilars. Nephrol Dial Transplant 2006;21(Suppl 5):v13–6.
14. U.S. Department of Health and Human Services. Food and Drug Administration. Clinical pharmacology data to support a demonstration of biosimilarity to a reference product. Available at: http://www.fda.gov/downloads/Drugs/GuidanceComplianceRegulatoryInformation/Guidances/UCM397017.pdf. Accessed April 16, 2016.
15. European Medicines Agency. Guideline on similar biological medicinal products, 2005. Available at: http://www.ema.europa.eu/docs/en_GB/document_library/scientific_guideline/2009/09/WC500003517.pdf. Accessed April 24, 2016.
16. Research C for DE and. Guidances (Drugs) - Biosimilars [Internet]. Available at: http://www.fda.gov/Drugs/GuidanceComplianceRegulatoryInformation/Guidances/ucm290967.htm. Accessed April 22, 2016.
17. Macdonald J. Biosimilar regulatory frameworks with room for convergence-what more is needed? Seoul (Korea): APEC Harmonization Center Biotherapeutics Workshop; 2013.
18. Dörner T, Strand V, Castañeda-Hernández G, et al. The role of biosimilars in the treatment of rheumatic diseases. Ann Rheum Dis 2013;72(3):322–8.
19. Feldman SR. Inflammatory diseases: integrating biosimilars into clinical practice. Semin Arthritis Rheum 2015;44(Suppl 6):S16–21.
20. Lee H. Is Extrapolation of the Safety and Efficacy Data in One Indication to Another Appropriate for Biosimilars? AAPS J 2013;16(1):22–6.
21. U.S. Food and Drug Administration. Guidance for industry: scientific considerations in demonstrating biosimilarity to a reference product (draft guidance). 2012. Available at: http://www.fda.gov.proxy.cc.uic.edu/downloads/Drugs/GuidanceComplianceRegulatoryInformation/Guidances/UCM291128.pdf. Accessed April 5, 2016.
22. Drugs@FDA: FDA Approved Drug Products [Internet]. Available at: https://www.accessdata.fda.gov/scripts/cder/drugsatfda/index.cfm?fuseaction=Search.Label_ApprovalHistory#labelinfo. Accessed June 2, 2016.
23. European Medicines Agency. Committee for Medicinal Products for Human Use (CHMP). Assessment report: Remsima (infliximab). 2013. Available at: http://www.ema.europa.eu/docs/en_GB/document_library/EPAR_-_Public_assessment_report/human/002576/WC500151486.pdf. Accessed May 2, 2016.
24. Isaacs JD, Cutolo M, Keystone EC, et al. Biosimilars in immune-mediated inflammatory diseases: initial lessons from the first approved biosimilar anti-tumour necrosis factor monoclonal antibody. J Intern Med 2016;279(1):41–59.
25. Jung SK, Lee KH, Jeon JW, et al. Physicochemical characterization of Remsima. MAbs 2014;6(5):1163–77.

26. Yoo DH, Hrycaj P, Miranda P, et al. A randomised, double-blind, parallel-group study to demonstrate equivalence in efficacy and safety of CT-P13 compared with innovator infliximab when coadministered with methotrexate in patients with active rheumatoid arthritis: the PLANETRA study. Ann Rheum Dis 2013;72(10):1613–20.
27. Nast A, Rosumeck S, Seidenschnur K. Biosimilars: a systematic review of published and ongoing clinical trials of antipsoriatics in chronic inflammatory diseases. J Dtsch Dermatol Ges 2015;13(4): 294–300.
28. Park W, Hrycaj P, Jeka S, et al. A randomised, double-blind, multicentre, parallel-group, prospective study comparing the pharmacokinetics, safety, and efficacy of CT-P13 and innovator infliximab in patients with ankylosing spondylitis: the PLANETAS study. Ann Rheum Dis 2013;72(10): 1605–12.
29. Yoo DH, Racewicz A, Brzezicki J, et al. A phase III randomized study to evaluate the efficacy and safety of CT-P13 compared with reference infliximab in patients with active rheumatoid arthritis: 54-week results from the PLANETRA study. Arthritis Res Ther 2016;18(1):82.
30. Park W, Yoo DH, Jaworski J, et al. Comparable long-term efficacy, as assessed by patient-reported outcomes, safety and pharmacokinetics, of CT-P13 and reference infliximab in patients with ankylosing spondylitis: 54-week results from the randomized, parallel-group PLANETAS study. Arthritis Res Ther 2016;18(1):25.
31. Amgen. Study to compare efficacy and safety of ABP 501 and 21 adalimumab (Humira®) in adults with moderate to severe plaque psoriasis. In: ClinicalTrials.gov [Internet]. Bethesda (MD): National Library of Medicine (US); 2000. Available at: http://ClinicalTrials.gov/show/NCT01970488. Accessed April 16, 2016.
32. Sandoz. Study to demonstrate equivalent efficacy and to compare safety of biosimilar adalimumab (GP2017) and humira (ADACCESS). In: ClinicalTrials.gov [Internet]. Bethesda (MD): National Library of Medicine (US); 2000. Available at: http://ClinicalTrials.gov/show/NCT02016105. Accessed April 16, 2016.
33. Sandoz. Study to demonstrate equivalent efficacy and to compare safety of biosimilar etanercept (GP2015) and enbrel (EGALITY). In: ClinicalTrials.gov [Internet]. Bethesda (MD): National Library of Medicine (US); 2000. Available at: http://ClinicalTrials.gov/show/NCT01891864. Accessed April 16, 2016.
34. Coherus. Comparison of CHS-0214 to enbrel (etanercept) in patients with chronic plaque psoriasis (PsO). In: ClinicalTrials.gov [Internet]. Bethesda (MD): National Library of Medicine (US); 2000. Available at: https://clinicaltrials.gov/ct2/show/NCT02134210?term=CHS-0214&rank=3. Accessed May 25, 2016.
35. Weise M, Bielsky M-C, De Smet K, et al. Biosimilars: what clinicians should know. Blood 2012;120(26): 5111–7.
36. Kay J. Biosimilars: a regulatory perspective from America. Arthritis Res Ther 2011;13(3):112.
37. American Academy of Dermatology. Position statement on generic therapeutic & biosimilar substitution. 2013. Available at: https://www.aad.org/Forms/Policies/Uploads/PS/PS-Generic%20Therapeutic%20and%20%20Biosimilar%20Substitution.pdf. Accessed April 24, 16.
38. Singh JA, Furst DE, Bharat A, et al. 2012 update of the 2008 American College of Rheumatology recommendations for the use of disease-modifying antirheumatic drugs and biologic agents in the treatment of rheumatoid arthritis. Arthritis Care Res (Hoboken) 2012; 64(5):625–39.

CHAPTER 15

Combination Therapies for Psoriasis

Anjali S. Vekaria, MD, Mark G. Lebwohl, MD

KEYWORDS

• Psoriasis • Combination • Acitretin • Cyclosporine • Methotrexate • Biologics • Etanercept • Adalimumab

KEY POINTS

- Combination therapies of biologics and systemic agents for psoriasis treatment can potentially enhance efficacy of treatment, increase onset of remission, and decrease side effects by allowing for dose reductions.
- Potential therapeutic combinations examined include methotrexate paired with biologics; cyclosporine paired with biologics; acitretin paired with biologics; or phototherapy paired with biologics.
- Randomized clinical trials, case series, and case reports chronicling these therapeutic combinations have demonstrated good safety and efficacy data, indicating an important future role for combination therapy in the treatment of psoriasis.

INTRODUCTION

Psoriasis is a chronic inflammatory disease that negatively affects approximately 2% of the US population[1] with significant impact on quality of life.[2] Approximately 20% of these patients have moderate-to-severe disease.[3] Its systemic effects include cardiovascular, metabolic, rheumatologic, and psychiatric comorbidities[4] with older studies showing 25% to 38% of patients with psoriasis dissatisfied with their traditional treatments.[5] Of those affected with psoriasis, 17% require treatment beyond traditional topical corticosteroids, such as phototherapy or systemic agents.[6] More traditional systemic treatments include methotrexate, cyclosporine, and acitretin with newer biologic treatments, such as ixekizumab, secukinumab, ustekinumab, adalimumab, etanercept, and infliximab, quickly becoming important players in the therapeutic arena. A new oral agent, apremilast, has also been in use since 2014, with a few case reports of its use in combination with other therapies.

As treatment methods progress for this chronic disease, clinicians have been forced to expand therapeutic regimens and explore new combination therapies for patients with recalcitrant disease or dose-related cumulative toxicity from traditional treatments.[3] Combination treatment of biologics with systemic agents, such as methotrexate, cyclosporine, and acitretin, can potentially enhance efficacy, hasten onset of remission, and decrease potential side effects by allowing for dose reductions (Table 15.1). When combining immunosuppressive agents, the possibility of additive immunosuppression should be considered, and the dosage and period of overlap of more than one immunosuppressive medication should be minimized. This chapter investigates different combination therapies with biologics and traditional oral treatments.

Methotrexate

Methotrexate is the most frequently used oral treatment for psoriasis and has been found to be significantly effective in randomized, controlled trials, open-label studies, and retrospective studies.[7–11] Combination therapy of methotrexate with biologics is an emerging field of treatment with many considerations. Importantly, combining biologic therapies with methotrexate has not been shown to increase the bone marrow toxicity or hepatotoxicity of

TABLE 15.1
Traditional treatments and biologics for combination therapies in patients with psoriasis

Combination Therapy	Source	Dosing	Comparisons	Study Type
Methotrexate + Ustekinumab	Puig,[13] 2012	Ustekinumab 90 mg (transient increase in injection frequency) + methotrexate 10 mg/wk	None	Case report
Methotrexate + Adalimumab	Philipp et al,[14] 2012	Standard dosing adalimumab + methotrexate 12.4 ± 4.5 mg/wk	None	Retrospective chart review
Methotrexate + Infliximab	Dalaker & Bonesronning,[31] 2009	3 mg/kg infliximab at week 0, 2, 6, then q 8 wk + methotrexate 7.5–15 mg/wk	None	Retrospective chart review
	Wee et al,[27] 2012	3 mg/kg or 5 mg/kg infliximab at week 0, 2, 6, then q 8 wk + methotrexate 5–20 mg/wk	None	Retrospective chart review
Methotrexate + Etanercept	Gottlieb et al,[3] 2012	Etanercept (50 mg twice weekly × 12 wk then 50 mg/wk × 12 wk) + methotrexate (7.5–15 mg/wk)	Etanercept monotherapy (50 mg twice weekly × 12 wk then 50 mg/wk × 12 wk)	Randomized, controlled trial
	Zachariae et al,[38] 2008	Etanercept (50 mg twice weekly × 12 wk then 25 mg twice weekly × 12 wk) + methotrexate (stable dosing × 3 mo)	Etanercept (50 mg twice weekly × 12 wk then 25 mg twice weekly × 12 wk) + methotrexate (stable dosing × 3 mo then 4 wk taper)	Randomized, controlled trial, open label
	Gelfand et al,[40] 2008	Etanercept (50 mg twice weekly × 12 wk, then continuous or interrupted etanercept 50 mg/wk × 12 wk) + stable dose of methotrexate	Etanercept monotherapy (50 mg twice weekly × 12 wk, then continuous or interrupted etanercept 50 mg/wk for 12 wk)	Randomized, controlled trial, open label
	Driessen et al,[17] 2008	Etanercept (50 mg twice weekly × 12 wk, then etanercept 25 mg/wk twice weekly × 12 wk) + methotrexate (2.5–35 mg/wk)	None	Case series
Cyclosporine + Etanercept	Yamauchi & Lowe,[18] 2008	Cyclosporine (200 mg BID until PASI-50), then etanercept (50 mg weekly while cyclosporine tapered)	None	Case series
	Lee et al,[46] 2010	Cyclosporine (200 mg daily) + etanercept (50 mg weekly)	None	Case series
Cyclosporine + Adalimumab	Karanikolas et al,[33] 2011	Cyclosporine (2.5–3.75 mg/kg/d) + Adalimumab (40 mg weekly)	Cyclosporine (2.5–3.75 mg/kg/d) monotherapy or adalimumab (40 mg weekly)	Nonrandomized, open-label clinical trial
Acitretin + Etanercept	Gisondi et al,[53] 2008	Etanercept (25 mg weekly) + oral acitretin (0.4 mg/kg daily)	Etanercept monotherapy (25 mg weekly) or oral acitretin (0.4 m/kg daily)	Randomized, controlled trial

Data from Refs.[3,13,14,17,18,27,31,33,38,40,46,53]

methotrexate. Although there is no published literature about the combination of methotrexate with the newer anti-interleukin-17 (IL-17) drugs, secukinumab or ixekizumab, one would expect the combination to be more effective than monotherapy with either agent.

Methotrexate and Ustekinumab

Ustekinumab is a human monoclonal immunoglobulin G antibody that binds to the p40 subunit of IL-12 and IL-23. Dosing is weight based with a 45-mg or 90-mg dose every 12 weeks for a patient weighing 100 kg or less or greater than 100 kg, respectively.[12] For patients who are not adequately treated with ustekinumab alone, combination therapy has been seen to be useful particularly in those suffering from psoriatic arthritis, as a bridging therapy, for palmoplantar disease control or for recalcitrant disease.[6]

The success of the combination of methotrexate and ustekinumab was highlighted in a case report of a patient who had failed therapy with psoralen and UV-A (PUVA), cyclosporine, infliximab, etanercept, and various combination therapies, including etanercept/methotrexate, etanercept/methotrexate/acitretin, adalimumab/efalizumab/cyclosporine, cyclosporine/efalizumab/cyclosporine/methotrexate, and cyclosporine/adalimumab. Responses to all these regimens and combinations had slowly lost their efficacy, usually after just a few months. Treatment with ustekinumab showed improvement within 1 month, although response was eventually lost as with the patient's other therapies. By adding methotrexate 10 mg to the regimen along with a slight increase in injection frequency, the patient regained response with persistent control.[13]

Methotrexate and Adalimumab

Adalimumab is a fully human monoclonal antibody approved for use with plaque psoriasis at a dose of 80 mg at week 0, 40 mg at week 1, and then 40 mg every other week. A retrospective chart review examined responses to combination therapy with standard dosing of adalimumab, without loading doses for some patients, and methotrexate dosing at 12.4 $\pm$ 4.5 mg per week.[14] In 27 of 32 patients, a very good to moderate response, defined as a Physician's Global Assessment (PGA) score of 0, 1, 2, or 3 was seen. In fact, a reduction in methotrexate dosage was possible in 5 patients. Combination therapy showed a good safety profile with AEs limited to mild infections, abdominal complaints, and diarrhea. Adalimumab was stopped in 1 patient due to recurrent infection; gastrointestinal effects were ameliorated with methotrexate dosage adjustments.[14] de Groot and colleagues[15] evaluated inflammatory markers in psoriatic lesional skin with decreased markers seen in combination therapy compared with methotrexate or adalimumab alone.

Data from clinical trials for rheumatoid arthritis show increased levels of adalimumab in patients treated with combination therapy as compared with adalimumab alone.[16] Thus, levels of adalimumab may be increased by an unknown mechanism when using it in combination with methotrexate. In fact, tumor necrosis factor-α (TNF-α) antagonists used with methotrexate have been approved for the use of rheumatologic diseases. Studies have also shown a decrease in antiadalimumab antibody formation in patients on combination therapy.[14]

Overall, larger trials are lacking, but positive results have been seen in multiple case series with psoriasis or psoriatic arthritis[6,17–32] as well as randomized trials for those with rheumatoid arthritis. Certainly, more data are needed to fully elucidate risks and benefits of this combination therapy.

Methotrexate and Infliximab

Infliximab, a TNF-α antagonist, is a chimeric monoclonal antibody shown to be effective at a dosage of 5 mg/kg for the treatment of psoriasis. Approved for combination usage of infliximab 3 mg/kg with methotrexate or infliximab 5 mg/kg with azathioprine in the treatment of rheumatoid arthritis and Crohn disease, respectively, such combination therapy for psoriasis is less common.[33]

A subanalysis in the IMPACT 2 (Infliximab Multinational Psoriatic Arthritis Controlled Trial 2) studied the efficacy of combination methotrexate (25 mg/wk or less with mean dosage 16.2 mg/wk) and infliximab. At week 54 of the trial, Psoriasis Area Severity Index (PASI)-75 was achieved in 53% of patients on combination therapy compared with 48% of patients on infliximab monotherapy. Safety profiles were similar between the 2 groups.[4]

A retrospective chart review was conducted on 23 patients with psoriasis treated with 3 mg/kg infliximab combined with intramuscular methotrexate (7.5–15 mg every week).[31] All patients had previously failed treatment with methotrexate, cyclosporine, or PUVA. Infliximab infusions were given at weeks 0, 2, 6, and then every 8 weeks. If patients maintained response after 6 months of treatment, infusion intervals were lengthened to 9 weeks up to 14 weeks. Most patients were given infusions every 8 to 10 weeks.

Twenty-one patients reached 50% improvement by week 14 of treatment. The remaining 3 patients continued with treatment with sustained improvement. Treatments effects included headache, dizziness, and thromboembolism in a patient with multiple other risk factors. Mild infections were also reported and treated successfully with standard therapy. No hepatotoxicity, which is traditionally seen with methotrexate therapy, was reported. To address loss of response, which has previously been reported with infliximab monotherapy after 1 year of treatment, treatment intervals were shortened or methotrexate dose was increased.[31]

Generally, it is advantageous that infliximab be dosed with concomitant methotrexate to inhibit the formation of antidrug antibodies. It is also thought that the concurrent dosing of methotrexate during the study reduces such immunogenicity. Another study by Wee and colleagues[27] showed the incidence of infusion reactions was much lower in those receiving infliximab with methotrexate than with those receiving only infliximab. Studies in both psoriatic arthritis and rheumatoid arthritis have established better patient outcomes using combination therapies with methotrexate. Lower doses of TNF-α antagonists are also more cost-effective for the patient. Infliximab has been associated with hepatosplenic T-cell lymphoma in inflammatory bowel disease patients treated concurrently with azathioprine. Thus, caution should be taken in using combination treatment and should not be first line because larger clinical trials are needed.[31]

Methotrexate and Etanercept

Etanercept is a TNF-α antagonist used for moderate-to-severe psoriasis at doses of 50 mg twice weekly for up to 3 months and then 50 mg once weekly.[3,34] Current recommendations for patients with psoriatic arthritis include the approved use of etanercept with methotrexate for those who have not responded to methotrexate alone.[3,35] In fact, long-term safety of this combination therapy has been established in patients with rheumatoid arthritis.[36]

Randomized, controlled trials have shown superior efficacy of etanercept and methotrexate therapy compared with etanercept monotherapy in psoriasis.[34] In the largest randomized, controlled trial (n = 478) lasting 24 weeks, Gottlieb and colleagues[3] dosed etanercept at 50 mg twice weekly for the first 12 weeks and then 50 mg/wk for 12 weeks with 1 group also receiving methotrexate dosed at 50 mg/wk and 7.5 to 15 mg/wk, respectively. Results showed 77.4% of patients in the combination group obtaining 75% disease improvement compared with 60.3% in the monotherapy group.[4,34] There were a higher number of adverse events (AEs) seen in the combination therapy group, 75%, as compared with the monotherapy group, 60%, with reported events being similar in the 2 groups.[4,37]

In a randomized, open-label, 24-week study, Zachariae and colleagues[38] chronicled adding etanercept to the treatment regimen of patients who had failed or had little effect from methotrexate for 3 months. Patients were randomized to either etanercept with methotrexate continued or etanercept with methotrexate eventually tapered and discontinued over a 4-week period. Etanercept was dosed at 50 mg twice weekly for 12 weeks and then 25 mg twice weekly for 12 weeks. Of the patients who had been on etanercept/methotrexate combination as compared with etanercept/methotrexate taper, 66.7% versus 37.0% were judged as "clear" or "almost clear." PASI-75 scores were also seen to be improved at both weeks 12 and 24 in the combination group. AEs were increased with statistically significant infectious AEs in the combination therapy group compared with the etanercept monotherapy group. Most AEs in either group were mild or moderate.[3,34] Mild-to-moderate hepatic enzyme elevation was seen in 17.9% and 12.9% of the etanercept/methotrexate taper and combination group, respectively.[4,39] Thus, etanercept and methotrexate combination therapy is a good treatment option with safety profiles generally being similar between the groups.

Finally, the EASE study (Etanercept Assessment of Safety and Effectiveness),[40] a multicenter, randomized, open-label trial, compared patients with psoriasis receiving continuous etanercept 50 mg twice weekly for 12 weeks, followed by continuous or interrupted etanercept 50 mg every week for 12 weeks. Those on a stable dose of methotrexate for 8 weeks before baseline were allowed to continue with results showing those on a combination treatment of etanercept and methotrexate were more likely to achieve a PGA score of 0 to 2 at week 24 compared with not being on methotrexate.[3,39,41] In fact, many of the patients were able to decrease their weekly methotrexate dosage or even eventually suspend its use.

Another small case series in high-need patients with psoriasis showed the efficacy of combination therapy for maximal therapeutic effect without significant difference in laboratory findings or AEs compared with methotrexate monotherapy.[17]

Pharmacologically, the greater response seen with combination therapy has yet to be explained. Studies of lesional and nonlesional skin with other combination therapies suggest increased targeting of inflammatory markers with such treatment compared with monotherapy alone.[39]

In fact, large rheumatologic studies, such as TEMPO (Trial of Etanercept and Methotrexate with Radiographic Patient Outcomes) and COMET (Combination of methotrexate and etanercept in active early rheumatoid arthritis), assessing etanercept and methotrexate combination therapy found no significant differences in terms of serious adverse events (SAE) reported or serious infections.[36,39,42]

Caution is advised because few trials have analyzed the potential for increased AEs with combination therapies. One exception, the CORRONA (Consortium of Rheumatology Researchers of North America) database for rheumatoid arthritis patients, found that combination therapy of methotrexate with TNF antagonists, particularly adalimumab, etanercept, and infliximab, was not associated with higher risk of infection compared with infection rates of monotherapy of any agent alone.[39,43] Finally, a Swedish registry for psoriatic arthritis patients found similar SAE rates for those on combination therapy compared with methotrexate alone.[39,44] Another source chronicled the potential use of etanercept with methotrexate coupled with subsequent tapering of methotrexate to a minimal effective dose. This combination lowered the risk of toxicity.[13] In fact, this combination therapy has been shown to be effective in rheumatoid arthritis, juvenile idiopathic arthritis, and psoriatic arthritis.[39,45]

Thus, etanercept and methotrexate combination therapy seems to be a successful alternative to treatment of recalcitrant disease with multiple studies and reports outlining its successful use.

Cyclosporine

There are limited studies on the use of cyclosporine with biologics. The information in later discussion highlights the data currently available on combination therapies with cyclosporine.

Cyclosporine and Etanercept

Yamauchi and Lowe[18] evaluated 8 patients who received cyclosporine 200 mg twice a day until reaching PASI-50, at which point etanercept was started at 50 mg weekly while cyclosporine was concomitantly tapered. This combination therapy maintained response during tapering as well as 12 weeks after tapering concluded. Lee and colleagues[46] administered cyclosporine 200 mg daily with etanercept 50 mg weekly to 7 patients until symptom improvement with subsequent dose reduction of both etanercept and cyclosporine. All 7 patients showed progress with PASI improvements at 94.9% after conditioning therapy lasting an average of 6.85 weeks and 93.2% after maintenance therapy lasting an average of 56.5 weeks. Finally, 1 small pilot study for patients with psoriatic arthritis (n = 11) added cyclosporine 3.0 mg/kg/d to those with inadequate dermatologic response to etanercept. Nine patients achieved PASI-75 by week 24 with AEs, including worsening of hypertension and elevated creatinine. Other combination therapy studies have evaluated patients already on cyclosporine treatment who require eventual cessation once disease control has been achieved with concomitant etanercept treatment.[18,19,39,47–49] Although few and small, these studies highlight the potential for cyclosporine and etanercept as effective combination therapy, although larger clinical trials are needed.

Cyclosporine and Adalimumab

The combination of cyclosporine and adalimumab was investigated in an open-label trial for patients with psoriasis and psoriatic arthritis refractory to methotrexate. This study showed a PASI-50 rate after 12 months of treatment in 95% of patients on combination therapy compared with an 85% and 65% PASI-50 rate in those receiving adalimumab and cyclosporine alone, respectively.[33] Another case series investigated 5 patients who transitioned without flare from cyclosporine to adalimumab with a cyclosporine taper ranging from 6 to 11 weeks.[4,50]

Cyclosporine and Apremilast

A recent case report highlighted the use of both cyclosporine and apremilast in a 45-year-old man who had previously failed or developed adverse reactions to methotrexate, phototherapy, ustekinumab, adalimumab, and etanercept.[51] Although taking certolizumab for joint pain, the patient was started on apremilast 30 mg twice daily. He eventually discontinued his certolizumab without return of joint symptoms but continued to have generalized psoriasis. He restarted cyclosporine at 100 mg twice a day, after a "cyclosporine holiday" due to 2 years of continuous dosing at 400 mg daily and achieved almost complete clearance. Thus, the patient was able to achieve a greater level of treatment success with combination therapy and a lower dose of cyclosporine than previously achieved. Although more data are certainly needed, this case report shows the potential use of combination therapy with apremilast.

Acitretin

Acitretin is an oral retinoid used as monotherapy in psoriasis treatment in both pustular and plaque psoriasis. Because acitretin monotherapy is not as effective as most other psoriasis treatments, it is usually prescribed in combination with other treatments, especially phototherapy.

Smith and colleagues[52] evaluated 15 patients in a retrospective chart review detailing combination therapy with acitretin and biologics. Overall, 29% showed complete clearance, 43% showed PASI 90, 14% showed PASI 75, and 7.1% showed no change. More data and clinical trials are certainly needed, but this study highlights the potential for therapeutic success with acitretin combination therapy.

Acitretin and Etanercept

A 24-week, randomized trial by Gisondi and colleagues[4,39,53] included 60 patients randomized to either combination etanercept (25 mg weekly) and oral acitretin (0.4 mg/kg daily) (n = 18), etanercept alone (25 mg twice weekly) (n = 22), or oral acitretin (0.4 mg/kg daily) alone (n = 20). At week 24, PASI-75 was seen in 44% of patients receiving combination therapy, 45% of patients receiving etanercept monotherapy, and 30% of patients with acitretin monotherapy. Body surface area improvement at week 24 was 78% in the combination group, 80% in the etanercept group, and 46% in the acitretin group. Safety profiles were the same in all 4 groups.[4,52,53] This study suggested using etanercept in combination with acitretin was equally as effective as using etanercept monotherapy. Of note, the etanercept monotherapy and combination therapy groups both had greater improvement than acitretin alone.[39] Other smaller clinical case series on the combination of etanercept and acitretin showed good disease control with no increase in AEs.[19,52,54] One study examined possible cases in which this combination would be recommended, such as in those with a history of nonmelanoma skin cancer in whom phototherapy would not be recommended.[55] Because acitretin has potential protective properties against the development of nonmelanoma skin cancer, it may warrant use in a patient with a history of nonmelanoma skin cancer.[52,56]

Acitretin and Apremilast

One case report of complete clearance of palmoplantar psoriasis in a 66-year-old woman was reported.[57] The patient had previously failed various topical corticosteroids, combination betamethasone dipropionate and calcipotriene ointment, and tazarotene 0.1% gel. She was subsequently started on systemic acitretin treatment at 10 mg daily, which was increased to 20 mg daily, combined with 10 months of biweekly excimer laser therapy. After 10 months, the patient was unable to continue excimer laser therapy and was started on apremilast with standard dosing escalation to 30 mg twice daily. After 3 months of combined acitretin and apremilast therapy, complete resolution of all symptoms was reported.

Biologics and Phototherapy

Etanercept in combination with narrowband UV-B (NBUVB) has been evaluated in multiple studies all showing a low rate of AEs. Kircik and colleagues[58] showed etanercept (50 mg twice weekly) combined with NBUVB (3 times per week) evaluated in 86 patients allowed for a PASI-75 rate of 84.0% at week 12, with PASI-90 and PASI-100 being achieved by 58.1% and 26%, respectively.

Park and colleagues[59] conducted a study during which 30 patients all received therapy with etanercept, 50 mg twice weekly, for 12 weeks, after which half received treatment with NBUVB 3 times per week for 12 weeks and a once weekly dose of 50 mg etanercept. At week 24, 53% of patients in the combination group had achieved PASI-75, whereas only 47% on monotherapy achieved similar results. Of note, it was found that combination therapy with etanercept did not show significant improvement compared with etanercept monotherapy.

Lynde and colleagues[60] studied etanercept, 50 mg per week, with NBUVB in 75 patients who had failed to reach PASI-90 improvement after 12 weeks of etanercept monotherapy. At week 16, of those patients adhering to thrice weekly phototherapy sessions, 43% reached PASI-90 improvement compared with 3% in the monotherapy group ($P<.05$).

In a 1-arm, open-label study, De Simone and colleagues[61] evaluated 33 patients receiving 50 mg weekly of etanercept and NBUVB 3 times weekly for 8 weeks, then followed by etanercept monotherapy for 4 weeks. After week 8, 15% of patients had achieved a PASI-90, and after week 12, 58% achieved a PASI-90.

Wolf and colleagues[62] evaluated the use of NBUVB in those patients failing to achieve PASI-75 after 6 weeks of etanercept monotherapy. Mean PASI reduction was 89% for the combination therapy group compared with 68% for those undergoing etanercept monotherapy ($P<.05$).

Bagel[63] evaluated the effectiveness of adalimumab with NBUVB in 20 patients with all receiving adalimumab, 80 mg at week 0 and then 40 mg every other week, and NVUVB 3 times weekly. At week 12, 95% of patients had reached PASI-75 with 55% achieving PASI-100.

From weeks 12 to 24, patients received no treatment, with 65% of patients maintaining their PASI-75.

In another study, Wolf and colleagues[64] treated 4 patients with standard dosing of adalimumab with half the body treated with 311-nm NBUVB once per week for 6 weeks. After 6 weeks, there was a statistically significant mean PASI reduction of 86% on the phototherapy-treated side compared with 53% on the untreated side.

Wolf and colleagues[65] also completed a similar study with ustekinumab therapy. Ten patients were treated with ustekinumab at weeks 0 and 4 along with 311-nm NBUVB 3 times per week. There was a statistically significant 82% reduction in PASI on the half also treated with phototherapy versus a 54% mean reduction in PASI score on the side without phototherapy.

Thus, phototherapy appears to be an effective adjunctive treatment to biologic treatment.

In summary, combination therapy achieves greater improvements in psoriasis. Ideally, combination therapy would allow dosage reduction of some individual treatments. Conversely, additive immunosuppression is a risk for increased malignancy and infection and should therefore be minimized.

REFERENCES

1. Famenini S, Wu JJ. Combination therapy with tumor necrosis factor inhibitors in psoriasis treatment. Cutis 2013;92(3):140–7.
2. Armstrong AW, Schupp C, Wu J, et al. Quality of life and work productivity impairment among psoriasis patients: findings from the National Psoriasis Foundation survey data 2003-2011. PLoS One 2012;7(12): e52935.
3. Gottlieb AB, Langley RG, Strober BE, et al. A randomized, double-blind, placebo-controlled study to evaluate the addition of methotrexate to etanercept in patients with moderate to severe plaque psoriasis. Br J Dermatol 2012;167(3):649–57.
4. Armstrong AW, Bagel J, Van Voorhees AS, et al. Combining biologic therapies with other systemic treatments in psoriasis: evidence-based, best-practice recommendations from the Medical Board of the National Psoriasis Foundation. JAMA Dermatol 2015;151(4):432–8.
5. Callis Duffin K, Yeung H, Takeshita J, et al. Patient satisfaction with treatments for moderate-to-severe plaque psoriasis in clinical practice. Br J Dermatol 2014;170(3):672–80.
6. Heinecke GM, Luber AJ, Levitt JO, et al. Combination use of ustekinumab with other systemic therapies: a retrospective study in a tertiary referral center. J Drugs Dermatol 2013;12(10):1098–102.
7. Montaudie H, Sbidian E, Paul C, et al. Methotrexate in psoriasis: a systematic review of treatment modalities, incidence, risk factors and monitoring of liver toxicity. J Eur Acad Dermatol Venereol 2011;25(Suppl 2):12–8.
8. Saurat JH, Stingl G, Dubertret L, et al. Efficacy and safety results from the randomized controlled comparative study of adalimumab vs. methotrexate vs. placebo in patients with psoriasis (CHAMPION). Br J Dermatol 2008;158(3):558–66.
9. Griffiths CE, Clark CM, Chalmers RJ, et al. A systematic review of treatments for severe psoriasis. Health Technol Assess 2000;4(40):1–125.
10. Heydendael VM, Spuls PI, Opmeer BC, et al. Methotrexate versus cyclosporine in moderate-to-severe chronic plaque psoriasis. N Engl J Med 2003;349(7): 658–65.
11. Carrascosa JM, de la Cueva P, Ara M, et al. Methotrexate in moderate to severe psoriasis: review of the literature and expert recommendations. Actas Dermosifiliogr 2016;107(3):194–206.
12. Langley RG, Lebwohl M, Krueger GG, et al. Long-term efficacy and safety of ustekinumab, with and without dosing adjustment, in patients with moderate-to-severe psoriasis: results from the PHOENIX 2 study through 5 years of follow-up. Br J Dermatol 2015;172(5):1371–83.
13. Puig L. Treatment of severe psoriasis. J Eur Acad Dermatol Venereol 2012;26(Suppl 5):17–8.
14. Philipp S, Wilsmann-Theis D, Weyergraf A, et al. Combination of adalimumab with traditional systemic antipsoriatic drugs—a report of 39 cases. J Dtsch Dermatol Ges 2012;10(11):821–37.
15. de Groot M, Picavet DI, van Kuijk AW, et al. A prospective, randomized, placebo-controlled study to identify biomarkers associated with active treatment in psoriatic arthritis: effects of adalimumab treatment on lesional and nonlesional skin. Dermatology 2012;225(4):298–303.
16. Humira (adalimumab) injection [prescribing infomation]. North Chicago (IL): Abbvie Inc.; 2013.
17. Driessen RJ, van de Kerkhof PC, de Jong EM. Etanercept combined with methotrexate for high-need psoriasis. Br J Dermatol 2008;159(2):460–3.
18. Yamauchi PS, Lowe NJ. Etanercept therapy allows the tapering of methotrexate and sustained clinical responses in patients with moderate to severe psoriasis. Int J Dermatol 2008;47(2):202–4.
19. Strober BE, Clarke S. Etanercept for the treatment of psoriasis: combination therapy with other modalities. J Drugs Dermatol 2004;3(3):270–2.
20. Strober BE. Successful treatment of psoriasis and psoriatic arthritis with etanercept and methotrexate in a patient newly unresponsive to infliximab. Arch Dermatol 2004;140:366.
21. Iyer S, Yamauchi P, Lowe NJ. Etanercept for severe psoriasis and psoriatic arthritis: observations on

combination therapy. Br J Dermatol 2002;146(1):118–21.

22. Langewouters AM, Van Erp PE, De Jong EM, et al. The added therapeutic efficacy and safety of alefacept in combination with other (systemic) antipsoriatics in refractory psoriasis. J Dermatolog Treat 2006;17(6):362–9.
23. Krueger GG, Gottlieb AB, Sterry W, et al. A multicenter, open-label study of repeat courses of intramuscular alefacept in combination with other psoriasis therapies in patients with chronic plaque psoriasis. J Dermatolog Treat 2008;19(3):146–55.
24. Heikkila H, Ranki A, Cajanus S, et al. Infliximab combined with methotrexate as long-term treatment for erythrodermic psoriasis. Arch Dermatol 2005;141:1607–10.
25. Takahashi MD, Castro LG, Romiti R. Infliximab, as sole or combined therapy, induces rapid clearing of erythrodermic psoriasis. Br J Dermatol 2007;157:828–31.
26. Warren RB, Brown BC, Lavery D, et al. Biologic therapies for psoriasis: practical experience in a U.K. tertiary referral centre. Br J Dermatol 2009;160(1):162–9.
27. Wee JS, Petrof G, Jackson K, et al. Infliximab for the treatment of psoriasis in the U.K.: 9 years' experience of infusion reactions at a single centre. Br J Dermatol 2012;167(2):411–6.
28. Kamili QU, Miner A, Hapa A, et al. Infliximab treatment for psoriasis in 120 patients on therapy for a minimum of one year: a review. J Drugs Dermatol 2011;10(5):539–44.
29. van den Reek JM, van Lumig PP, Kievit W, et al. Effectiveness of adalimumab dose escalation, combination therapy of adalimumab with methotrexate, or both in patients with psoriasis in daily practice. J Dermatolog Treat 2013;24(5):361–8.
30. Barland C, Kerdel FA. Addition of low-dose methotrexate to infliximab in the treatment of a patient with severe, recalcitrant pustular psoriasis.' Arch Dermatol 2003;139:949–50.
31. Dalaker M, Bonesronning JH. Long-term maintenance treatment of moderate-to-severe plaque psoriasis with infliximab in combination with methotrexate or azathioprine in a retrospective cohort. J Eur Acad Dermatol Venereol 2009;23(3):277–82.
32. Kirby B, Marsland AM, Carmichael AJ, et al. Successful treatment of severe recalcitrant psoriasis with combination infliximab and methotrexate. Clin Exp Dermatol 2001;26(1):27–9.
33. Karanikolas GN, Koukli EM, Katsalira A, et al. Adalimumab or cyclosporine as monotherapy and in combination in severe psoriatic arthritis: results from a prospective 12-month nonrandomized unblinded clinical trial. J Rheumatol 2011;38(11):2466–74.
34. Busard C, Zweegers J, Limpens J, et al. Combined use of systemic agents for psoriasis: a systematic review. JAMA Dermatol 2014;150(11):1213–20.
35. Goldsmith DR, Wagstaff AJ. Etanercept: a review of its use in the management of plaque psoriasis and psoriatic arthritis. Am J Clin Dermatol 2005;6(2):121–36.
36. Emery P, Breedveld FC, Hall S, et al. Comparison of methotrexate monotherapy with a combination of methotrexate and etanercept in active, early, moderate to severe rheumatoid arthritis (COMET): a randomised, double-blind, parallel treatment trial. Lancet 2008;372(9636):375–82.
37. Cather JC, Crowley JJ. Use of biologic agents in combination with other therapies for the treatment of psoriasis. Am J Clin Dermatol 2014;15(6):467–78.
38. Zachariae C, Mork NJ, Reunala T, et al. The combination of etanercept and methotrexate increases the effectiveness of treatment in active psoriasis despite inadequate effect of methotrexate therapy. Acta Derm Venereol 2008;88(5):495–501.
39. Foley PA, Quirk C, Sullivan JR, et al. Combining etanercept with traditional agents in the treatment of psoriasis: a review of the clinical evidence. J Eur Acad Dermatol Venereol 2010;24(10):1135–43.
40. Gelfand JM, Kimball AB, Mostow EN, et al. Patient-reported outcomes and health-care resource utilization in patients with psoriasis treated with etanercept: continuous versus interrupted treatment. Value Health 2008;11(3):400–7.
41. Moore A, Gordon KB, Kang S, et al. A randomized, open-label trial of continuous versus interrupted etanercept therapy in the treatment of psoriasis. J Am Acad Dermatol 2007;56(4):598–603.
42. van der Heijde D, Klareskog L, Landewe R, et al. Disease remission and sustained halting of radiographic progression with combination etanercept and methotrexate in patients with rheumatoid arthritis. Arthritis Rheum 2007;56(12):3928–39.
43. Greenberg JD, Reed G, Kremer JM, et al. Association of methotrexate and tumour necrosis factor antagonists with risk of infectious outcomes including opportunistic infections in the CORRONA registry. Ann Rheum Dis 2010;69(2):380–6.
44. Kristensen LE, Gulfe A, Saxne T, et al. Efficacy and tolerability of anti-tumour necrosis factor therapy in psoriatic arthritis patients: results from the South Swedish Arthritis Treatment Group register. Ann Rheum Dis 2008;67(3):364–9.
45. Mease PJ, Goffe BS, Metz J, et al. Etanercept in the treatment of psoriatic arthritis and psoriasis: a randomised trial. Lancet 2000;356(9227):385–90.
46. Lee EJ, Shin MK, Kim NI. A clinical trial of combination therapy with etanercept and low dose

cyclosporine for the treatment of refractory psoriasis. Ann Dermatol 2010;22(2):138–42.
47. D'Angelo S, Cutro MS, Lubrano E, et al. Combination therapy with ciclosporin and etanercept in patients with psoriatic arthritis. Ann Rheum Dis 2010;69:934–5.
48. Ortiz A, Yamauchi PS. A treatment strategy for psoriasis: transitioning from systemic therapy to biologic agents. Skinmed 2006;5(6):285–8.
49. Kress DW. Etanercept therapy improves symptoms and allows tapering of other medications in children and adolescents with moderate to severe psoriasis. J Am Acad Dermatol 2006;54:S126–8.
50. Gattu S, Wu JJ, Koo J. Can adalimumab make a smooth and easy transition from cyclosporine a reality? a case series of successful transitions. Psoriasis Forum 2009;15(2):33–5.
51. Sasaki JL, Zhu TH, Austin A, et al. Apremilast and cyclosporine combination therapy for a patient with both psoriasis and psoriatic arthritis: a case report. Journal of Psoriasis and Psoriatic Arthritis 2016;1(2):70–2.
52. Smith EC, Riddle C, Menter MA, et al. Combining systemic retinoids with biologic agents for moderate to severe psoriasis. Int J Dermatol 2008;47(5):514–8.
53. Gisondi P, Del Giglio M, Cotena C, et al. Combining etanercept and acitretin in the therapy of chronic plaque psoriasis: a 24-week, randomized, controlled, investigator-blinded pilot trial. Br J Dermatol 2008; 158(6):1345–9.
54. Conley J, Nanton J, Dhawan S, et al. Novel combination regimens: biologics and acitretin for the treatment of psoriasis–a case series. J Dermatolog Treat 2006;17(2):86–9.
55. Hodulik SG, Zeichner JA. Combination therapy with acitretin for psoriasis. J Dermatolog Treat 2006; 17(2):108–11.
56. Lebwohl M, Tannis C, Carrasco D. Acitretin suppression of squamous cell carcinoma: case report and literature review. J Dermatolog Treat 2003; 14(Suppl 2):3–6.
57. Colao R, Yanofsky VR, Lebwohl MG. Successful treatment of palmoplantar psoriasis using combination acitretin and apremilast: a case report. Journal of Psoriasis and Psoriatic Arthritis 2016;1(2):66–9.
58. Kircik L, Bagel J, Korman N, et al. Utilization of narrow-band ultraviolet light B therapy and etanercept for the treatment of psoriasis (UNITE): efficacy, safety, and patient-reported outcomes. J Drugs Dermatol 2008;7(3):245–53.
59. Park KK, Wu JJ, Koo J. A randomized, 'head-to-head' pilot study comparing the effects of etanercept monotherapy vs. etanercept and narrowband ultraviolet B (NB-UVB) phototherapy in obese psoriasis patients. J Eur Acad Dermatol Venereol 2013; 27(7):899–906.
60. Lynde CW, Gupta AK, Guenther L, et al. A randomized study comparing the combination of nbUVB and etanercept to etanercept monotherapy in patients with psoriasis who do not exhibit an excellent response after 12 weeks of etanercept. J Dermatolog Treat 2012;23(4):261–7.
61. De Simone C, D'Agostino M, Capizzi R, et al. Combined treatment with etanercept 50 mg once weekly and narrow-band ultraviolet B phototherapy in chronic plaque psoriasis. Eur J Dermatol 2011; 21(4):568–72.
62. Wolf P, Hofer A, Legat FJ, et al. Treatment with 311-nm ultraviolet B accelerates and improves the clearance of psoriatic lesions in patients treated with etanercept. Br J Dermatol 2009; 160(1):186–9.
63. Bagel J. Adalimumab plus narrowband ultraviolet B light phototherapy for the treatment of moderate to severe psoriasis. J Drugs Dermatol 2011;10(4): 366–71.
64. Wolf P, Hofer A, Weger W, et al. 311 nm ultraviolet B-accelerated response of psoriatic lesions in adalimumab-treated patients. Photodermatol Photoimmunol Photomed 2011;27(4):186–9.
65. Wolf P, Weger W, Legat FJ, et al. Treatment with 311-nm ultraviolet B enhanced response of psoriatic lesions in ustekinumab-treated patients: a randomized intraindividual trial. Br J Dermatol 2012;166(1): 147–53.

CHAPTER 16

Investigational Therapies for Psoriasis

Peter W. Hashim, MD, MHS, Mark G. Lebwohl, MD

KEYWORDS

• Janus kinase • Tumor necrosis factor-α • Interleukin-17 • Interleukin-23

KEY POINTS

- Investigational therapies aim to inhibit the specific immunologic mechanisms behind plaque psoriasis without widely affecting the normal immune system.
- Pathways targeted by investigational therapies include Janus kinase, tumor necrosis factor-α, interleukin-17, and interleukin-23.
- Phase II and phase III clinical trials have demonstrated strong safety and efficacy data for several agents, indicating an important future role in treating moderate-to-severe psoriasis.

INTRODUCTION

Enhanced insight into the immunogenetic mechanisms behind plaque psoriasis has led to the development of multiple new systemic therapies. These treatments include drugs targeting Janus kinase (JAK), tumor necrosis factor-α (TNF-α), interleukin (IL)-17, and IL-23 pathways (Table 16.1). Clinical trials are currently underway to examine the safety and efficacy of these agents in moderate-to-severe patients. The treatments discussed have demonstrated promising results in phase II or phase III trials and may play an important role in future treatment algorithms.

Tofacitinib

Tofacitinib is an oral JAK1/JAK3 inhibitor currently approved for rheumatoid arthritis at a dose of 5 mg twice daily. The current label includes a black box warning for serious infection and malignancy. It is under investigation for chronic plaque psoriasis. In a phase IIb, randomized, placebo-controlled trial, treatment outcomes were examined by Papp and colleagues[1] using twice a day doses of 2 mg, 5 mg, or 15 mg. At week 12, the proportion of patients who experienced 75% or greater reduction in the Psoriasis Area and Severity Index (PASI-75) was compared with the placebo group. PASI-75 responses were achieved in 25.0% of patients receiving the 2-mg dose, 40.8% of those receiving the 4-mg dose, and 66.7% of those receiving the 15-mg dose, compared with 2.0% in patients with placebo ($P<.001$ for each comparison to placebo). Infections were the most common adverse events, seen in 22.4% of the 2-mg dosing group, 20.4% of the 5-mg dosing group, 38.7% in the 15-mg dosing group, and 32% in the placebo group. Of note, 15-mg dosing was associated with statistically significant decreases in hemoglobin (−0.52 g/dL vs −0.14 g/dL with placebo; $P<.05$), hematocrit, and red blood cell counts as well as transient decreases in neutrophil count.[13]

Rapid and significant improvements in itch severity have been demonstrated with tofacitinib.[14] In patient-reported surveys using 5-mg and 10-mg twice a day dosing, reductions in the itch severity index (ISI) were evident as early as 2 or 3 days after treatment initiation. Among patients with a baseline ISI 1 or greater (indicating the presence of itch), treatment with tofacitinib provided a statistically significant reduction in pruritus ($P<.05$) by day 6 and through all 12 weeks of treatment.

A phase III, noninferiority trial between tofacitinib and high-dose etanercept was conducted by Bachelez and colleagues.[2] After 12 weeks, PASI-75 responses were achieved in 39.5% (130/329) of patients receiving 5 mg of tofacitinib twice a day and 63.6% (210/330) of patients receiving tofacitinib 10 mg twice a day, compared with 58.8% (197/335) of those receiving etanercept

TABLE 16.1
Summary of clinical trials

Primary Agent	Target	Source	Dosing	Comparisons	Study Length (wk)
Tofacitinib	JAK1/JAK3	Papp et al,[1] 2012	Tofacitinib, 2–15 mg twice daily	Placebo	12
		Bachelez et al,[2] 2015	Tofacitinib, 5–10 mg twice daily	Etanercept, 50 mg twice weekly or placebo	12
Certolizumab	TNF-α	Reich et al,[3] 2012	CZP, 400 mg at week 0, then 200–400 mg q 2 wk	Placebo	12
		Mease et al,[4] 2014	CZP, 200 mg q 2 wk or 400 mg q 4 wk	Placebo	24
Brodalumab	IL-17R	Nakagawa et al,[5] 2016	Brodalumab, 70–210 mg Q2W	Placebo	12
		Papp et al,[6] 2014	Brodalumab, 140–210 mg Q2W	None	120
		Mease et al,[7] 2014	Brodalumab, 140–280 mg Q2W	Placebo	12, then 40 wk open label extension with 280 mg q 2 wk
		Lebwohl et al,[8] 2015	Brodalumab, 140–210 mg Q2W	Ustekinumab 45–90 mg (standard weight-based dosing) or placebo	12, then extension with brodalumab 210 mg q 2 wk or 140 mg q 2 wk, q 4 wk, or q 8 wk, or ustekinumab (standard dosing)

Guselkumab	IL-23p19	Sofen et al,[9] 2014	Guselkumab, single dose of 10–300 mg	Placebo	24
		Gordon et al,[10] 2015	Guselkumab, 5 mg at weeks 0 and 4 and then q 12 wk, 15 mg q 8 wk, 50 mg at weeks 0 and 4 and then q 12 wk, 100 mg q 8 wk, or 200 mg at weeks 0 and 4 and then q 12 wk	Adalimumab (standard dosing) or placebo	16, then extension through week 40 (placebo patients transitioned to guselkumab 200 mg Q8W)
Tildrakizumab	IL-23p19	Papp et al,[11] 2015	Tildrakizumab 5–200 mg at weeks 0 and 4 and then q 12 wk	Placebo	52, then 20 wk follow-up
Risankizumab	IL-23p19	Krueger et al,[12] 2015	Risankizumab single dose of 0.01, 0.05, 0.25, 1, 3, or 5 mg/kg intravenously, 0.25 or 1 mg/kg subcutaneously	Placebo	12

Data from Refs.[1–12]

50 mg twice weekly, and 5.6% (6/107) of those receiving placebo. Thus, relative to etanercept 50 mg twice weekly, noninferiority was demonstrated with 10-mg dosing of tofacitinib, but not with 5-mg dosing. The rate of adverse events was similar across all groups.

Certolizumab Pegol

Certolizumab pegol (CZP) is a PEGylated monoclonal antibody to TNF-α approved for the treatment of Crohn disease, rheumatoid arthritis, and psoriatic arthritis. In a phase II trial conducted by Reich and colleagues,[3] subcutaneous doses of CZP 200 mg and CZP 400 mg were compared with placebo. PASI-75 responses were achieved in 75% (44/59) of patients in the CZP 200-mg group (*P*<.001 vs placebo), 83% (48/58) of patients in the CZP 400-mg group (*P*<.001 vs placebo), and 7% (4/59) of patients in the placebo group. The Physician's Global Assessment (PGA) score was measured as clear or almost clear in 53% of patients receiving 200 mg and 72% of patients receiving 400 mg, relative to 2% in controls (*P*<.001 for each treatment group compared with placebo). Adverse events occurred at comparable rates across the 3 groups.

The efficacy of CZP has also been demonstrated in treating psoriatic arthritis. In a phase III, placebo-controlled trial of 409 patients, Mease and colleagues[4] examined American College of Rheumatology 20% (ACR20) responses for doses of 200 mg every 2 weeks or 400 mg every 4 weeks. After 12 weeks of treatment, ACR20 responses were significantly greater in patients treated with CZP 200 mg (58.0%) or 400 mg (51.9%) relative to placebo (24.3%; *P*<.001 for each treatment group vs placebo).

ANTI-IL-17 AGENTS

IL-17, a proinflammatory cytokine involved in host defense against monilial infection, plays an important role in the pathogenesis of plaque psoriasis. The IL-17 group of molecules includes 6 ligands (A through F) and 5 receptors (RA through RE). Secukinumab, an IL-17A antagonist, was recently approved for the treatment of moderate-to-severe plaque psoriasis in adult patients eligible for systemic therapy. At present, 2 other biologic drugs that target the IL-17 signaling pathway have been investigated through phase III trials: ixekizumab and brodalumab. Most recently, ixekizumab was approved for psoriasis.

Brodalumab

In contrast to ixekizumab, brodalumab targets the IL-17 pathway through its receptor, rather than ligand. In a phase II study by Nakagawa and colleagues[5] involving 151 Japanese patients, brodalumab was subcutaneously administered at weeks 1, 2, 4, 6, 8, and 10 at doses of either 70 mg, 140 mg, or 210 mg. Higher response rates were seen at higher doses; in the 37 patients receiving 210 mg, PASI-75, PASI-90, and PASI-100 responses were achieved by 94.6%, 91.9%, and 59.5% of subjects, respectively, compared with 7.9%, 2.6%, and 0%, respectively, in the 38-person placebo group (*P*<.001 for each comparison of treatment to placebo).

Through 120 weeks of an open-label extension study by Papp and colleagues,[6] the long-term efficacy and safety of brodalumab were evaluated in 181 patients. A dosage of 140 mg every 2 weeks was administered in patients weighing less than 100 kg, compared with 210 mg every 2 weeks for heavier patients or those who demonstrated inadequate responses. At week 120, PASI-75, PASI-90, and PASI-100 response rates were 86%, 70%, and 51%, respectively. Nasopharyngitis, upper respiratory tract infections, and arthralgias were the most frequent adverse events.

Brodalumab has also demonstrated utility in the treatment of psoriatic arthritis. In a phase II, placebo-controlled trial by Mease and colleagues,[7] 168 patients were randomized to 140 mg, 280 mg, or placebo. At week 12, ACR20 response rates were significantly higher in the 140-mg group (37%) and 280-mg group (39%) relative to placebo (18%; *P*<.05 for each treatment group vs placebo).

Lebwohl and colleagues[8] compared brodalumab and ustekinumab in the treatment of moderate-to-severe plaque psoriasis through 2 phase III, placebo-controlled trials: AMAGINE-2 and AMAGINE-3. Patients were assigned to brodalumab doses of either 140 mg or 210 mg every 2 weeks or to standard weight-based doses of ustekinumab. At week 12, dosing with 140 mg of brodalumab led to significantly higher PASI-100 response rates than ustekinumab in the AMAGINE-3 study (27% vs 19%; *P*<.05) but not in AMAGINE-2 (26% vs 22%; *P* = .08). However, for patients receiving 210 mg of brodalumab, PASI-100 response rates were significantly higher relative to ustekinumab in both trials (44% vs 22% in AMAGINE-2; 37% vs 19% in AMAGINE 3; *P*<.001 in both studies). Patients in the 210-mg brodalumab group also improved nearly twice as rapidly as those in the ustekinumab group, achieving PASI-75 responses in a median time of only 4 weeks. Of note, candidiasis occurred more frequently with brodalumab than with ustekinumab or placebo, possibly due to the impact of

IL-17 on host defense. Also noteworthy is the announcement by Amgen of its decision to not pursue marketing of brodalumab because of a small number of suicides in subjects treated in the development program for this drug.

ANTI-IL-23 AGENTS

Selective targeting of the IL-23 cytokine has become an emerging treatment approach for plaque psoriasis. IL-23 plays an important role in driving Th17 cell differentiation and producing the T-cell–mediated immune dysregulation seen in psoriasis. The cytokine is composed of 2 subunits: IL-23p19 and IL-12/23p40. Although IL-23p19 is unique to IL-23, IL-12/23p40 is shared by IL-23 and IL-12. The utility of targeting the IL-12/23p40 subunit has been established by the ability of ustekinumab to significantly lower psoriasis disease activity.[15,16] However, studies now support the theory that such demonstrated efficacy is largely due to inhibitory effects on IL-23, rather than IL-12.[17,18] These results have led to heightened interest in targeting the IL-23p19 subunit. Three agents that have shown promise in clinical trials—guselkumab, tildrakizumab, and risankizumab—are discussed.

Guselkumab

Guselkumab is a human antibody that inhibits IL-23p19. In a phase I, randomized trial of 24 patients by Sofen and colleagues,[9] guselkumab doses of 10 mg, 30 mg, 100 mg, and 300 mg were compared with placebo. At week 12, PASI-75 response rates in the guselkumab treatment groups were 50% (10-mg dosing), 60% (30- and 100-mg dosing), and 100% (300-mg dosing), versus 0% in the placebo group. The frequency of adverse events was comparable between patients receiving guselkumab and placebo.

Gordon and colleagues[10] compared guselkumab to adalimumab in a 52-week, phase II, randomized, placebo-controlled trial. Several guselkumab dosing regimens were examined: 5 mg at weeks 0, 4 and every 12 weeks afterward, 15 mg every 8 weeks, 50 mg at weeks 0, 4 and every 12 weeks afterward, 100 mg every 8 weeks, or 200 mg at weeks 0, 4, and every 12 weeks afterward. These groups were compared with standard dosing adalimumab and placebo. At week 18, the proportion of patients with a PGA score of 0 (clear) or 1 (almost clear) was significantly higher with guselkumab 50 mg (79%), 100 mg (86%), and 200 mg (83%) compared with adalimumab (58%) (*P*<.05 for all comparisons). These increased responses were maintained through week 40. There were no significant differences between therapy regimens with regards to adverse events, serious adverse events, or infections.

Tildrakizumab

Papp and colleagues[11] evaluated tildrakizumab, an anti-IL-23p19 monoclonal antibody, in a 355-person phase IIb, randomized, placebo-controlled trial. At week 16, PASI-75 responses were 33% in patients receiving 5 mg, 64% in those receiving 25 mg, 66% in those receiving 100 mg, and 74% in those receiving 200 mg, versus 4% in placebo (*P*≤.001 for each comparison to placebo). The sole difference in adverse events between treatment groups and placebo was a higher frequency of hypertension with tildrakizumab, although most of the affected subjects were noted to have hypertension or borderline hypertension at baseline.

Risankizumab

Risankizumab, which targets IL-23p19, was examined in a phase I study by Krueger and colleagues.[12] Subjects (n = 31) were randomized to single treatment with escalating doses of risankizumab (0.01, 0.05, 0.25, 1, 3, or 5 mg/kg intravenously, 0.25 or 1 mg/kg subcutaneously), which were compared with placebo (n = 8). At week 12, PASI-75, PASI-90, and PASI-100 response rates for patients receiving risankizumab (all doses) were 87% (*P*<.001 vs placebo), 58% (*P*<.05 vs placebo), and 16% (*P* = .590 vs placebo), respectively. All subjects achieved a PGA rating of clear or almost clear at weeks 12 and 24. Rates of adverse events were similar between treatment and placebo groups.

SUMMARY

Current data from clinical trials suggest that several emerging systemic therapies for moderate-to-severe plaque psoriasis are safe and efficacious. These agents benefit from mechanisms targeting the underlying immunologic processes without broadly interrupting the normal immune system. The treatment landscape for psoriasis continues to change rapidly, and further investigation brings the hope of improved management for this debilitating disease.

REFERENCES

1. Papp KA, Menter A, Strober B, et al. Efficacy and safety of tofacitinib, an oral Janus kinase inhibitor, in the treatment of psoriasis: a Phase 2b randomized placebo-controlled dose-ranging study. Br J Dermatol 2012;167(3):668–77.

2. Bachelez H, van de Kerkhof PC, Strohal R, et al. Tofacitinib versus etanercept or placebo in moderate-to-severe chronic plaque psoriasis: a phase 3 randomised non-inferiority trial. Lancet 2015;386(9993):552–61.
3. Reich K, Ortonne JP, Gottlieb AB, et al. Successful treatment of moderate to severe plaque psoriasis with the PEGylated Fab' certolizumab pegol: results of a phase II randomized, placebo-controlled trial with a re-treatment extension. Br J Dermatol 2012; 167(1):180–90.
4. Mease PJ, Fleischmann R, Deodhar AA, et al. Effect of certolizumab pegol on signs and symptoms in patients with psoriatic arthritis: 24-week results of a phase 3 double-blind randomised placebo-controlled study (RAPID-PsA). Ann Rheum Dis 2014;73(1):48–55.
5. Nakagawa H, Niiro H, Ootaki K, Japanese Brodalumab Study Group. Brodalumab, a human anti-interleukin-17-receptor antibody in the treatment of Japanese patients with moderate-to-severe plaque psoriasis: efficacy and safety results from a phase II randomized controlled study. J Dermatol Sci 2016;81(1):44–52.
6. Papp K, Leonardi C, Menter A, et al. Safety and efficacy of brodalumab for psoriasis after 120 weeks of treatment. J Am Acad Dermatol 2014;71(6): 1183–90.e3.
7. Mease PJ, Genovese MC, Greenwald MW, et al. Brodalumab, an anti-IL17RA monoclonal antibody, in psoriatic arthritis. N Engl J Med 2014;370(24): 2295–306.
8. Lebwohl M, Strober B, Menter A, et al. Phase 3 studies comparing brodalumab with ustekinumab in psoriasis. N Engl J Med 2015;373(14):1318–28.
9. Sofen H, Smith S, Matheson RT, et al. Guselkumab (an IL-23-specific mAb) demonstrates clinical and molecular response in patients with moderate-to-severe psoriasis. J Allergy Clin Immunol 2014; 133(4):1032–40.
10. Gordon KB, Duffin KC, Bissonnette R, et al. A phase 2 trial of guselkumab versus adalimumab for plaque psoriasis. N Engl J Med 2015;373(2):136–44.
11. Papp K, Thaci D, Reich K, et al. Tildrakizumab (MK-3222), an anti-interleukin-23p19 monoclonal antibody, improves psoriasis in a phase IIb randomized placebo-controlled trial. Br J Dermatol 2015;173(4): 930–9.
12. Krueger JG, Ferris LK, Menter A, et al. Anti-IL-23A mAb BI 655066 for treatment of moderate-to-severe psoriasis: safety, efficacy, pharmacokinetics, and biomarker results of a single-rising-dose, randomized, double-blind, placebo-controlled trial. J Allergy Clin Immunol 2015;136(1):116–24.e7.
13. Strober B, Buonanno M, Clark JD, et al. Effect of tofacitinib, a Janus kinase inhibitor, on haematological parameters during 12 weeks of psoriasis treatment. Br J Dermatol 2013;169(5):992–9.
14. Mamolo C, Harness J, Tan H, et al. Tofacitinib (CP-690,550), an oral Janus kinase inhibitor, improves patient-reported outcomes in a phase 2b, randomized, double-blind, placebo-controlled study in patients with moderate-to-severe psoriasis. J Eur Acad Dermatol Venereol 2014;28(2):192–203.
15. Papp KA, Langley RG, Lebwohl M, et al. Efficacy and safety of ustekinumab, a human interleukin-12/23 monoclonal antibody, in patients with psoriasis: 52-week results from a randomised, double-blind, placebo-controlled trial (PHOENIX 2). Lancet 2008; 371(9625):1675–84.
16. Leonardi CL, Kimball AB, Papp KA, et al. Efficacy and safety of ustekinumab, a human interleukin-12/23 monoclonal antibody, in patients with psoriasis: 76-week results from a randomised, double-blind, placebo-controlled trial (PHOENIX 1). Lancet 2008;371(9625):1665–74.
17. Lee E, Trepicchio WL, Oestreicher JL, et al. Increased expression of interleukin 23 p19 and p40 in lesional skin of patients with psoriasis vulgaris. J Exp Med 2004;199(1):125–30.
18. Chan JR, Blumenschein W, Murphy E, et al. IL-23 stimulates epidermal hyperplasia via TNF and IL-20R2-dependent mechanisms with implications for psoriasis pathogenesis. J Exp Med 2006;203(12): 2577–87.

Index

O

P

R

Printed and bound by CPI Group (UK) Ltd, Croydon, CR0 4YY
03/10/2024
01040303-0001